SAUNDERS
EQUINE
FORMULARY

Content Strategist: *Robert Edwards*
Content Development Specialist: *Catherine Jackson/Nicola Lally*
Senior Project Manager: *Beula Christopher*
Designer: *Christian J. Bilbow*
Illustrator: *Lesley Frazier*

SAUNDERS
EQUINE
FORMULARY
Second Edition

DEREK C. KNOTTENBELT
OBE, BVM&S, DVM&S, DipECEIM, MRCVS
Philip Leverhulme Hospital
University of Liverpool
Liverpool, UK

FERNANDO MALALANA
DVM, DipECEIM, FHEA, MRCVS
Philip Leverhulme Hospital
University of Liverpool
Liverpool, UK

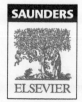

SAUNDERS

ELSEVIER

Edinburgh London New York Oxford Philadelphia St Louis Sydney Toronto 2015

ELSEVIER
SAUNDERS

First edition: 2006
Second edition: 2015

ISBN 978-0-7020-5109-8
EISBN 978-0-7020-5424-2

British Library Cataloguing in Publication Data
A catalogue record for this book is available from the British Library

Library of Congress Cataloging in Publication Data
A catalog record for this book is available from the Library of Congress

Notices
Knowledge and best practice in this field are constantly changing. As new research and experience broaden our understanding, changes in research methods, professional practices, or medical treatment may become necessary.

Practitioners and researchers must always rely on their own experience and knowledge in evaluating and using any information, methods, compounds, or experiments described herein. In using such information or methods they should be mindful of their own safety and the safety of others, including parties for whom they have a professional responsibility.

With respect to any drug or pharmaceutical products identified, readers are advised to check the most current information provided (i) on procedures featured or (ii) by the manufacturer of each product to be administered, to verify the recommended dose or formula, the method and duration of administration, and contraindications. It is the responsibility of practitioners, relying on their own experience and knowledge of their patients, to make diagnoses, to determine dosages and the best treatment for each individual patient, and to take all appropriate safety precautions.

To the fullest extent of the law, neither the Publisher nor the authors, contributors, or editors, assume any liability for any injury and/or damage to persons or property as a matter of products liability, negligence or otherwise, or from any use or operation of any methods, products, instructions, or ideas contained in the material herein.

 your source for books,
journals and multimedia
in the health sciences

www.elsevierhealth.com

  Working together
to grow libraries in
developing countries

www.elsevier.com • www.bookaid.org

The
Publisher's
policy is to use
paper manufactured
from sustainable forests

Printed in Great Britain
Last digit is the print number: 10 9 8 7 6 5 4 3

CONTENTS

PREFACE TO SECOND EDITION

The *Saunders Equine Formulary* has become a standard "must have in the car" book for equine practitioners and those who only see a few horses from time to time. Its distribution has been world-wide and we hope that it will continue to prove to be a useful aid to high-quality equine practice internationally. We have maintained its handy nature and its concise format so that information is readily available and useable advice and support can be easily accessed.

I am particularly pleased to welcome Fernando Malalana to the co-authorship of the Second Edition. I hope that he will be able to carry the baton of this little book into the future. I am also very grateful to him for undertaking the update so enthusiastically and so thoroughly.

Inevitably in the modern world, new drugs have come onto the market and others have disappeared from production and we have tried to update this aspect of the book in particular. The process of outdating and new drugs will mean that gradually there will be changes—the reader is encouraged to deface the book by deleting things that disappear and writing in new information! The book is there to be used and it's best when it is dirty and worn out! Of course, we recognise that many drugs used in equine practice have no licence for equine use because there is no commercial logic in seeking a licence for a minority species. It therefore becomes even more important that their use is fully understood and that they are used correctly.

We have also updated the diagnostic tests and procedures sections and the various appendices which have proven so useful over the life of the First Edition.

We would like particularly to thank the following for their contributions to the book—without their special help we would really struggle to keep up with all the changes that have taken place: Alex Dugdale, David Bardell and Caroline Argo deserve special mention.

The dedication of this book to the memory of Clare Harrison remains—she still lives within many of us; a happy, outgoing, and energetic veterinary student whose memory continues to inspire students at Liverpool University. It is little consolation to Victoria and Roger, I am sure, but Clare remains in my heart to this day, even as the years roll by and the world keeps turning.

DEREK C. KNOTTENBELT, OBE, BVM&S, DVM&S, DipECEIM, MRCVS

Part 1 VITAL SIGNS, NORMAL VALUES

REFERENCE VALUES

Abnormalities of physiological parameters (vital signs, haematological or biochemical parameters) are frequently used to assist the diagnosis and management of disease but there are important considerations to be taken into account before they can be relied upon. Hitherto, the term 'normal value' has been used to indicate that the measured parameter is within the reference range for a pool of apparently normal horses. There are always valid criticisms of defined normal values in view of individual variations within the natural/normal population distribution. The term 'reference value' is now used widely so that the implication of normality is not emphasised. An apparently normal individual animal may have values that fall outside the accepted 95% confidence limits and abnormal ones may fall within the normal range. However, the clinician is usually able to select the samples required and assess the validity of the results on the basis of the clinical features and the reference values provided by the laboratory.

Many commercial laboratories have pathologists who may be qualified and able to provide interpretive assistance, but without provision of a complete range of information it is unreasonable to expect this. Therefore, all requests for laboratory testing should be accompanied by as much clinical and historical information as can reasonably be provided. This also provides the pathologist with added information, which might bias or alter the tests that are performed. Clinicians can seldom be effective or convincing specialist pathologists!

Commercial and 'in-house' laboratories must ensure that they are subjected to proper and regular quality control assessments. This serves to ensure the quality and, therefore, the validity, of the results of assays. Failure to do this opens the door for misinterpretation at best and litigation at worst. Misleading laboratory results can also jeopardise the well-being of the patient and are in any case a complete waste of time, effort and money. Organisations exist to provide quality control assessments and these provide a vital service to the profession and the owners of animals who have a right to expect quality and value for their money (Fig. 1.1).

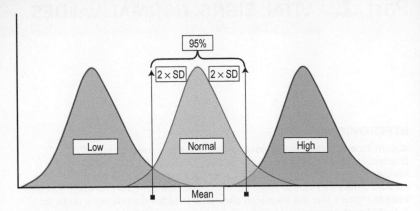

Fig. 1.1 Distribution curves for a haematological or biochemical parameter showing the 'normal' reference range in the middle, an 'abnormally low' range to the left and an 'abnormally high' range to the right. It can be seen that there are (large) areas of overlap such that a normal horse can have an apparently abnormal result while an abnormal one might easily have a normal value. This makes interpretation a critical factor in clinical practice. The more distant the value from the normal the more likely it is to be abnormal, but these values are unlikely to create major problems for the clinician. It is the subtle differences that are the challenge. In many cases, the trends in values are more helpful than the single 'snapshot' estimation. This applies, in particular, to conditions where the clinical signs are not themselves pathognomonic, e.g. liver disease.

Statistical analysis of the results of profile v individual laboratory examinations shows that where a single test is performed the chances of the result being an error are low, but where six parameters are measured there is a 50% chance that one of them will be outside the reference range. The greater the number of tests performed the greater the chance of abnormal findings (in otherwise normal horses!).

Notes:
- The reference values shown in this section are those that are accepted in the Department of Veterinary Pathology, University of Liverpool. The values may differ from those in other laboratories and may also be varied from time to time in the light of ongoing developments and experience in clinical pathology. For example, estimation of creatine kinase (CK) can be made at different temperatures and so a value that seems low or high from one laboratory may appear to be normal when compared to the reference range from another.
- The laboratory should provide their own 'reference values' on every report, although the lab should not report on the findings unless this is based on a full history and is the opinion of a qualified and experienced clinical pathologist.

Normal Vital Signs

The normal vital signs for horses will vary according to the circumstances, e.g. transport, exercise and mental status. External and internal factors may influence them and due note should always be made of the circumstances under which they are obtained. There are some circumstances when abnormalities can be masked by temporary or intermittent physiological alterations in vital signs. There are physiological/natural variations that are the result of breed, age and stage of training.

Table 1.1 Reference ranges for the basic vital signs in horses.

	Pulse rate (b/min)	Respiration rate (b/min)	Temperature (rectal) (°C)	Capillary refill time (seconds)
Foal (newborn)	100–128	14–15	38.5–39.5	<2
Foal (7 days)	80–120	14–16	38.0–39.0	<2
Foal (3 months)	60–100	14–15	37.5–38.0	<2
Pony	45–55	12–15	37.5–38.0	<2
Thoroughbred (resting)	35–45	12–15	37.5–38.0	<2
Thoroughbred (fit)	25–40	10–15	37.5–38.5	<2

SAMPLE COLLECTION

Not only is the correct anticoagulant essential for accurate laboratory analysis, but also it is essential that the tubes are filled correctly.

Note:
- Check anticoagulant requirements with laboratory before obtaining samples. Consider effects of transport on samples, particularly when this involves postal services.

Table 1.2 Sample collection requirements for the range of parameters measured from blood.

Tube: Parameter	FIO$_x$	Citrate	LiHep	Plain	Affected by
Haematology	√	0	0	±	0	L H
Clotting	0	0	√	0	0	L H
Glucose	0	√	0	0	0	S
Phosphate	0	√	0	0	±	H
Urea	0	0	±	±	√	H
Proteins	0	0	±	±	√	L H
Fibrinogen	0	0	±	√	0	
Serum amyloid A	0	0	0	±	√	L H
Bilirubin	±	0	±	±	√	H
Cholesterol	0	0	0	±	√	
Triglycerides	0	0	0	±	√	L
Creatinine	0	0	0	±	√	L H
Lactate	Mixture of FIO$_x$+EDTA – check with lab (assay immediately)					
Copper	0	0	0	±	√	H
Electrolytes	0	0	0	0	√	
Blood gases	0	0	0	√	0	L H
Bicarbonate	0	0	0	√	0	L H S
Ammonia	Special requirements – check with lab first (assay immediately)					
Enzymes	0	0	0	±	√	S
Hormones	0	0	0	√	√	

H, affected by haemolysis; L, affected by lipaemia; S, immediate separation. Samples marked: √, best; ±, acceptable; 0, unacceptable.

Haematology

Table 1.3 Reference ranges for haematologic parameters

Parameter (units)	0–3 weeks	Pony/mare	TB	TB (fit)
Haemoglobin (g/L) Range	130 110–150	120 90–140	125 110–180	145 120–180
Haematocrit (L/L) Range	0.38 0.31–0.45	0.36 0.30–0.42	0.40 0.35–0.46	0.42 0.37–0.45
RBC ($\times 10^{12}$/L) Range	9.9 8.0–11.0	10.0 8.8–12.6	10.5 8.5–12.5	10.8 8.5–12.9
MCV (fl)	41–49			
MCHC (g/L) (%)	310–370 (31–36%) (max value = saturated)			
MCH (pg)	13–18			
RBC diameter (μm)	5–6			
Platelets ($\times 10^9$/L)	240–550			
WBC TOTAL ($\times 10^9$/L)	6.0–12.0 (often slightly higher in yearlings)			
Neutrophils ($\times 10^9$/L) (%)[a]	2.7–6.7 (higher in foals) (45–55%)			
Lymphocytes ($\times 10^9$/L) (%)[a]	1.5–5.5 (n:L: 1.2:1.0) (35–50%)			
Eosinophils ($\times 10^9$/L) (%)[a]	0.1–0.6 (0–5%)			
Monocytes ($\times 10^9$/L) (%)[a]	0.0–0.2 (0–3%)			
Bone marrow M:E ratio	0.5:1.0–1.5			

Note:
(i) Stab/unsegmented neutrophils are not usually present in normal blood.
(ii) Normoblasts very rarely appear in peripheral/circulating blood even in profound anaemia.
(iii) Reticulocytes (as identified by supravital staining) are not present.
(iv) Early erythrocytes may show Heinz bodies, but are best recognised by increased cell volume.
[a]Differential counts should not be expressed in percentage terms – this can be grossly misleading.

Derived values

These parameters are derived from the red cell values and include:

1. MCHC (mean cell haemoglobin concentration):

   - This is the average proportion of haemoglobin in the average red cell.

   - This value cannot exceed about 36 because this represents the saturation point. Laboratory errors, etc., will, however, often reveal a value of slightly above this (up to 38 can probably be accepted).

   - However, anything beyond this value represents a problem that should be explored. It could be caused by technical problems or result from haemolysis deriving either from intravascular haemolysis (pathological) or *in vitro* (resulting from technical errors of collection, storage and handling).

   - Whenever the value exceeds 36–38, the blood haemoglobin should be remeasured and the haemoglobin concentration should be measured in the plasma. The haematocrit should also be repeated.

   $$\text{MCHC (g/L)} = \frac{\text{Haemoglobin (g/L)}}{\text{Haematocrit}} \times 10$$

2. MCV (mean cell volume):

   - This is a measure of the average volume of one red cell (erythrocyte).

   - An average volume is not really an easy index to interpret and so the appearance of the red cells on the smear must be examined to see if there are many small cells and many large ones or whether the distribution of the size of the red cells is normal.

   - Modern laser cell counters provide an accurate measure of the size distribution and this is a very valuable aid to the interpretation of the red cells parameters.

   $$\text{MCV (fl)} = \frac{\text{Haematocrit (L/L)} \times 10}{\text{Red cell count} \left(\times 10^9 / \text{L}\right)}$$

3. MCH (mean cell haemoglobin) – actual weight of haemoglobin in the average red cell:

   - MCH is seldom used because it is derived from the two most inexact measurements, i.e. haemoglobin and red cell counts. It is not considered here, as it has no material advantage over MCHC and considerable problems of accuracy.

Many clinical pathologists regard the MCHC and the MCV as the most sensitive indicators of red cell normality. However, errors of calculation can result in significant errors of judgement. The most common errors arise from the following:

- Technical problems associated with collection of blood samples (including partial or extensive clotting or haemolysis during or after collection).

- Failure to take account of the very high erythrocyte sedimentation rate of horse blood. For this reason, blood samples should always be handled correctly from the moment of collection.

- During preparation for cell counting or other haematological analysis the sample should be continuously mixed, preferably on an automatic rotating mixer.

For example:

1. Lysis of red cells results in a low haematocrit reading but a normal haemoglobin concentration – this results in an elevation of MCHC above the natural maximum/saturated value of 36–38% (often well above 40). This value, therefore, can be used as an index of the technical aspects of red cell measurement. MCHC values greater than 36–38% should be viewed with caution. Repeated testing is probably indicated.

2. A haematocrit tube that is filled from the top of a sample that has been left to stand even for only a minute or two will have fewer red cells (and, therefore, a lower haematocrit reading). The 'corresponding' haemoglobin concentration might be obtained from a similar sample a few moments later (low haemoglobin/haematocrit/red cell count) or may be taken from the bottom of the blood collection tube (high haemoglobin/haematocrit). In either case there will be a serious distortion of the values, potentially resulting in a significant error of interpretation.

Plasma and Serum Biochemistry

(i) Plasma/serum proteins

It is important to ensure the correct choice of collection tubes/anticoagulants when deciding what parameters are needed. See P. 6, Table 1.2 for ideal/acceptable collection tubes.

Table 1.4 Reference values for blood protein concentrations	
Parameter (units)	Normal value/range
Total protein serum (g/L) Plasma (g/L)	62.5–70.0 65–73
Albumin (g/L)	30–36
Globulin (g/L)	17.0–40.0 (8–32 in newborn)
α-Globulin (total) (g/L) α_1-Globulin α_2-Globulin	8.0–13.0 2.0–4.0 6.0–13.0
β-Globulin (total) (g/L) β_1-Globulin β_2-Globulin	8.0–15.0 7.0–13.0 6.0–10.0
γ-Globulin (g/L)	7.0–14.0 (note foal IgG ex colostrum)
Fibrinogen (plasma) (g/L)	1.5–3.0[a]
Albumin:globulin ratio	A/G×100=100%; A:G: 1:1
Serum amyloid A (SAA) (u/L)[b]	0–20

[a]Check method of estimation as the estimated values can vary widely with heat precipitation/subtraction methods.
[b]Measured by electroimmunoassay.

(ii) Globulins

Table 1.5 Globulin distribution in plasma of normal horses

Globulin fraction	Major components	Function
α_1	α_1-Lipoprotein α_1-Anti-trypsin α_1-Glycoprotein Caeruloplasmin	Lipid/hormone transport Proteinase inhibitor Copper transport
α_2	α_2-Macroglobulins α_2-Glycoproteins Haptoglobulin	Proteinase inhibitor Haemoglobin Binding/peroxidase
β_1	β_1-Lipoprotein Transferrin Complement (3/4/5)	Lipid transport Iron transport Complement factors
β_2	IgG (T) IgA Fibrinogen	Antibodies Antibodies Coagulation
γ	IgG IgM	Antibodies Antibodies

After Blackmore and Brobst (1981) Biochemical Values in Equine Medicine, AHT, Newmarket.

INTERPRETIVE COMMENT ON PROTEIN DISTRIBUTION AS CALCULATED FROM ELECTROPHORESIS

The interpretation of protein profiles forms an important part of clinical pathology, but the clinical status of the horse MUST be taken into account during the assessment of the significance of the findings.

Table 1.6 Plasma protein variations in some pathological disease states

Condition		Albumin	α-Globulin	β-Globulin	γ-Globulin
Infection	Viral	Normal	Normal	Elevated	Normal
	Acute	Normal (low)	Elevated	Normal	(Elevated later)
	Chronic	Normal	Elevated	Elevated	Elevated
Parasitism		Low	Elevated	Elevated	Normal
Hepatic disease		Low	Normal	Normal	Elevated

After Taylor FGR, Hillier MH (1977) Diagnostic Techniques in Equine Medicine, WB Saunders, London.

Table 1.7 Interpretive values for serum amyloid A protein (SAA) in newborn foals

	Serum amyloid A (u/L)
Normal	0–20
Non-infective acute phase response (trauma/prematurity)	20–100
Infective response	>200

After Chavvatte PM, Pepys MB, Roberts B, Ousey JC, McGladdery AJ, Rossdale PD (1992) Measurement of serum amyloid A protein (SAA) as an aid to differential diagnosis of infection in newborn foals. Proceedings of 6th International Conference – Equine Infectious Diseases, R&W Publications, Newmarket.

(iii) Non-protein biochemistry
The correct sample must be taken for the selected parameters. See P. 6, Table 1.2 for ideal/acceptable tubes.

Table 1.8 Reference values for non-protein biochemical parameters in normal horses.

Parameter (units)	Normal value/range
Ammonia (mmol/L)	<40
Bile acids (μmol/L)	10.0–20.0
Bilirubin (total) (μmol/L)	24.0–50.0 (up to 120 if starved >24 h)
Conjugated (direct) (μmol/L)	4.0–15.0
Unconjugated (indirect) (μmol/L)	5–35
Cholesterol (mmol/L)	2.5–3.5
Creatinine (μmol/L)	90.0–200.0
Glucose (mmol/L)	3.5–6.0
Lactate (mmol/L)	0.6–1.9 (Slightly lower in arterial blood)
Phosphate (inorganic) (mmol/L)	1.0–2.0 (Higher in young: up to 4.0)
Triglycerides (mmol/L)	0.1–0.8
Urate (mmol/L)	50–60
Urea (mmol/L)	3.5–8.0

(iv) Electrolyte and mineral parameters

It is important to ensure the correct choice of collection tubes/anticoagulants when deciding what parameters are needed. See P. 6, Table 1.2 for ideal/ acceptable tubes.

Table 1.9 Reference values for plasma electrolyte parameters in normal horses

Parameter (units)	Normal value/range
Calcium (total) (mmol/L)	2.5–4.0
Calcium (ionised) (mmol/L)	1.5–1.8
Chloride (mmol/L)	90.0–105.0
Copper (µmol/L)	19.0–28.0
Iodine (total) (nmol/L)	400–900
Protein bound (mg/L)	1.5–2.5
Iron (µmol/L)	25.0–30.0
Iron binding cap (total) (µmol/L)	40.0–80.0
Unbound (µmol/L)	35–45
Iron saturation (%)	25–50
Ferritin (µg/L)	60–360
Magnesium (mmol/L)	0.6–1.0
Potassium (mmol/L)	3.5–5.5
Potassium (red cell) (mmol/L)	75.0–104.0
Selenium (µmol/L)	>1.5
Sodium (mmol/L)	134.0–143.0
Osmolality (mosmol/L/mmol/L)	279–296
Calcium:phosphate ratio	2–5

Note:
● The anaemia of chronic inflammation is possibly the most common form of chronic, slowly progressive anaemia in horses. Diagnostic confirmation of this state is problematical. However, an iron profile can be helpful and can confirm the diagnosis when considered along with the presenting clinical signs and other haematological and biochemical parameters.

Table 1.10 Reference values for iron parameters in normal horses and variations encountered in anemia of chronic inflammation

	Reference	Anaemia of chronic inflammation
Plasma iron (µmol/L)	25–30	Reduced
Iron binding cap (total) (µmol/L) Unbound iron (µmol/L) Iron saturation (%)	40.0–80.0 35–45 25–50	Reduced
Transferrin	Not yet established	Decreased per cent saturation
Ferritin (µg/L)	60–360	Elevated

(v) Vitamins/hormones (excluding sex hormones)

Ensure correct choice of collection tubes/anticoagulants when deciding what parameters are needed. See P. 6, Table 1.2 for ideal/acceptable tubes.

Table 1.11 Reference values for vitamins and (non-sex) hormones in blood of normal horses

Parameter (units)	Normal value/range
Cortisol (nmol/L)	25.0–155.0 (marked diurnal variations)
Insulin (µIU/mL)	5.0–36.0
Parathormone (pmol/L)	60.0–80.0
Tri-iodothyronine (T_3) (nmol/L)	0.5–2.0
Thyroxine (T_4) (nmol/L)	4.0–40.0 (high in neonate)
Vitamin A (pg/mL)	20–175
β-carotene (mg/L)	150–400
Folate (ng/mL)	7.0–13.0
Vitamin B_{12} (pg/mL)	>1000
Vitamin E (µmol/L) (α-tocopherol)	>4.6

(vi) Acid–base balance

Table 1.12 Reference values for acid-base electrolyte parameters in normal horses

	Arterial	Venous
pH	7.35–7.41	7.36–7.43
pCO_2	37.00–43.00	45.00–49.00
pO_2	73.00–98.00	36.00–47.00
HCO_3^{2-} (mmol/L)	22.50–26.50	22.30–25.00
Base excess	0.00 to +4.00	–2.00 to +1.50
Anion gap (meq/L)	6–15	
Metabolic fluid requirement = 50 mL/kg/day		

The fluid requirement can be calculated from the formula:

$$\text{Defict (litres)} = \frac{\text{Bodyweight (kg)} \times \text{Dehydration (\%)}}{100}$$

The bicarbonate deficit in acidosis can be calculated from the formula:

$$\text{Bicarbonate deficit (mL of 8.4\% molar)} = 0.3 \times \text{Base excess} \times \text{Bodyweight (kg)}$$

Comments
- Bicarbonate should only be administered when metabolic acidosis is known to be present, i.e.:
  - (a) base excess is negative;
  - (b) pH is acidic;
  - (c) plasma bicarbonate is low.
- Bicarbonate is contraindicated in respiratory acidosis.

(vii) Enzymes
The estimation of serum/plasma enzymes usually relies upon dynamic assays, so the correct sample must be obtained and the sample must be handled correctly to ensure that enzymes are not degraded by the manipulations. Ensure correct choice of collection tubes/anticoagulants when deciding what parameters are needed. See P. 6, Table 1.2 for ideal/acceptable tubes.

Table 1.13 Reference values for plasma/serum enzymes in normal horses

Parameter (units)	Normal value/range
Alkaline phosphatase (ALP) (IU/L)	<250 (higher in young)
Amylase (IU/L)	75–150
Arginase (IU/L)	0–14
Aspartate aminotransferase (IU/L)	80–250
Creatine kinase (IU/L)	<50
γ-Glutamyl transferase (γGT) (IU/L)	<40
Glutamate dehydrogenase (GLDH) (IU/L)	<6
Glutathione peroxidase (GsHPx) (m/mL RBC)	30–70
Intestinal alkaline phosphatase (IALP) (IU/L)	<30
Lactate dehydrogenase (LDH) (IU/L)	76–400 (higher in young)
LDH_1 (IU/L) (% of total)	6–48 (8–12)
LDH_2 (IU/L) (% of total)	15–120 (20–30)
LDH_3 (IU/L) (% of total)	26–180 (35–45)
LDH_4 (IU/L) (% of total)	10–80 (12–20)
LDH_5 (IU/L) (% of total)	1–20 (1–5)
Inositol (sorbitol) dehydrogenase (IDH/SDH) (IU/L)	<2[a]

[a]IDH (SDH) has a very short half-life in vitro and in vivo (~2 h).

Comments
● Alanine aminotransferase (ALT/SGPT) estimation is of no practical/ diagnostic value for a horse.

INTERPRETIVE COMMENTS ON ENZYME PROFILES FOR HORSES

- The interpretation of plasma enzyme changes depends upon the distribution of the enzymes in the tissues that are damaged by a specific disorder.

- Intracellular enzymes are released into the blood stream when cells are either disrupted or where there is an increased permeability without necessarily incurring cell destruction.

- Specific organs have specific distributions of enzymes so it is possible to identify the extent and type of damage from a careful interpretation of enzyme profiles. However, some enzymes are not as specific as others. Combinations of enzyme assays can be helpful in discriminating between the various organs (Tables 1.14–1.16).

Table 1.14 The distribution of the various common, diagnostically useful enzymes in the various body tissues

Enzyme \ Organ	Liver	Pancreas	Muscle	Kidney	Gut	Brain	Bone
Alkaline phosphatase (ALP)	♦			♦	♦[a]		♦
Amylase		♦					
Aspartate transaminase (AST)	♦		♦				
Creatine kinase (CK)			♦			♦	
Gamma glutamyl transferase (GGT)	♦	♦		♦			
Glutamate dehydrogenase (GLDH)	♦						
Lactate dehydrogenase (LDH)	♦	♦	♦	♦	♦	♦	
Inositol (sorbitol) dehydrogenase (IDH/SDH)	♦						
Ornithine carbamoyl transferase (OCT)	♦						

[a] *Intestinal alkaline phosphatase is measured at a different pH to the total value in plasma.*

Table 1.15 The distribution of the enzymes in the major body tissues

Enzyme	Specificity rating[a]	Stability rating[b]	Comments
Alkaline phosphatase (ALP)	Bone Intestine (ileum) Biliary tree Kidney	High	ISO enzymes increase specificity but are not often measured apart from intestinal ALP
Amylase	Pancreas	High	
Aspartate transaminase (AST)	Liver Skeletal muscle Cardiac muscle	High	Good screening enzyme used to support differential detection of tissue damage
Creatine kinase (CK)	Muscle Brain	Moderate	Isoenzymes helpful for brain measure in CSF
Gamma glutamyl transferase (GGT)	Liver Kidney	High	For kidney measure in urine
Glutamate dehydrogenase (GLDH)	Liver	Moderate	Index of nuclear (profound) damage
Lactate dehydrogenase (LDH)	All tissues	Moderate	Isoenzyme profile important (see p. 21)
Inositol (sorbitol) dehydrogenase (IDH/SDH)	Liver	Low	Very labile Highly specific to liver
Ornithine carbamoyl transferase (OCT)	Liver	Low	Very labile Few labs perform this

[a]Specificity rating relates the extent to which the enzyme is specifically indicative of damage to a particular organ. Enzymes that have multiple organ distributions are likely, therefore, to have a low specificity, although paired enzyme tests may enable the specificity to be increased significantly.
[b]Stability rating relates to the extent to which stored (or posted) samples remain stable for analysis. A low rating means that the test is likely (or certain) to be affected by storage or delays between collection and analysis.

Table 1.16 The relative activities of the major systemic enzymes as a proportion of the organ with the most activity (marked 100% in BOLD)

Organ	Enzyme					
	ALP	AST	CK	IDH	GLDH	GGT
Brain	2	9	28	3	0	1
Myocardium	1	59	70	4	1	1
Skeletal muscle	1	**100**	**100**	0	1	1
Spleen	9	7	2	0	2	1
Liver	7	62	22	**100**	**100**	17
Pancreas	21	41	9	4	3	71
Kidney	**100**	13	1	19	7	**100**
Ileum	22	5	0	3	0	1
Colon	4	3	0	3	0	1

For abbreviations see Table 1.15.
After Gerber H (1969) Equine Veterinary Journal 1:129–139.

Note:
- Table 1.16 is included to demonstrate the distribution of enzymes in the various tissues of the horse and to illustrate the importance of understanding the role of the enzyme in the diagnostic process. For example, although GGT is highest in the kidney tissue, blood levels are not increased in renal disease simply because the enzyme escapes into the lumen of the nephron; therefore, urinary GGT will be a significant aid to diagnosis in these cases.

LACTATE DEHYDROGENASE (LDH) ISOENZYME PROFILE

- Total LDH is probably of limited value in horses unless it is accompanied by an isoenzyme profile because elevations can be due to broad increases or a more dramatic increase in one or two of the isoenzymes.

- Laboratories should be expected to perform an isoenzymes profile in the event of significant elevations in total LDH so that meaningful diagnostic information can be provided. A simple elevation of the total LDH is probably meaningless without a breakdown of the relative distribution of the isoenzymes. However, where this is provided the results can be very helpful.

Table 1.17 The distribution of the lactate dehydrogenase isoenzymes in various organs

Isoenzyme	Organ specificity
1	Heart muscle Brain Testis
2	Non-locomotor muscle Heart Brain Kidney Bone Thyroid
3	All major organs All non-locomotor muscles
4	Intestine Liver Skin
5	Locomotor muscles Liver Intestine Skin

(viii) Blood coagulation

● Collect blood into buffered or unbuffered Na citrate; other anticoagulants are not acceptable.

Table 1.18 Reference values for blood coagulation parameters in normal horses

Platelet count (×10⁹/L)	75–305
Plasma fibrinogen (g/L)	<4[a]
Prothrombin time (PT) (One Stage PT) (seconds)	12–15
Activated prothrombin time (APT) (seconds)	9–12
Activated partial prothrombin time (APTT) (seconds)	45–70
Activated clotting time (seconds)	120–190
In vitro clotting time (minutes)	5–7
Bleeding time (in vivo) (minutes)	2–3
Fibrin degradation products (FDPs) (mg/mL)	<0.20
Plasminogen (% of pooled normal equine plasma)	65–155
Protein C (µg/L)	90–120
Antithrombin III (% of pooled normal equine plasma)	63–131
Clot retraction time (hours at room temperature)	1–2

[a]The value for plasma fibrinogen varies slightly with the method of estimation. The reference value stated here is that accepted for use with the heat precipitation method. When subtraction (total plasma protein less serum protein) method is used the value may be lower.

Notes:

- Prothrombin time is the time required for fibrin formation after the addition of tissue thromboplastin and calcium to citrated plasma. Prolongation indicates deficiency in the extrinsic or common pathways (see below).

- Activated partial thromboplastin time is the time required for the formation of a fibrin clot after addition of a contact activator, phospholipids and calcium to citrated plasma. Prolongation indicates deficiency in the extrinsic or common pathways. Disseminated intravascular coagulopathy, warfarin toxicity, vitamin K deficiency and inherited prekallikrein deficiency may be involved.

- Activated clotting time is a measure of the intrinsic and common pathways. It is dependent on platelet phospholipid for activation. Platelet deficiencies (numbers or function) will result in a prolongation of the ACT in the presence of normal coagulation factors.

- Fibrin degradation products are the result of intravascular fibrinolysis. These compounds are intensely anticoagulant and increases are associated with disseminated intravascular coagulopathy or primary fibrinolysis (especially within the major body cavities).

Comments

- Blood coagulation tests are important in horses because there are several disorders that can be differentiated by selective use of coagulation tests. Most of these tests are performed in specially equipped laboratories and the tests require citrated blood samples taken in precisely the correct proportion of nine parts of blood to one part of citrate.

- Special clotting test tubes are available. Specimens should be delivered to the laboratory within 4 hours of collection.

- If postal delays are inevitable, a sample from a normal horse should be sent at the same time.

- *The extrinsic clotting pathway:* This is initiated by tissue thromboplastin (factor III) released from damaged tissue. This pathway is usually tested by use of the *one-stage prothrombin time*.

    Extensions in prothrombin time will be found in vitamin K deficiency (warfarin toxicosis), advanced liver failure and late disseminated intravascular coagulopathy (DIC).

- *The intrinsic pathway:* This is initiated by platelet-derived thromboplastin released as a result of vascular collagen exposure. The *activated partial thromboplastin time* (APTT) tests this pathway. An indication of this pathway's efficiency can also be gained from the *in vitro* clotting time (see below).

  An extended APPT result indicates a defect of whole blood coagulation and is found in disseminated intravascular coagulopathy (DIC) or specific deficits in clotting factors (e.g. Factor VIII haemophilia).

- In vitro *clotting time:* This is measured by collecting a fresh blood sample and immediately placing it in a plain (clotting) tube. The tube is maintained at or near 37 °C and is turned every 30 seconds to check for coagulation. The test is a crude method of assessing the extrinsic clotting cascade as it relies solely on platelet-derived thromboplastin.

- In vivo *bleeding time:* This is a simple, approximate test that evaluates the capillary platelet aspect of clotting. A small clipped area of skin or a visible mucous membrane such as the inside of the lip is punctured with a medical stylet and is then blotted every 15 seconds until there is no further blood on the paper. The time taken for the disappearance of the blood spot is the *in vivo* bleeding time. It is, therefore, an index of the overall status of clotting – the so-called final common pathway.

  Clot retraction time is a crude indicator of platelet defects (either in number or function). A blood sample is drawn into a plain (clotting) tube and the time taken for the clot to retract from the walls of the vessel is measured. It is prolonged when platelet numbers are low or function is poor (Fig. 1.2).

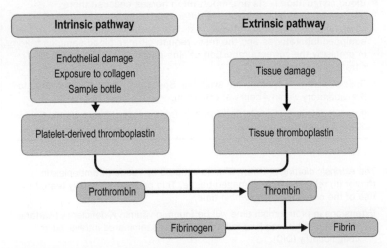

Fig. 1.2 A simple scheme of the main clotting pathways. Each component is a highly complex process that relies on several bioactive mediators.

(ix) Cerebrospinal fluid

- COLLECT INTO PLAIN (Sterile) AND EDTA TUBES.
- If a bacteriological culture is required, collect immediately into biphasic (blood) culture medium.

Table 1.19 Reference values for cerebrospinal fluid parameters in normal horses

Colour	Water clear
Cisternal pressure	150–300 mmH$_2$O
Refractive index	1.334–1.335
pH	7.4
Cell count (total)	<0.005×10^9/L
Cell distribution	Neutrophils/small lymphocytes only
Glucose	50–60% of blood glucose
Pandy's test (globulins)[a]	NEGATIVE
Protein (total)	<1.0 g/L
Creatine kinase[b]	<2 IU/L
Aspartate transaminase (AST)	20 IU/l
Lactic dehydrogenase (LDH)	<8 IU/L

[a]Pandy's test using concentrated phenol.
[b]CK may be higher (30–50 IU/L) in foals 7 days old.

Comments

- Cells in cerebrospinal fluid degenerate very fast and the low numbers mean that special methods need to be used. The laboratory will usually provide suitable guidance.
- Assay should be performed within 15 minutes if possible.

(x) Synovial fluid

- The collection of synovial fluid should always be treated as an aseptic procedure with full precautions being taken. There is no justification at all for sampling from any synovial structure in a non-aseptic manner even when the structure is known to be infected.
- Contamination with blood is relatively common and makes subsequent interpretation difficult.
- COLLECT INTO PLAIN (sterile) AND EDTA TUBES.
- If a bacterial culture is required, collect immediately into BLOOD CULTURE TUBES (biphasic medium essential).

Table 1.20 Reference values for synovial fluid parameters in normal horses

Appearance	Clear, non-turbid, pale yellow
Volume	Variable with joint
Viscosity (stringing test)	POSITIVE
Erythrocytes	NIL
Leucocyte count (total)	$<0.5\times10^9$/L
Total protein	<18 g/L

Correction formula for blood contaminated samples:

$$\text{White cell count of synovial fluid} = \frac{\text{Haematocrit of synovial fluid (\%)} \times \text{Total leucocyte count}}{\text{Haematocrit of blood (\%)}}$$

Note:
- This correction is simply a means of providing a guide, but it can still be problematical.

Comments
- Serum/plasma can easily be mistaken for synovial fluid and more critically vice versa – normal synovial fluid clots with acetic acid!
- Blood contamination can arise during centesis or from internal joint/synovial trauma.

(xi) Peritoneal fluid

Normally, there is a very small volume of peritoneal and pleural fluid (25 and 10 mL, respectively) so it is sometimes very difficult to obtain a suitable sample from a normal body cavity. Furthermore, contamination with blood is more significant if the volume is low. Collection technique is important and repeated punctures should be avoided. A full knowledge of the likely anatomy is helpful in identifying the best site for puncture. In the event that fluid is not obtained, a simultaneous ultrasonographic examination may help to identify a pocket of fluid that can be sampled safely and easily:

- COLLECT INTO PLAIN (sterile) AND EDTA TUBES.
- If a culture is required, collect immediately into biphasic (blood) culture medium.

Table 1.21 Reference values for peritoneal fluid parameters in normal horses

Colour	Clear, pale yellow, non-clotting
Protein (g/L)	<20
Leucocyte count (total) ($\times 10^9$/L)	<1
Total red cell count	Negligible
Creatinine (μmol/L)	160–200
Urea (mmol/L)	3.5–6.5
Lactate (mol/L)	<2

Comments

- Peritoneal fluid with the same PCV/haematocrit as jugular blood is probably from a blood vessel.
- Peritoneal fluid with a very high PCV/haematocrit is likely to have come from the spleen.
- Peritoneal fluid with a PCV/haematocrit slightly less than jugular blood may indicate peritoneal bleeding.
- Peritoneal fluid with very low PCV/haematocrit is probably the result of a strangulating or infarctive lesion.

(xii) Urine
● COLLECT INTO STERILE CONTAINERS

Note:
● It is important to ensure that bottles, etc., are clean and free from sugar contamination so new, sterile containers should be used where possible.

Table 1.22 Reference values for urinealysis in normal horses

pH	7.5–9.5
Colour	Clear or cloudy/turbid
Deposit	Carbonate crystals
Blood	NEGATIVE
Specific gravity	1.020–1.060
Gamma glutamyl transferase (GGT) (IU/L)[a]	0–5

[a]*Note that gamma glutamyl transferase (GGT) is not released into blood in significant amounts from damaged tubular cells. Serum concentrations will not be affected by even severe tubular necrosis.*

Table 1.23 Reference values and specificity for urinary enzyme parameters in horses

Enzyme	Reference values	Specificity
Alkaline phosphatase (ALP) (IU/L)	0–28	Proximal tubule Values over 28 are significant Diurnal variations
Gamma glutamyl transferase (GGT) (IU/L)	0–5	Proximal tubule Values over 20 are significant Diurnal variations
Lactate dehydrogenase (LDH) (IU/L)	0–12	Distal tubule Renal papillary necrosis

Comments

- Equine urine frequently contains heavy calcium carbonate deposits. This imparts a cloudy appearance to the urine. The first flow of urine is often clear as the urine is voided from the supernatant in the bladder. The final flow may be yellow and a thick creamy consistency. The extent of calcium carbonate in urine depends largely on the diet. Diets that contain high levels of calcium, such as alfalfa, induce a much higher urine calcium carbonate.

- Normal horse urine may be mucoid in appearance due to the secretions of mucus cells in the renal pelvis. This may cause a positive protein result on a urine dipstick or on full biochemical assay for protein.

- GGT and urine creatinine should be measured together to take account of the variations in enzyme concentrations which occur with a period of increased/decreased diuresis.

- Urinary GGT is a useful indicator of renal damage. The concentrations of the enzyme are very high but do not appear in blood as a result of renal tubular cell damage.

(xiii) Faecal analysis

Equine faeces provide several important diagnostic clues in disease conditions. Rational anthelmintic programmes should employ specific targeted therapy to avoid the unnecessary use of drugs and minimise the potential for resistance development:

1. Routine worm egg count:
   - Qualitative and quantitative worm egg counts relying on egg flotation are performed routinely in parasitological laboratories. Quantitative tests employ a counting chamber technique (McMaster chamber) and a saturated salt solution. A strongyle egg count greater than 100 eggs per gram of faeces is usually accepted as being significant.
   - Differentiation of worm eggs within the strongyle family is difficult and relies on special culture methods.
   - The severity of infestation with cyathostomins is not proportional to the worm egg count. Arrested third-stage larvae may cause many more problems than adult worms.
   - An ELISA blood test has been developed[1] that gives a proportional response to the severity (number of parasites) in equine *Anoplocephala perfoliata* infestation.

Note:
   - The response to anthelmintic treatment is often taken to indicate drug efficacy, but worm egg output is variable in any case. Nevertheless, failure to reduce the egg count following treatment may support the diagnosis of drug-resistant parasites.

2. Faecal occult blood test:
   - Almost all apparently normal horses will have slight intestinal blood loss; this probably indicates that there is a degree of sub-clinical intestinal pathology in many otherwise healthy horses. This can be detected simply by mixing a single faecal pellet (up to around 25 g of faeces) in a litre of water and testing the fluid with a urine dipstick to see if the blood square shows changes consistent with haemoglobin or red blood cells. This *ortho*-toluidine test is highly sensitive and any more than a slightly positive blood result indicates abnormal intestinal bleeding. A commercially available validated test that selectively measures hemoglobin and albumin is available (SUCCEED, Freedom Health USA). Severe parasitism, gastric or other intestinal ulceration, clotting disorders and neoplasia may cause large increases in the faecal occult blood. Non-steroidal anti-inflammatory drugs will invariably induce significant intestinal blood loss. Severe bleeding in the upper intestinal tract is usually manifest also as patent melaena, i.e. dark, tarry blood-stained faeces. Bleeding in the small colon is usually more obviously red.

---

[1] *Diagnosteq*, University of Liverpool, Leahurst, Neston, Wirral, CH64 7TE, UK.

3. Bacterial culture:

- Bacterial culture is unreliable from single swabs inserted into the rectum or collection of stale faeces from the environment. It is better practice to submit a sample of freshly voided faeces (or freshly collected faeces from the rectum). Usually the bacterial culture is problematical and, in cases where salmonella is suspected, at least five separate samples should be taken at 12–24-hour intervals. The faeces may be placed directly into enrichment media. Where clostridia are suspected then anaerobic culture will be required and the specimen needs to be placed in a meat broth directly on collection.

4. Rotavirus test:

Several tests are available to detect Rotavirus in faeces from foals:

- Direct electron microscopy on a freshly collected sample.

- Enzyme-linked immunosorbent assay (ELISA) for the antigen in faeces (*Rotazyme*, Abbott Laboratories, North Chicago, Illinois, USA).

- Latex agglutination Test *(Virogen Rotatest*, Wampole Labs, Cranbury, New Jersey, USA).

5. Tests for sand:

- Sand colic is a common problem that is sometimes difficult to diagnose clinically. A specimen of faeces is mixed with water and allowed to stand for up to 2 hours. Sand precipitates to the bottom and is easily felt or even seen in some cases. It may be necessary to encourage the passage of the sand with psyllium or laxatives if the sample is initially negative and the diagnosis is still suspected.

REPRODUCTIVE DATA

The horse is a seasonal (polyestrous) breeder, with a spring and summer breeding season. The timing of the breeding season is different between the northern and southern hemispheres.

Mare

Table 1.24 Reproductive data for normal mares

Oestrous cycle length	21 days is normal average 17–24 day oestrous cycle range is normal 'fertile' cycle range 13–25 days (maximal range recorded)
Oestrus	2–7 days (average 4 days)
Ovulation	24–48 h *before* end of behavioural oestrus
Gestation length	Normal range = 332–342 Maximum range for viable foal is 320–400 days 320–360 days (normal = 335–340 days) Most horse stud farms use 335 days to derive a predicted foaling date

Plasma hormone concentrations

Interpret hormone concentrations from single blood/urine samples with caution! Many sources of variation exist. Exact values may differ with breed and age as well as with reproductive status. The normal range of hormone concentrations associated with reproductive states may differ between laboratories. The following tables of values are intended only as guides to sample collection times and choice of analysis requested.

Ensure correct choice of collection tubes/anticoagulants when deciding what parameters are needed. See P. 6, Table 1.2 for ideal/acceptable collection tubes.

Table 1.25 Reference values for reproductive hormone concentrations in normal mares

Reproductive status		Oestrone conjugated (total) (ng/mL)	Progesterone (nmol/L)	eCG[a] (PMSG)
Follicular phase	Early oestrus	<6.0	<3.0 (<1 ng/mL)	−ve
	Late oestrus	<6.0	<3.0 (<1 ng/mL)	−ve
Luteal phase		<6.0	>12 (>6 ng/mL)	−ve
Pregnancy 8–25 days		<6.0	>13–57	−ve
40–100 days		<4.0	>10.0	+ve[b]
100–150 days		<6.0	<1.0	−ve
200–300 days		>2	<1.0	−ve
300-term		<2–4	<1.0	−ve

[a]Equine chorionic gonadotrophin.
[b]False-negatives may occur before 60 days and after 90 days.

Pregnane secretion increases during the final approximately 30 days pre-partum. As most P4 assays cannot distinguish these compounds from P4, laboratories may report increased concentrations at this time.

Granulosa theca cell tumour

Table 1.26 Hormone concentrations consistent with a diagnosis of granulosa theca cell tumour

	Oestrone (pg/mL)	Progesterone (ng/mL)	Testosterone (nmol/L)	Inhibin (ng/mL)
Granulosa cell tumour	<1	<1	0.5 (>50 pg/mL)	>0.7

Notes:
- Testosterone concentrations are significant but not diagnostic.
- Values over 100 pg/mL are often associated with stallion-like behaviour.

Urinary hormone concentrations

Table 1.27 Reference ranges for urinary oestrogen concentrations during reproductive events in normal horses

	Total urinary oestrogens (nmol/L)
Luteal phase	<500
Follicular phase	600–3000
Pregnancy (over 100 days)	>3000

Prediction of Foaling Date from Service Date

Note:
- A calculated foaling date is not prescriptive in the horse simply because of the variations in gestation length. Nevertheless, it does provide a focus date for the foaling. Mares often have normal foals up to 20 days either side of the expected date.

Table 1.28 Prediction of foaling date chart

SERVE	Jan	1	3	5	7	9	11	13	15	17	19	21	23	25	27	29	31
FOAL		Dec 7	9	11	13	15	17	19	21	23	25	27	29	31	Jan 2	4	6
SERVE	Feb	1	3	5	7	9	11	13	15	17	19	21	23	25	27	29	
FOAL		Jan 7	9	11	13	15	17	19	21	23	25	27	29	31	Feb 2	4	
SERVE	Mar	1	3	5	7	9	11	13	15	17	19	21	23	25	27	29	31
FOAL		Feb 4	6	8	10	12	14	16	18	20	22	24	26	28	Mar 2	4	6
SERVE	Apr	1	3	5	7	9	11	13	15	17	19	21	23	25	27	29	
FOAL		Mar 7	9	11	13	15	17	19	21	23	25	27	29	31	Apr 2	4	
SERVE	May	1	3	5	7	9	11	13	15	17	19	21	23	25	27	29	31
FOAL		Apr 6	8	10	12	14	16	18	20	22	24	26	28	30	May 2	4	6
SERVE	Jun	1	3	5	7	9	11	13	15	17	19	21	23	25	27	29	
FOAL		May 7	9	11	13	15	17	19	21	23	25	27	29	31	Jun 2	4	
SERVE	Jul	1	3	5	7	9	11	13	15	17	19	21	23	25	27	29	31
FOAL		Jun 6	8	10	12	14	16	18	20	22	24	26	28	30	Jul 2	4	6
SERVE	Aug	1	3	5	7	9	11	13	15	17	19	21	23	25	27	29	31
FOAL		Jul 7	9	11	13	15	17	19	21	23	25	27	29	31	Aug 2	4	6
SERVE	Sep	1	3	5	7	9	11	13	15	17	19	21	23	25	27	29	
FOAL		Aug 7	9	11	13	15	17	19	21	23	25	27	29	31	Sep 2	4	
SERVE	Oct	1	3	5	7	9	11	13	15	17	19	21	23	25	27	29	31
FOAL		Sep 6	8	10	12	14	16	18	20	22	24	26	28	30	Oct 2	4	6

Signs of impending parturition

The majority of thoroughbred foals' pregnancies are closely monitored and so an expected foaling date can be reasonably predicted. Nevertheless, there is a wide range of 'normal' gestation length and some mares will habitually foal either early or late. In paddock-bred mares, the service date and, therefore, the foaling date may not be known and then there is a danger that foaling will take place unexpectedly.

Regular observation of the mare may allow an owner to identify changes that indicate the proximity of foaling and so the attending veterinarian can be informed in reasonable time. Although most foalings are normal and occur without any interference, it is helpful to know when a mare is about to foal so that careful observation may take place.

The natural signs of impending parturition include:

1. Increased abdominal size (usually noticeable from around 8 months of gestation).

2. Pelvic relaxation with a prominent tail base as the pelvic ligaments become slack. This sign usually occurs within 2–4 days of parturition.

3. Udder development usually takes place in the last 2 days, although the teats may become longer and some udder development may occur over the 2 weeks before foaling.

4. Teat 'waxing' (wax-candles) are usually indicative of impending foaling within 24 hours (this feature is unpredictable).

5. Milk/colostrum ejection/leakage. In a mare with a normal gestational length this usually means the onset of first-stage labour. This means that foaling should take place within 2–3 hours.

Notes:
- Premature lactation is a worrying sign indicative of placental inflammation or foetal stress; it must never be ignored in any pregnant mare that is not at full term.
- Excessive leakage may mean that colostral deprivation will occur in the foal.

6. Milk calcium concentration of over 10 mmol/L indicates that parturition is pending (usually less than 24 hours).

7. Restlessness with repeated flank watching (very similar to milder spasmodic forms of colic!) and repeated lying down and rising. These signs usually indicate onset of stage 1 labour, i.e. within a few hours of birth.

8. Behavioural changes (isolation, inappetence and sweating) usually indicate delivery is imminent (within 2–3 hours).

Stallion
Semen characteristics

Table 1.29 Reference values for parameters in semen obtained from normal stallions.

	Range	Average
Volume (mL)	50–200	50
Gel-free volume (mL)	20–80	45
pH	7.3–7.7	7.4
Sperm/mL ($\times 10^9$)	100–500	200
Sperm/ejaculate ($\times 10^9$)	2–20	10
Progressively motile sperm (%)	0–95	55
Normal morphology (%)	30–90	55

Values are intended as estimates only.
Ejaculate parameters vary considerably between breeds, seasons and frequency of ejaculation.

Part 2 DIAGNOSTIC TESTS

Several part pages have been deliberately left blank to allow the reader to add any useful comments/tips which he/she observes during execution of the procedures themselves and any new helpful tips which are learned along the way! New tests and new interpretations are being developed and these should be learned by referring to current journals.

Combined Intravenous Glucose and Insulin Test

This test is a measure of blood glucose homeostasis and is used to diagnose insulin resistance (IR) in horses as part of the diagnosis of Equine Metabolic Syndrome (EMS).

Procedure

1. The horse can receive its normal feed the evening before but no food is to be given on the morning of the test and as the test is taking place.
2. Insert (with aseptic precautions) IV cannula with tap/plug. Flush carefully with heparin saline before and after each sampling, taking care to discard the first 5 mL of blood.
3. Obtain a blood sample for baseline glucose and insulin measurements.
4. Inject 150 mg/kg of glucose, immediately followed by 0.1 IU/kg of regular insulin.
5. Blood glucose concentrations are measured on blood samples directly using a glucometer or taken into fluoride oxalate anticoagulant at 1, 5, 15, 25, 35, 45, 60, 75, 90, 105, 120, 135 and 150 minutes post-infusion.
6. Blood is also collected at 45 minutes after infusion for insulin determination. Blood glucose concentration is plotted against time.

Result

In normal animals, blood glucose concentrations should return to *below* the baseline concentration after 45 minutes.

Insulin concentration greater than 100 μIU/mL at 45 minutes is interpreted as an indication of insulin resistance (Fig. 2.1).

Comments
- Hypoglycaemia is a potential complication of the test, although it is rarely encountered. If clinical signs of hypoglycaemia are observed, such as weakness and/or muscle fasciculations or if blood glucose concentration falls below 2.2 mmol/L, administer 60 mL of 40% glucose solution. The test will of course then be abandoned.

41

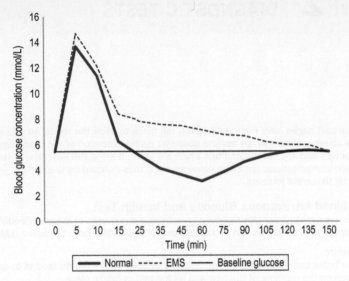

Fig. 2.1 Combined glucose insulin test showing the responses in a normal and in a horse affected with equine metabolic syndrome (insulin resistance).

Glucose/Xylose Absorption Test

Procedure

1. Starve the horse for 12 hours before and during test.

2. Insert (with aseptic precautions) IV cannula with tap/plug. Flush carefully with heparin saline before and after each sampling, taking care to discard the first 5 mL of blood.

3. Collect blood samples into fluoride oxalate anticoagulant. Alternatively the blood glucose can be measured directly using a glucometer at 30 and 15 minutes (time −30 and −15 minutes) before starting and at the time of dosing (time 0) sample at the time of dosing prior to start (STAT samples) (best if unstressed) (in-dwelling IV cannula).

4. Administer 1 g glucose/kg bodyweight as 20% solution by stomach tube.

5. Take blood samples (using fluoride oxalate anticoagulant) immediately after glucose administration and at 30-minute intervals for 3 hours.

6. Determine blood glucose concentration of each sample and plot concentration against time (−60 to +180 minutes) to produce a graph.

7. Calculate relative maximum concentration (base level is the mean of the first three samples, i.e. those taken before any glucose absorption) and the time of peak concentration.

Comments

- Accuracy of time is important! Either sample accurately at 30-minute intervals or record the precise time of sampling relative to the start of the test for later plotting.

- Xylose absorption test is identical but uses 5 g xylose/kg bodyweight given as 5% solution by stomach tube. Xylose is difficult to estimate, but it is not affected by endogenous glucose metabolism so it is theoretically more accurate.

- Check with lab before sending samples (fluoride oxalate anticoagulant is essential).

Result

Normal glucose/xylose absorption = peak at 90 – 120 minutes at 2 × basal concentration

Alterations from normal indicated by poor (low) peak value or prolonged time to peak (or both). Flat or delayed peak curves are suggestive of failure of small intestinal absorption of glucose (Fig. 2.2).

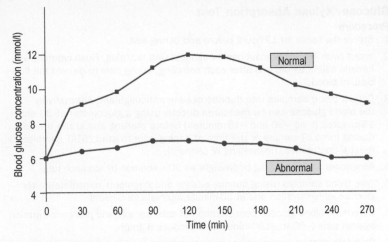

Fig. 2.2 Blood glucose values (mmol/L) for normal glucose absorption (♦—♦) and an abnormal absorption curve (●—●) obtained from a case of diffuse intestinal lymphosarcoma.

Comments

● Feeding and stress should be avoided during the test.

● Water must be available at all times during the test.

● There is merit in sampling at the time a catheter is placed (30 minutes before the test starts) because nasogastric intubation may be resented and cause a stress-related elevation in the initial (stat) sample taken at time zero. The resting value can be taken as the mean of the first two pre-treatment samples.

● Sampling every 30 minutes is the gold standard, but sampling every hour from the 120-minute point can reduce the number of samples taken without having a material effect on the test interpretation.

Assessing the Immunological Status of Foals

The foal is born immunologically naïve and has no effective immunity at birth. Survival and, more specifically, resistance to neonatal septicaemic infection, relies heavily upon effective passive transfer of immune globulins via the colostrum. The quality of the available colostrum must be excellent and the foal must obtain an effective volume of this within 1–3 hours of birth. The same mechanisms that are responsible for colostral (IgG) absorption are also the main portals of entry of infection into the blood stream and so early colostral ingestion and prevention of ingestion of infective bacteria form the cornerstones of neonatal medicine:

- Testing foals' blood for circulating IgG at 20–24 hours has become routine in good-quality breeding farm management, but testing at this stage allows very little (if any) time for corrective measures to be taken. By 12–18 hours, the intestinal absorption of colostral antibody is virtually zero and so corrective measures taken after this stage must involve intravenous plasma.

- An effective test can be performed at 12 hours using a rapid testing method such as the zinc sulphate test, the latex agglutination test or the CITE tests.

- The value of a test performed at 12–24 hours can be immense. While most septicaemic foals show signs of illness at 24–48 hours of age, the extent of infection can be critical at 12–24 hours.

Zinc sulphate turbidity test

The zinc sulphate turbidity test is a simple test that can be very useful.[1,2] It measures the approximate concentration of IgG in serum or plasma to establish the immune status of foals.

PROCEDURE

1. Prepare 250 mg $ZnSO_4 \cdot 7H_2O$ in 1 L freshly boiled water (to remove CO_2).

2. Place 6-mL aliquots of the zinc sulphate solution into sealed 7–10 mL vacuumed collection tubes (plain). It is useful to use a syringe attached to a fine needle, which is inserted through the bung into the vacuum (this leaves an air-free space over the solution and retains a slight vacuum in the tube). Tubes prepared in this way remain useful for several months without risk of carbon dioxide contamination and consequent cloudiness.

3. Add 0.1 mL serum or plasma (collect with a 1 mL insulin syringe from the sedimented blood).

4. Mix by repeated inversion of the tube.

5. Wait 10 minutes (qualitative) or 60 minutes (quantitative).

6. Measure against calibrated barium sulphate standards or 'printing test' (see below).

---

[1]Le Blanc MM (1990) Chapter 16: Immunologic considerations. In: *Equine Clinical Neonatology.* AM Koterba, WH Drummond, PC Kosch, eds. Lea & Febiger, Philadelphia, pp. 275–294.
[2]Le Blanc MM (1990) A modified zinc sulfate turbidity test for the detection of immune status in newly born foals. *Journal of Equine Veterinary Science* 10:36–40.

INTERPRETATION

Qualitative result: Obvious turbidity developed in 10 minutes = positive result, i.e. adequate immunoglobulin content.

Beware of possible CO_2 absorption into solution giving cloudiness!

If you can JUST read the print through the zinc sulphate solution tube after adding the plasma, the globulin level is approximately as shown opposite to each size of print below.

Zinc sulphate turbidity test = <3 g/L

Zinc sulphate turbidity test = 3–6 g/L

Zinc sulphate turbidity test = 6–8 g/L

Zinc sulphate turbidity test = 8–10 g/L

Zinc sulphate turbidity test = >10 g/L

Comments
- Significant difference between serum and plasma especially in foals with elevated plasma fibrinogen (i.e. those which are sick, so misleading results might be obtained!).
- Subjective assessment by observing for obvious cloudiness/turbidity of solution after 10 minutes (equates to adequate passive transfer).
- Quick, accurate and cheap (commercial kits are available).
- Accuracy less in low levels (<4 g/L); tends to overestimate in this lower range.
- Easy 'in field' method using pre-prepared tubes with vacuum (avoids atmospheric carbon dioxide contamination).
- Useful to test mare's serum at the same time (ideally turbidity should be same as or greater than the mare's serum).
- The test gives false-positive results with haemolysed serum.
- Can be quantified using spectrophotometer, but for this it requires a properly standardised calibration graph.

Notes:
- Haemolysis gives distorted (falsely elevated) results.
- Serum is used rather than plasma as distorted results may be obtained if the plasma fibrinogen is elevated. Serum is slower to obtain than plasma. Therefore, rapid testing could be delayed.
- Alternative sodium sulfite turbidity test is easy and cheap, but it is probably too unpredictable for everyday use. Furthermore, there is no need to use it if the other tests are available.

Single radial immunodiffusion (SRID)
- Specific immunoglobulin assay performed in agar gel.[3]
- Kits are commercially available.[4-7] Similar kits are available for IgM estimation.
- Home/practice prepared kits are less predictable and must be calibrated.
- The kit can also be used to quantify colostrum quality using whey fraction (minimal acceptable levels 100 g/L of unfractionated/unseparated colostrum).
- Plasma or serum can be used.
- Not applicable stableside as the test needs 24 hours; compromised foals may be dangerously low for 24 hours longer than they might otherwise.
- Accurate (wide range from 0 to 30 g/L), quantitative, but expensive.
- Useful accurate confirmation test.

Electrophoresis and biochemical protein estimation
- Total serum protein can be accurately determined by the Biuret reaction or using a refractometer but this is an unreliable indicator of globulin status because of the wide range of 'normal' concentrations of total protein in pre-suckle foals.
- Individual plasma proteins ($\alpha_{1/2}$, $\beta_{1/2}$, γ globulins and albumin) determined from electrophoresis and scanning by densitometer provide a very accurate estimation, but the process is time consuming and needs special equipment.
- A combination of laboratory estimation and electrophoresis can be a useful confirmation of stableside results obtained from other methods.

Latex agglutination
- Polystyrene particles (latex beads) used to visualise the reaction between antibody and specific protein.[8]
- Specific equine immunoglobulin (IgG) antiserum coated onto latex reagent and mixed with sample under test.

---

[3]Rumbaugh GE et al. (1978) Measurement of neonatal equine immunoglobulins for assessment of colostral immunoglobulin transfer: Comparison of single radioimmunodiffusion with zinc sulfate turbidity test, serum protein electrophoresis, refractory for total serum protein and sodium sulfite precipitation test. *Journal of the American Veterinary Medical Association* 172:321–325.

[4]Aglutinade Equine Colostrum Test® (Ab-Ag Laboratories, 11 Victoria Street, Littleport, Cambs, CB6 1LU, UK).

[5]ICN Immunobiologicals, PO Box 1200, Lisle, Illinois 60532, USA.

[6]VMRD Inc., PO Box 502, Pullman, WA 99163, USA.

[7]Veterinary Immunogenic Ltd, USA and Penrith, UK.

[8]Kruse-Elliot K, Wagner DC (1984) Failure of passive antibody transfer in the foal. *Compendium of Continuing Education for the Practising Veterinarian* 6:702–706.

- Positive agglutination occurs within 15 minutes with quantitative capability.
- Some kits are only useful for plasma and others only serum. ENSURE THAT THE CORRECT SPECIMEN IS USED.

> **Comments**
> - Very expensive commercial kits available.[9]
> - Technically simple and rapid.
> - High accuracy around or below 4 g/L, but above this it is poor (may miss marginal deficiencies around 6 g/L).
> - Not affected by haemolysis and whole blood can be used in some kits.
> - Can be performed stableside or in stud office.

Concentration immunoassay technology test (CITE test)

- This is a rapid (8–10 minutes to completion) and reliable test that can easily be performed with practice facilities.[10] It does require accurate pipetting (suitable pipettes are included in the commercial pack).
- The instructions on the commercial kits must be followed accurately.

> **Note:**
> - Accuracy is close to the definitive methods. Standards provide reliable quality and technical controls. The test is relatively expensive but its convenience makes this a minor consideration. The test is less affected by haemolysis than most others.

Glutaraldehyde coagulation

- Chemical (analytical) grade 25% glutaraldehyde solution is used and this forms an insoluble precipitate when mixed with basic proteins.[11,12] The test is rather crude, but it is very inexpensive and very reliable. Any haemolysis may result in overestimated IgG. The method should be quality checked against the SRID test (above).
- Prepare a 10% solution of glutaraldehyde in deionised (pure) water.
- Add 50 µL glutaraldehyde to 5 mL of serum and start clock.
- Measure time for clotting of serum to develop.

---

[9]Haver-Lockhart, Shawnee, Kansas, USA.
[10]IDEXX Ltd, Portland ME; USA and UK.
[11]Clabough DL, Conboy S, Roberts MC (1989) Comparison of four screening techniques for the diagnosis of equine neonatal hypogammaglobulinaemia. *Journal of the American Veterinary Medical Association* 194:1717–1720.
[12]Madigan JE (1997) Assessment of passive immunity. Chapter 9. *Manual of Equine Neonatal Medicine*, 3rd edn. Live Oak Publishing, Woodland, USA, pp. 36–40.

INTERPRETATION
- Clotting in less than 10 minutes = IgG >8.0 g/L.
- Clotting in 60 minutes = IgG concentration 4.0–8.0 g/L.

Immunoturbidometry
Immunoprecipitate measured by optical instruments. These are accurate and rapid but unnecessarily complicated for practical situations. Their main use lies in research and quality control/calibration of other methods.

Remember
- There is no transplacental immune globulin transfer so the foal is immunologically naïve at birth.
- Passive transfer is the most significant (only) source of immune globulin in the newborn foal.
- The foetus has some immunological competence from 6 months' gestation, but only starts to produce significant antibodies at birth. It takes >14 days to produce any effective active humoral protection and establishment of normal cellular responses may take longer.
- The mare concentrates IgGs into udder in last 3 weeks of gestation in preparation for colostrum production.

Assessment of Colostrum Quality
- Colostrum should be checked at the earliest possible stage and in any case before the foal has nursed. A 5-mL aliquot is usually all that is required.
- The physical appearance of the secretion will often provide a good guide of quality. Thick, sticky yellow secretion is likely to be good quality.
- Gentle warming to 65 °C or so will cause good-quality colostrum to clot strongly. This test can easily be performed in a teaspoon held over a lighter flame for a few seconds.
- Good-quality colostrum should have a specific gravity of >1.060 and contain at least 300 g/L of IgG.
- The specific gravity of the colostrum can be measured with a colostrometer.[13]
- Recent developments enable the use of small volumes (5–10 mL) of colostrum.

---

[13]Massey RE, LeBlanc MM, Klapstein EF (1991) Colostrum feeding of foals and colostrum banking. *Proceedings of the American Association of Equine Practitioners,* 36.

Colostral quality can also be measured quantitatively using a variety of commercially available kits[14] including:

Colostrocheck

- Samples clotting within 3 minutes of mixing with reagents in tube have >60 g/L IgG.
- Samples clotting 3–10 minutes after mixing have 40 g/L IgG.

These test kits are simple to perform and help to identify mares with poor-quality colostrum. Owners can easily perform them stableside.

Cryptorchidism Test

Serum oestrone sulphate

- For horses >3 years of age.
- Single sample of clotted blood necessary.
- Normal values: <0.02 ng/mL for geldings, 0.1–10 ng/mL for cryptorchids and >10 ng/mL for stallions.

hCG stimulation test

- In horses <3 years old and donkeys of any age.
- Obtain a clotted blood sample (plain tube).
- Administer 6000 IU human chorionic gonadotrophin intravenously.
- Obtain a second clotted blood sample 30–120 minutes later.
- Samples are submitted for testosterone analysis.

Testosterone concentrations used to identify the endocrinologic status of castrated (gelding) and cryptorchid horses following the administration of hCG.			
hCG stim. test	Gelding	Crytorchid	Stallion
Resting testosterone	<0.15 nmol/L	0.3–4.3 nmol/L	5–30 nmol/L
Second testosterone	<0.2 nmol/L	1.0–12.9 nmol/L	

Water Deprivation Test

- Water deprivation tests are used to identify renal failure and to differentiate psychogenic polydipsia from neurological (central) and nephrogenic (renal) diabetes insipidus.
- These tests MUST NOT be performed in horses that are azotaemic or that show evidence of any dehydration.
- It is essential that an accurate bodyweight is taken and tested during the procedure.

---

[14]GAMMA-CHECK-C ® (Veterinary Immunogenics Ltd, Carlton Hill, Penrith, Cumbria, UK).

Procedure

1. Take a blood sample and submit for routine haematology, total protein and albumin and urea and creatinine.
2. Weigh the horse accurately.
3. Remove water from the stable in the evening (so that the tests can be performed on the following morning). Sometimes feed is removed, but this is not likely to affect the test materially. Concentrate and salty foods must not be given, however.
4. Empty the bladder by catheterisation and determine urine specific gravity.
5. Weigh the horse and obtain urine and blood samples at 4–8-hour intervals.

Note:
- The test should be stopped if the horse shows an ability to concentrate urine (SG rising above 1.025) or if weight loss reaches 5% or if any overt evidence of azotaemia or dehydration develops.

Interpretation

- Normal horses show rapid urine concentration with SG rising above 1.025.
- Horses with psychogenic polydipsia also show normal concentration ability.
- A low or suboptimal SG suggests diabetes insipidus or renal medullary washout (see below).
- If urine does not concentrate at 24 hours to SG >1.025 an extended modified (partial water deprivation test is advisable) (see below).

Comments
- Renal medullary washout is due to excessive drinking in the absence of pathology and is due to the loss of osmotic gradient within the renal tubules. In this case, it is possibly better to perform a partial water deprivation test. Water intake is restricted to 40–45 mL/kg/day for several days, fed in small volumes frequently throughout the day. This will usually restore the gradient and the urine SG will rise to >1.025 and the associated polydipsia will usually resolve.
- Increase in SG >1.025 suggests psychogenic polydipsia while failure to concentrate >1.025 suggests diabetes insipidus.
- An ADH response test is then indicated (see below).

Vasopressin (Antidiuretic Hormone) Challenge Test

This test is used to distinguish neurogenic diabetes insipidus from nephrogenic diabetes insipidus.

Procedure

1. The bladder is emptied by catheterisation.
2. Bodyweight is recorded.

3. Blood and urine samples are obtained prior to the start of the test.
4. EITHER: 0.2 IU of exogenous ADH (vasopressin: Pitressin synthetic) is administered IM; OR: 60 IU ADH is administered IM every 6 hours over a 24-hour period.
5. Urine and blood samples are taken every 4–6 hours and bodyweight checked.

Interpretation
● In normal horses and those with central diabetes insipidus, urine SG should increase to over 1.025 within 4–12 hours of the start of the test.
● Horses affected with nephrogenic diabetes insipidus show little or no response to the ADH indicating that the renal tubular resorption of water is incapable of responding to the hormone.

Renal Clearance Ratios
1. Creatinine clearance ratio
This is proportional to GFR if renal function is normal.

PROCEDURE
1. Collect total 24-hour urine output.
2. Determine creatinine concentration and volume of urine.

Creatinine clearance ratio, glomerular filtration rate (assuming normal kidney function). GFR is traditionally measured by inulin clearance (a starch-like polymer of fructose which passes readily through the renal glomerular membrane and which is neither secreted nor absorbed by the renal tubules) or by 24-hour endogenous creatinine clearance:

$$\text{Creatinine clearance ratio} = \frac{[\text{Creatinine}]_{\text{SERUM}}}{[\text{Creatinine}]_{\text{URINE}}}\%$$

(Normal = 1.0 – 2.0 mL/kg/min)

2. Electrolyte clearance ratio
PROCEDURE
1. Obtain simultaneous venous blood (clotted) and urine (preferably by catheterisation).
2. Submit for creatinine and electrolyte clearances.
3. Remember that urinary creatinine may be expressed in mmol/L rather than µmol/L, as it will be for serum! (If you forget this, the results will look wildly off!)
4. The same principle can be applied to any metabolite including cortisol for pituitary–adrenal disorders such as equine Cushing's disease:

$$\text{Clearance}[X](\%) = \frac{[\text{Creatinine}]_{\text{SERUM}}}{[\text{Creatinine}]_{\text{URINE}}} \times \frac{[X]_{\text{URINE}}}{[X]_{\text{SERUM}}} \times 100\%$$

Table 2.1 Normal clearance ratios	
Na^+	0.1–1.0%
K^+	15–65.0%
Ca^{2+}	1.5–3.5%
pO_4^{3-}	0.0–0.5%
Cl^-	0.05–1.5%

Comments

● Simultaneously obtained urine and plasma samples can be used to obviate the need to collect 24-hour urine output. However, the accuracy of the analysis is dependent on normal renal function.

● If renal function is not normal the test is invalid (renal creatinine clearance ratio not normal).

● Values may show diurnal variation – results should be used as a guide rather than an absolute indicator.

● Diet has been shown to be a major influence on the results so interpretation can be very difficult.

3. Excretion factors

$$\frac{\text{Urine concentration (mmol)}}{\text{Urine specific gravity } 0.997} \times 0.04$$

Calcium excretion = 15μmol/mosmol (micromoles per milliosmole)
phosphate excretion = 15μmol/mosmol

Diagnostic Tests for Pituitary Pars Intermedia Dysfunction (PPID or Cushing's Disease)

Basal plasma ACTH

PROCEDURE

1. Collect EDTA plasma, preferably in plastic blood collection tube.

2. Chill the sample within 3 hours of collection.

3. Separate plasma by centrifugation.

4. Samples should be submitted to the lab chilled or frozen.

INTERPRETATION

- Reference range depends on methodology and laboratory.

- Typically an ACTH concentration <35 pg/mL is considered normal.

- There are circannual variations in plasma ACTH concentrations. In the autumn, ACTH concentration increases more in PPID than in normal horses so the period between August and October may represent the best time of the year to test for PPID.

Overnight dexamethasone suppression test

The ability of a small dose of exogenous dexamethasone to suppress the secretion of ACTH from the pituitary gland is tested by this method.

PROCEDURE

1. A plain (clotted) blood sample is obtained between 4 and 6 pm.

2. Administer 40 μg/kg dexamethasone intramuscularly.

3. Second clotted blood sample is obtained 19–20 hours later.

4. Samples are submitted for cortisol assay.

INTERPRETATION

- Normal horses show a suppression of serum cortisol levels to less than 10% of the resting cortisol concentration.

- In cases of PPID, the depression is much less (often negligible).

Note:
- There is a theoretical risk of inducing laminitis by the administration of the dexamethasone (even though the dose is very small – usually around 20 mg). The test should not be used in horses that have had laminitis or which are clinically affected at the time or are otherwise prone to develop laminitis.

Thyrotropin-releasing hormone response

The test relies upon there being an aberrant response of the pituitary adenoma to TRH and the release of ACTH in response to this. The mechanism for the test is not well understood.

PROCEDURE
1. Collect a serum sample.
2. Inject 1 mg thyrotropin-releasing hormone (TRH) intravenously.
3. Obtain serum samples at time 15, 30 and/or 60 minutes.
4. Submit specimens for cortisol assay.

INTERPRETATION
- Normal horses show minimal or absent responses.
- Horses affected with pituitary-dependent hyperadrenocorticism show an abnormal elevation of cortisol of 30–50% at 30 minutes and will remain elevated at 60 minutes.

Comments
- TRH is expensive and may be difficult to obtain.
- This test is preferred by some clinicians because of a perceived lower risk of inducing laminitis compared to the dexamethasone suppression test.

Combined dexamethasone suppression test/TRH stimulation test
PROCEDURE
1. Collect serum between 8 and 10 am and immediately after administer 40 μg/kg dexamethasone intramuscularly.
2. Collect serum 3 hours later and then administer 1 mg TRH intravenously.
3. Collect a follow-up serum sample 30 minutes after TRH administration.
4. Collect a final serum sample 24 hours after the dexamethasone injection.

INTERPRETATION
- Plasma cortisol >1 μg/dl at 24 hours post dexamethasone injection or >66% increase in cortisol levels 3 hours after TRH administration suggests PPID.

Schirmer Tear Test

Tear production in the horse is high compared to other species but the large majority of the aqueous component of the pre-corneal tear film is lost by evaporation from the surface of the eye. The Schirmer test provides information about the volume of tears that are being produced. The options are excessive tearing (as in painful, injured or infected eyes) or reduced (as in *keratoconjunctivitis sicca*).

Procedure

1. Either a standard Schirmer tear test strip or a 65 cm length (×4–6 mm wide) piece of Whatman Number 1 Filter Paper can be used. In the latter case, a bend or a small notch is placed about 5 mm from one end.

   - The Schirmer test strip has a notch that should be placed level with the eyelid margin.
   - The fold on the homemade paper serves the same purpose and measurement is made from these points.

2. The paper is introduced into the lower conjunctival sac so that the mark/fold or notch is at the eyelid margin, behind the lower lid and the eye allowed to close.

3. The paper is left *in situ* for 1 minute exactly and the distance the wetness has advanced down the paper is measured accurately.

4. The result is expressed as mm/minute.

Interpretation

- Normal tear production results in a distance of 12–28 mm/minute.

- Less than 10 mm/min is consistent with inadequate tear production while values over 35 mm indicate excessive tear production.

- Horses with obstructed tear ducts (in the absence of any conjunctival infection or inflammation) will usually have normal tear production.

  The patency of the nasolacrimal duct is tested by instilling a dye (usually fluorescein) into the conjunctival sac and examining the floor of the ipsilateral nostril for the dye some 10–15 minutes later.

  (Note that this is much later than in many other species.)

> **Comment**
> Topical local anaesthetic is not used and medications should be withdrawn for some hours prior to the test.

Phenylephrine Equine Dysautonomia (Grass Sickness) Test

The clinical diagnosis of equine dysautonomia (grass sickness) can be very difficult. However, the phenylephrine eye (ptosis reversal) test can be an effective diagnostic aid. The test is particularly useful in the field situation where sophisticated facilities may not be available.

Procedure

1. Prepare a 0.5% solution of adrenaline (epinephrine) by diluting 1 mL of a 10% solution with 19 mL sterile saline.
2. Assess the degree of ptosis (drooping of the upper eyelids) in both eyes by carefully viewing from the front.
3. Add 0.5 mL of the 0.5% solution to the conjunctival sac of one eye only.
4. Reassess the eyelash angle (degree of ptosis) in both eyes after 30 minutes.

Interpretation

Positive result (i.e. the horse has equine dysautonomia (grass sickness)) if the angle of the treated eye is normalised, i.e. the eyelashes are lifted and the palpebral fissure is widened (the degree of ptosis is reduced) when compared to the untreated eye (see Fig. 2.3).

> **Comment**
> The test must not be performed on a horse that has received acepromazine or an alpha-2 adrenoreceptor agonist drug in the previous 6–8 hours.

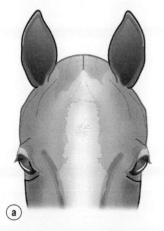 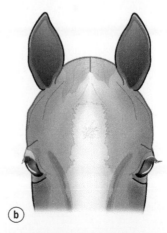

(a)   (b)

Fig. 2.3 Prior to application of the phenylephrine the eyelids of most grass sickness cases are uniformly drooped (ptosis) (a). Following application of phenylephrine to one eye the treated eyelid returns to a more normal position. The difference between the eyelid positions is usually very noticeable (b).

Alpha-2 Adrenoreceptor Agonist Test for Horner's Syndrome

Horner's syndrome is a rare condition in horses associated with impaired autonomic function in the region of the head and neck. The signs are less obvious in the horse than some other animals and usually there is sweating, ptosis, mydriasis and corneal dryness associated with the affected side. Intravenous injection of an alpha 2-adrenoreceptor agonist such as romifidine to an affected horse will cause the sweating signs to transfer from the affected side to the normal side.

Procedure

1. Identify the difference in temperature between the two sides of the horse's face by careful palpation or with the help of a thermal camera.

2. Inject a sedative dose (75 μg/kg) of romifidine (Sedivet, Boehringer Ingelheim, UK) intravenously.

3. Wait 12–15 minutes.

4. Reassess temperature of the two sides in the same way.

Interpretation

Positive result (i.e. Horner's syndrome is present) if the warmth and sweating of the affected side is reduced and there is increased sweating and warmth on the unaffected side.

Part 3

INDEX OF DRUGS USED IN EQUINE MEDICINE

**THE USE OF VETERINARY MEDICINAL PRODUCTS
GUIDELINES ON HORSE MEDICINES AND HORSE
PASSPORTS
PRESCRIPTIONS
PRESCRIPTION ABBREVIATIONS**

SECTION 1
DRUGS ACTING ON THE CENTRAL NERVOUS SYSTEM
- (a) Sedatives and anxiolytics
- (b) Analgesics
- (c) Anaesthetic agents
- (d) Muscle relaxants
- (e) Opioid antagonists
- (f) Parasympathomimetics
- (g) Parasympatholytics
- (h) Sympathomimetics
- (i) Sympatholytics
- (j) Anticonvulsants

SECTION 2
DRUGS ACTING ON THE CARDIOVASCULAR SYSTEM
- (a) Angiotensin converting enzyme (ACE) inhibitors
- (b) Anti-arrhythmic drugs
- (c) Cardiac glycosides
- (d) Anticholinergics
- (e) Vasodilators
- (f) Shock treatments

SECTION 3
DRUGS ACTING ON THE RESPIRATORY SYSTEM
- (a) Bronchodilators
- (b) Antihistamines
- (c) Antitussives
- (d) Mucolytics
- (e) Respiratory stimulants
- (f) Corticosteroids
- (g) Antimicrobials

SECTION 4
DRUGS ACTING ON THE URINARY TRACT
- (a) Diuretics
- (b) Other drugs
- (c) Antimicrobials

SECTION 5
DRUGS ACTING ON THE GASTROINTESTINAL TRACT
- (a) Antacids/anti-ulcer drugs
- (b) Intestinal stimulants
- (c) Intestinal sedatives/antispasmodics
- (d) Laxatives/cathartics
- (e) Antidiarrhoeals

SECTION 6
HORMONES/STEROIDS AND NON-STEROIDAL ANTI-INFLAMMATORY DRUGS
- (a) Sex steroids (drugs used to manipulate equine reproduction)
- (b) Anabolic steroids
- (c) Adrenal corticoids
- (d) Non-steroidal anti-inflammatory drugs
- (e) Pituitary suppression drugs
- (f) Others

SECTION 7
ANTI-INFECTIVE DRUGS
- (a) Antiviral drugs
- (b) Antibacterials
- (c) Compound antibacterials
- (d) Antifungal agents
- (e) Antiprotozoal drugs
- (f) Anthelmintics
- (g) Ectoparasiticides

SECTION 8
BLOOD-MODIFYING AGENTS
HAEMOSTASIS
- (a) Anticoagulants (*in vivo*)
- (b) Coagulants
- (c) Haematinics
- (d) Immunosuppressive drugs
- (e) Miscellaneous
- (f) Vitamin preparations
- (g) Electrolytes/fluids

SECTION 9
VACCINES/ANTISERA

SECTION 10
MISCELLANEOUS DRUGS/MEDICATIONS AND OTHER MATERIALS
- (a) Local anaesthetics
- (b) Eye preparations

SUSPECTED ADVERSE REACTIONS TO DRUGS USED IN THE HORSE

INDEX OF DRUGS USED IN EQUINE MEDICINE

THE USE OF VETERINARY MEDICINAL PRODUCTS

(Reproduced from the *RCVS Guide to Professional Conduct*, 2012.)

The responsible use of veterinary medicines for therapeutic and prophylactic purposes is one of the major skills of a veterinary surgeon and crucial to animal welfare and the maintenance of public health.

Classification of veterinary medicines

The main authorised veterinary medicines are the following:

a. Prescription-only Medicine – Veterinarian; abbreviated to POM V.

b. Prescription-only Medicine – Veterinarian, Pharmacist, Suitably Qualified Person (SQP); abbreviated to POM VPS.

c. Non-Food Animal – Veterinarian, Pharmacist, Suitably Qualified Person; abbreviated to NFA-VPS.

d. Authorised Veterinary Medicine – General Sales List; abbreviated to AVM-GSL.

Prescription of veterinary medicines

Veterinary surgeons and those veterinary nurses who are also SQPs should prescribe responsibly and with due regard to the health and welfare of the animal.

POM V medicines must be prescribed by a veterinary surgeon, who must first carry out a clinical assessment of the animals under his or her care. (See below for RCVS interpretations.)

POM VPS medicines may be prescribed in circumstances where a veterinary surgeon has carried out a clinical assessment and has the animals under his or her care. However, the Veterinary Medicines Regulations provide that POM VPS may be prescribed in circumstances where the veterinary surgeon, pharmacist or SQP has made no clinical assessment of the animals and the animals are not under the prescriber's care.

NFA-VPS medicines may be supplied in circumstances where the veterinary surgeon or SQP is satisfied that the person who will use the product is competent to do so safely and intends to use it for the purpose for which it is authorised.

Veterinary surgeons have additional responsibilities with the prescription or supply of POM V and POM VPS and the supply of AVM-GSL medicines.

There are five schedules of controlled drugs under the Misuse of Drugs Regulations 2001, each subject to a variety of different controls, including, for example: schedule 1 – possession requires a Home Office licence; schedule

2 – drugs obtained and supplied must be recorded in a register for each drug; schedule 2 and 3 – prescriptions are subject to additional requirements; and, schedule 4 and 5 – drugs are subject to fewer controls. Veterinary surgeons should take extra care when prescribing controlled drugs, to ensure that the medicines are used only for the animals under treatment.

Under his care
The Veterinary Medicines Regulations do not define the phrase 'under his care' and the RCVS has interpreted it as meaning that:

a. the veterinary surgeon must have been given the responsibility for the health of the animal or herd by the owner or the owner's agent

b. that responsibility must be real and not nominal

c. the animal or herd must have been seen immediately before prescription or,

d. recently enough or often enough for the veterinary surgeon to have personal knowledge of the condition of the animal or current health status of the herd or flock to make a diagnosis and prescribe

e. the veterinary surgeon must maintain clinical records of that herd/flock/individual.

What amounts to 'recent enough' must be a matter for the professional judgement of the veterinary surgeon in the individual case.

A veterinary surgeon cannot usually have an animal under his or her care if there has been no physical examination; consequently a veterinary surgeon should not treat an animal or prescribe POM V medicines via the Internet alone.

Clinical assessment
The Veterinary Medicines Regulations do not define 'clinical assessment' and the RCVS has interpreted this as meaning an assessment of relevant clinical information, which may include an examination of the animal under the veterinary surgeon's care.

Diagnosis
Diagnosis for the purpose of prescription should be based on professional judgement following clinical examination and/or post mortem findings supported, if necessary, by laboratory or other diagnostic tests.

Choice of medicinal products
The selected product should be authorised for use in the UK in the target species for the condition being treated and used at the manufacturer's recommended dosage.

If there is no suitable authorised veterinary medicinal product in the UK for a condition in a particular species, a veterinary surgeon may, in particular to avoid unacceptable suffering, treat the animal in accordance with the 'cascade'.

If there is no medicine authorised in the UK for a condition affecting a non-food-producing species, the veterinary surgeon responsible for treating the animal(s) may, in particular to avoid unacceptable suffering, treat the animal(s) in accordance with the following sequence:

a. a veterinary medicine authorised in the UK for use in another animal species or for a different condition in the same species or, if there is no such product:

b. either:

    i. a medicine authorised in the UK for human use or

    ii. in accordance with an import certificate (see the guidance note issued by the Veterinary Medicines Directorate [VMD]), a medicine authorised for veterinary use in another Member State

or, if there is no such product:

c. a medicine prepared extemporaneously by a veterinary surgeon, a pharmacist or a person holding an appropriate manufacturer's authorisation, as prescribed by the veterinary surgeon responsible for treating the animal.

A decision to use a medicine which is not authorised for the condition in the species being treated where one is available should not be taken lightly or without justification. In such cases, clients should be made aware of the intended use of unauthorised medicines and given a clear indication of potential side effects. Their consent should be obtained in writing. In the case of exotic species, most of the medicines used are unlikely to be authorised for use in the UK and owners should be made aware of and consent to, this from the outset.

When it is necessary to have a product prepared as an extemporaneous preparation, in the first instance it is recommended that the veterinary surgeon contacts a manufacturer holding an authorisation that permits them to manufacture such products (commonly referred to as Specials Manufacturers [ManSA]. See the list of Specials Manufacturers held by the Medicines and Healthcare products Regulatory Agency.).

Specials Manufacturers may already have experience preparing the product in question and will have the necessary equipment to prepare and check the quality of the product.

Horses declared 'not for human consumption' under the horse passport scheme are regarded as non-food-producing animals for the purposes of these provisions.

The prescribing cascade – food-producing animals

If there is no medicine authorised in the UK for a condition affecting a food-producing species, the veterinary surgeon responsible for treating the animal(s) may use the cascade options (see Choice of medicinal products, p. 64), except that the following additional conditions apply:

a. The treatment in any particular case is restricted to animals on a single holding.

b. Any medicine imported from another Member State (option b[ii]) must be authorised for use in a food-producing species in the other Member State.

c. The pharmacologically active substances contained in the medicine must be listed in the table in the Annex to Regulation (EU) No. 37/2010 (this table replaces Annexes I, II or III of Council Regulation [EEC] 2377/90).

d. The veterinary surgeon responsible for prescribing the medicine must specify an appropriate withdrawal period.

e. The veterinary surgeon responsible for prescribing the medicine must keep specified records.

f. See Fig. 3.1.

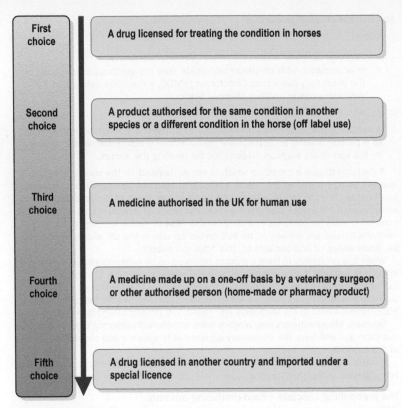

Fig. 3.1 The cascade system applicable to the UK.

First choice
A drug licensed for treating the condition in horses

Second choice
A product authorised for the same condition in another species or a different condition in the horse (off label use)

Third choice
A medicine authorised in the UK for human use

Fourth choice
A medicine made up on a one-off basis by a veterinary surgeon or other authorised person (home-made or pharmacy product)

Fifth choice
A drug licensed in another country and imported under a special licence

Antimicrobial and anthelmintic resistance

The development and spread of antimicrobial resistance is a global public health problem that is affected by use of these medicinal products in both humans and animals. Veterinary surgeons must be seen to ensure that when using antimicrobials they do so responsibly and be accountable for the choices made in such use. Resistance to anthelmintics in grazing animals is serious and on the increase; veterinary surgeons must use these products responsibly to minimise resistance development.

Responsibilities associated with the prescription and supply of medicines

A veterinary surgeon or SQP who prescribes POM VPS veterinary medicinal product or supplies a NFA-VPS veterinary medicinal product and a veterinary surgeon who prescribes a POM V veterinary medicinal product must:

a. before he/she does so, be satisfied that the person who will use the product is competent to use it safely and intends to use it for a use for which it is authorised

b. when he/she does so, advise on the safe administration of the veterinary medicinal product

c. when he/she does so, advise as necessary on any warnings or contraindications on the label or package leaflet and

d. not prescribe (or in the case of a NFA-VPS product, supply) more than the minimum quantity required for the treatment.

The Veterinary Medicines Regulations do not define 'minimum amount' and the RCVS considers this must be a matter for the professional judgement of the veterinary surgeon in the individual case.

Veterinary medicinal products must be supplied in appropriate containers and with appropriate labelling.

Administration

A medicine prescribed in accordance with the cascade may be administered by the prescribing veterinary surgeon or by a person acting under their direction. Responsibility for the prescription and use of the medicine remains with the prescribing veterinary surgeon.

Registration of practice premises

Practice premises from which veterinary surgeons supply veterinary medicinal products (except AVM-GSL medicines) must be registered with the RCVS as 'veterinary practice premises', in accordance with the Veterinary Medicines Regulations (Paragraph 8 of Schedule 3).

Premises likely to be considered as 'veterinary practice premises' are those:

a. from which the veterinary surgeons of a practice provide veterinary services and/or

b. advertised or promoted as premises of a veterinary practice and/or

c. open to members of the public to bring animals for veterinary treatment and care and/or

d. not open to the public, but which are the base from which a veterinary surgeon practises or provides veterinary services to more than one client and/or

e. to which medicines are delivered wholesale, on the authority of one or more veterinary surgeons in practice.

Main and branch practice premises from which medicines are supplied are veterinary practice premises and must be registered with the RCVS.

Storage of medicines

All medicines should be stored in accordance with manufacturers' recommendations whether in the practice or in a vehicle. If it is stipulated that a medicine be used within a specific time period, it must be labelled with the opening date, once broached.

Drugs controlled under the Misuse of Drugs Act and the 2001 Regulations, as amended, must be stored properly, so that there is no unauthorised access. There should be no direct access by members of the public (including family and friends); and, staff and contractors employed by the practice should be allowed access only as appropriate. Veterinary surgeons should take steps to ensure that members of staff with access to controlled drugs are not a danger to themselves or others, when they join the practice and at times when they may be vulnerable.

Veterinary surgeons should keep a record of premises and other places where they store or keep medicinal products, for example, practice vehicles and homes where medicinal products are kept for on-call purposes. The record should be held at the practice's main 'veterinary practice premises' in accessible form.

Associations with other suppliers of medicines

A veterinary surgeon who is associated with retail supplies of POM VPS, NFA-VPS or AVM-GSL veterinary medicinal products (or makes such supplies) should ensure that those to whom the medicines are supplied or may be supplied, are informed of:

a. the name and qualification (veterinary surgeon, pharmacist or SQP) of any prescriber

b. the name and qualification (veterinary surgeon, pharmacist or SQP) of the supplier and

c. the nature of the duty of care for the animals.

Similar safeguards should be put in place by a veterinary surgeon who is associated with retail supplies of POM V veterinary medicinal products by pharmacists.

Ketamine

Ketamine may be the subject of misuse and, therefore, should be stored in the controlled drugs cabinet and its use recorded in an informal register.

Suspected adverse reactions to veterinary medicines

The Suspected Adverse Reaction Surveillance Scheme (SARSS) for veterinary medicines is operated by the VMD (telephone number for SARSS 01932/338427, fax 336618). All suspected adverse reactions should be reported using the yellow form (MLA 252A Rev. 09/11). Supplies should be held in the practice and may be obtained by return of post using the telephone or fax number. Serious reactions (death or prolonged severe clinical signs) are mentioned specifically in the European Directives and companies marketing products are required to report them to the SARSS. Further information is available from the VMD.

Obtaining medicines

Veterinary surgeons should ensure that medicines they supply are obtained from reputable sources and in accordance with the legislation, particularly where medicines are imported or manufactured overseas.

GUIDELINES ON HORSE MEDICINES AND HORSE PASSPORTS

(Issued by the Veterinary Medicines Directorate, September 2011.)

Horses and other equidae are considered to be food-producing species in the European Union (EU). Veterinary medicines used to treat animals, including horses, fall within the scope of Directive 2001/82, as amended and the national legislation that transposes the EU legislation into national law. The VMR transpose Directive 2001/82/EC into UK law.

In accordance with Commission Regulation 504/2008, horses can be declared as either intended for human consumption (food-producing horse) or not intended for human consumption (non-food-producing horse) in the horse passport. This declaration determines what products can be administered to the animal and, therefore, consideration of what medicines may be used must be taken.

Horse passports

All horses and ponies are required to have a passport identifying the animal. All horses born after July 2009 must be microchipped.

Horse passports contain information relating to:

horse's appearance, which is illustrated in a diagram called a 'silhouette'
microchip details
age
breed/type
all the medications administered (if the animal has been declared 'intended for human consumption').

Medicines for horses

All horses should be treated with veterinary medicinal products (VMPs) which have a UK marketing authorisation (MA) for use in horses as the first choice. However, if there is no suitable authorised product available, the veterinary surgeons may prescribe a medicine under the cascade for use in the animals under his care.

Under the cascade, a horse that is signed off from the food chain can be treated with any veterinary medicine authorised in the UK to treat another animal species or another condition in the horse. If there is no suitable veterinary medicine authorised in the UK, a UK-authorised human medicine or veterinary medicine authorised in another Member State (MS) may be imported for use with permission from the VMD. The last option is to prescribe a medicine specially prepared for that animal by a veterinarian, a pharmacist or a person holding a manufacturing authorisation or a medicine imported from a Third Country.

The prescribing cascade, explained above, also applies to food-producing horses. However, a food-producing horse can only be treated with a veterinary medicine that contains pharmacologically active substance(s) listed in Table 1 of Regulation EU 37/2010 for use in a food-producing species and a suitable withdrawal period should be set by the responsible veterinary surgeons.

Commission Regulation 1950/2006 established, in accordance with Directive 2001/82, a list of substances essential for the treatment of equidae: this is European legislation that allows the use of certain substances in horses (declared as food- or non-food-producing in the passport) under the use of the cascade and with a statutory withdrawal period of 6 months.

If any substance which is *not* contained within Table 1 (the Allowed List) of Regulation EU 37/2010 or on the list of Essential Substances, such as phenylbutazone, is administered to an animal, that animal must be permanently excluded from the food chain and the passport declaration should be completed at Part II of Section IX by the owner or horse keeper or by the veterinary surgeon who administers the product. If the owner/keeper does not sign Part II of Section IX, the veterinary surgeon must do so.

Record keeping requirements

According to Commission Regulation No 504/2008, all vaccines administered by a veterinary surgeon must be recorded in the horse passport regardless of whether or not the horse is intended for human consumption.

There is no statutory requirement to record any other medicines in the non-food horse's passport; however, veterinary surgeons have record-keeping obligations for all prescription medicines under the VMR.

Any substance on the essential substances list administered to a food-producing horse must be recorded in the passport. Recording medicines administered under the cascade in the passport is optional.

In addition to the Horse Passport Regulations, there are other record-keeping obligations within the VMR that apply to keepers of horses intended for human consumption and to veterinary surgeons, pharmacists and SQPs supplying medicines for horses. These are set out within the body of the guidance document, but in summary, records of use for medicines of all distribution categories must be kept for all horses that have been declared as 'intended for slaughter for human consumption' in the horse passport or have Part II of Section IX unsigned. It is not a legal requirement for the record to be kept in the medicines pages of the horse passport, but it is acceptable for this to be done if preferred by the owner or keeper. Alternatively, a separate written record must be kept.

PRESCRIPTIONS

There is considerable pressure to remove the right to dispense from veterinary surgeons and if we are to retain this right then we have a duty to ensure that our standards are at least as high as any pharmacy (and preferably higher). Prescription writing is frequently cited as being an area in which we perform poorly as a profession.

Medicines should only be prescribed when they are necessary and in all cases the benefit of the medication should be weighed against the risk/harm that might be involved. The owner of the horse should be carefully advised in all cases before a drug is administered or prescribed. In this way, problems can be minimised and 'best practice' in the use of drugs applied. Factors that contribute to difficulties with medications prescribed for horses include the following:

1. Prescriptions not collected or not used in spite of dispensation

2. Purpose of medication is not clear to the owner and instructions for administration are not absolutely clear

3. Unrealistic expectation that the owner can/will administer the drug in the correct way

4. Perceived lack of efficacy for any reason at all including an error of drug selection or unexpected problems (e.g. a horse with diarrhoea may not absorb orally administered drugs as well as one without)

5. Real or perceived side effects detected/reported by the owner but not addressed by the dispensing veterinary surgeon

6. Unattractive formulations (e.g. suspensions that are hard to mix or particularly smelly drugs or thick injectable materials that cannot easily pass through a needle that the horse will tolerate) that make administration difficult

7. Complex instructions and advice that are imparted verbally or written instructions that are incomprehensible by the layperson (e.g. use of complex words and expressions).

When handling or dispensing drugs due attention must be paid to possible Health and Safety aspects. For example, some drugs may cause serious problems (e.g. chloramphenicol can cause aplastic anaemia) in humans and so appropriate care must be taken to explain the use and care of the drug. Suitable protective gloves may be required at the time. Drugs MUST be kept out of reach of children at all times and ideally should be kept in a totally safe place away from human food or drink.

Advice should be given on the safe disposal of unused drugs; ideally all unused drugs should be returned to the dispenser for disposal.

Good prescription principles include the following:

1. Write legibly with indelible ink and sign with your normal signature and your qualifications, including the bracketed 'Veterinary Surgeon' – even if on practice paper. Add printed details of your name (even if using practice paper).

2. Use approved names for drugs IN CAPITAL LETTERS – **DO NOT ABBREVIATE.**

3. State duration of treatment (where known) and if not known give pharmacist some chance of helping (i.e. add 'Repeat ...n... times' but do not comment 'Repeat as necessary').

4. Write out microgram/nanogram. DO NOT ABBREVIATE THESE – abbreviations are not always instantly recognisable and there should be no debate about the statement of dose.

5. Always put a 0 before a decimal point. For example, 0.3 milligrams NOT .3 mg.

6. GIVE PRECISE INSTRUCTIONS concerning ROUTE of administration and DOSE rate (either overall or 'per kg' – if per kg is used make sure pharmacist knows weight of animal or he/she won't know how much to dispense).

7. Any alterations invalidate the prescription – rewrite in its entirety – do not attempt to sign alterations – it is not valid.

8. **Prescriptions for Schedule 2 and 3 Controlled Drugs MUST be entirely written in longhand by the prescribing veterinary surgeon.**

It is NOT acceptable under any conditions to use typewriting or the handwriting of any other person.

If in any doubt, phone and speak to the pharmacist first – he/she will always attempt to help as far as possible and they have knowledge of available formulations, tablet sizes, etc., and which might be most suitable. This applies particularly to those drugs which are not in common equine usage and which the veterinary surgeon considers provide the best therapeutic options for the well-being of the patient. Pharmacists who receive prescriptions that are clearly wrong in some aspect will return them to the prescriber for correction – this is both time consuming and an embarrassment.

Computer-generated prescriptions are becoming more common. The prescription must include the date, patient's name, clients name and address. The prescription must be printed in English with NO ABBREVIATIONS AT ALL. The name and address of the prescriber must be printed completely and the signature MUST be handwritten.

Comment:
- Most drugs have established withdrawal times.
- These MUST be considered when using drugs to treat horses intended for human consumption.
- Any drug without a withdrawal time should be used with caution in any animal intended for human consumption.

Notwithstanding these comments, veterinary surgeons are reminded of their responsibilities regarding the use of drugs in 'food-producing animals' with respect to minimum acceptable residues and drug clearance times prior to slaughter. Apart from personal safety, the primary concern for the veterinary surgeon is for the patient – all other considerations (cost, disposal, withdrawal times, etc.) are secondary.

PRESCRIPTION ABBREVIATIONS

ac	before feeding	pc	after feeding
ad(s)	right ear (left)	po	by mouth
au	both ears	prn	as needed
ad lib	free access	qd	every day
amp	ampoule	qid	four times daily
aq	water	qod	every other day
bid	twice daily	q 4 h	every (4) hours
c	with	qA	sufficient quantity
cap(s)	capsule(s)	rep	repeat
circ	about/approximately	s	without
disp	dispense	sid	once daily
et	and	sig	instruction/label
ext	extract	solve	dissolve
g	gram	sol'n	solution
gtt(s)	drop(s)	SC	subcutaneous(ly)
id	the same	SS	half
IM (im)	intramuscular(ly)	stat	immediately
IV (iv)	intravenous(ly)	susp	suspension
m	mix	tabs	tablets
meg (ng)	microgram	tbs	tablespoon
mg	milligram	tid	three times daily
ml	millilitre	tr	tincture
non rep.	do not repeat	tsp	teaspoon
o.d.(s)	right eye (left)	Ut dict	as directed
o.m.	every morning	(s)	left
o.n.	every evening/night	(d)	right
o.u.	both eyes		

Notes:
- Avoid using the specific administration abbreviations qd, qod, id, sid, bid, tid because they may be confused with other abbreviations and are almost unknown outside the veterinary profession.
- If you are in any doubt, write out plain directions in longhand!

INDEX OF DRUGS USED IN EQUINE MEDICINE

Section 1
Drugs acting on the central nervous system

(a) Sedatives and Anxiolytics

Definitions:

Sedative: An agent that produces a mental calming effect, characterised by sleepiness in addition to a disinterest in the environment. Animals, however, are still momentarily arousable by sufficiently large stimuli so precautions should still be taken when handling sedated animals.

Anxiolytic/Tranquilliser/Neuroleptic/Ataractic: A drug that produces a mental calming effect characterised by reduced anxiety and a lack of concern for or interest in, the environment. The effects are not predictably dose-dependent and in some cases higher doses induce lesser or untoward effects.

Neuroleptanalgesia: Altered state of consciousness and inhibited responses induced by a combination of a tranquilliser and an opioid analgesic.

These definitions are not in themselves of much value but they do identify that the drugs chosen may be expected to have different types and extents of effect.

Acepromazine maleate
Injectable form (10 mg/mL) no longer available in UK but can be imported from France (5 mg/mL) under Special Import Certificate.
    POM V

Indications:

- Restraint.
- Control of excitement.
- Premedication.
- Examination of penis.

Presentations: 5 mg/mL 50 mL multidose bottles for injection. 35 mg/mL paste for oral administration.

Dose: Injection: 0.01–0.1 mg/kg IV/IM/SC (for premedication, use doses in the lower half of the dose range). Animal should be left quietly until effects become apparent. Effects become apparent within 10–20 minutes of IV dosing, but may take up to 40 minutes for peak effect, especially following IM administration.

Notes:

Contraindicated in Hypotensive Conditions
- Acute hypotension due to acepromazine may be treated with phenylephrine or noradrenaline (norepinephrine) and/or rapid IV fluids.
- May cause penile prolapse/priapism/paraphimosis (especially stallions).
- Significant drug interactions with quinidine sulphate (cardiac depression/hypotension).

NB: 2 mg/kg solution for small animals also available (CHECK CONCENTRATION OF SOLUTION BEING USED).

Detomidine
POM V

Indications:
- Sedation and analgesia (visceral > somatic), with muscle relaxant effects.
- Premedication.

Presentations: Solution for IV/IM injection 10 mg/mL (5 and 20 mL multidose vial); 7.6 mg/mL gel for oral transmucosal (sublingual) delivery.

Dose: 0.005–0.08 mg/kg IV/IM; 40 μg/kg sublingual delivery.

Note:
- Pyrexic horses may become tachypnoeic after detomidine administration. This response has been suggested to be due to the anti-pyretic action of α_2 agonists and may represent an attempt by the animal to 'pant' in order to cool down.

Standing sedation for 500 kg horse: detomidine 10 μg/kg + butorphanol 0.025 mg/kg IV, e.g. 0.5 mL detomidine with 1.25 mL butorphanol solution.

Useful IM combination for needle-shy or flighty animals: detomidine 20 μg/kg + butorphanol 0.05 mg/kg + acepromazine 0.03 mg/kg, combined together for IM administration. Butorphanol can be replaced with morphine (0.2–0.3 mg/kg) if a painful procedure is planned.

Table 3.1 Detomidine			
Level of sedation	Dosage (μg/kg)	Onset (minutes)	Duration (hours)
Light	10–20	3–5	0.5–1
Medium	20–40	2–5	0.5–1
Heavy	40–80	1–5	0.5–2

Notes:

- Peak effect 5 minutes after IV administration.
- Duration of action dose-dependent but around 60–90 minutes.
- Marked bradycardia with first- and second-degree A-V blocks, common.
- Ataxia more marked at higher doses and may be more pronounced when combined with an opioid.
- Diuresis and sweating are common side effects.
- IM dose 1.5–2× IV dose.
- Intractable horses can be sedated with sub-lingual high dose and be prepared to wait – effect may take some 40–90 minutes.
- **Beware when using with sympathomimetic amines.**
- **Not licensed for use in pregnant mares as no safety data is available. However, no good evidence exists for any teratogenic or ecbolic effects.**
- **DO NOT ADMINISTER IV ALONGSIDE potentiated sulphonamides (sulfonamides) (possible fatal dysrhythmias).**
- Maximal effects obtained when horse is left quiet after administration.
- May be combined with an opioid (butorphanol, buprenorphine, morphine or methadone) for good standing sedation.
- For field anaesthesia, use 10–20 μg/kg, preferably in *combination with an opioid, followed by ketamine at 2.2 mg/kg administered 5–10 minutes later (i.e. when sedation is maximal).

Administer detomidine first. After 5 minutes [peak effect of detomidine], administer the opioid. Wait another 5 minutes until anaesthetic induction.

Fluphenazine
POM V

Indication: Long-acting phenothiazine (duration of action up to 6 weeks).

Presentation: 2.5 and 25 mg/mL solution for injection.

Dose: 0.05–0.08 mg/kg IM.

Notes:

- Severe neurological signs can develop: restlessness, muscle rigidity, muscle spasms.
- If adverse signs develop, administer diphenhydramine 0.5–1 mg/kg IV q 24–48 h.

Romifidine
POM V

Indications:

- Sedation and analgesia (visceral > somatic) with muscle relaxant effects.
- Premedication.

Presentation: 10 mg/mL (20 mL multidose vial) for injection.

Dose: 40–120 μg/kg IV (slow).

Table 3.2 Romifidine			
Sedation effect	Dose rate (μg/kg)	Dose volume (mL/100 kg)	Duration (hours)
Light sedation	40	0.4	0.5–1.0
Moderate sedation	80	0.8	0.5–1.5
Deep sedation	120	1.2	>3

Notes:

- Peak effect 5 minutes after IV administration.
- Duration of action dose-dependent, but >80 minutes for higher doses.
- Marked bradycardia with first- and second-degree A-V blocks, common.
- Usually less ataxia than the other α_2 agonists, but may still occur and can be more marked if combined with an opioid.
- Diuresis and sweating are common side effects.
- For field anaesthesia, use 50–100 μg/kg, preferably in *combination with an opioid, followed by ketamine at 2.2 mg/kg 5–10 minutes later.
- Not licensed for use in pregnant mares as no safety data is available. However, no good evidence exists for any teratogenic or ecbolic effects.
- May be combined with an opioid (butorphanol, buprenorphine, morphine or methadone), for good standing sedation.

Per 100 kg: 0.6 mL romifidine + 0.2 mL butorphanol gives good sedation for diagnostic procedures.

Administer romifidine first. After 5 minutes [peak effect of romifidine], administer the opioid. After another 5 minutes, induce anaesthesia.

Xylazine
POM *V*

Indications:

- Sedation and analgesia (visceral > somatic) with muscle relaxant effects.
- Premedication.

Presentations:

- 20 mg/mL (20 mL multidose vial) for injection.
- 100 mg/mL (10 mL multidose vial) for injection.
- 500 mg dry powder (10 mL single-dose vial) + diluent.

Dose: 0.25–1.1 mg/kg IV (slow).

Notes:

- Peak effect 3 minutes after IV administration.
- Duration of action somewhat dose-dependent but commonly 10–20 minutes.
- Marked local reaction/unreliable effect if administered IM (2–3× IV dose).
- Bradycardia with first- and second-degree heart block is common following administration.
- Ataxia more marked at higher doses and may be more pronounced when combined with an opioid.
- Diuresis and sweating are commonly observed.
- Not licensed for use in pregnant mares as no safety data is available. However, no good evidence exists for any teratogenic or ecbolic effects.
- Check concentration of solution available to ensure correct dose administered.

DO NOT USE AS PREMEDICANT FOR QUINALBARBITAL (SECOBARBITAL)/ CINCHOCAINE EUTHANASIA.

(b) Analgesics

1. Non-steroidal anti-inflammatory drugs (NSAIDs): drugs that inhibit formation of prostaglandins and thromboxanes from arachidonic acid with anti-inflammatory properties, that are not steroids. Classically, these drugs have anti-inflammatory, analgesic and anti-pyretic effects.

2. Opioids: drugs that work in a similar manner to morphine (synthetic or non-synthetic). Opioids exert their effects by binding to special opioid receptors in the CNS and periphery. Classic properties: analgesia, sedation (sometimes).

3. NMDA receptor antagonists – ketamine. In sub-anaesthetic doses mostly analgesic and antihyperalgesic properties; especially useful in chronic pain situations.

4. α_2 agonists: work on α_2 receptors which are widely distributed throughout the body. Have analgesic properties but because of sedative and cardiovascular

effects, are rarely used as primary analgesics. The analgesia they provide is, however, an advantage in the perioperative setting and they may be considered as part of a multimodal analgesic protocol for treatment of more long-standing painful conditions, when they are usually administered by continuous intravenous infusion. Analgesia, as well as sedation, can be antagonised with atipamezole.

5. Local anaesthetics: see p. 215.

Opioids
BUTORPHANOL TARTRATE
POM V/CD (S-IV)

Indications:

- Relief of musculoskeletal and visceral pain (colic).
- With sedative/anxiolytic for standing chemical restraint.

Presentation: 10/50 mL multidose bottle, 10 mg/mL for injection.

Dose: 0.05–0.2 mg/kg IV/IM/SC. Lower doses are used when combined with α_2 agonists for sedation/restraint.

> **Notes:**
> - Duration of action approximately 45–60 minutes.
> - Not as good analgesic properties as other opioids.
> - Expensive.

Side effects:

- Increased locomotor activity ('box-walking' behaviour) has been described, especially if high doses are given to non-painful animals.
- Potent antitussive.

Contraindications:

- Lower respiratory tract conditions associated with copious mucus production.
- As with all opioids, relatively contraindicated in patients with head trauma/increased intracranial pressure where even slight respiratory depression may lead to sufficient hypercapnia to further increase intracranial pressure.

BUPRENORPHINE HYDROCHLORIDE
POM V/CD (S-III)

Indications:

Analgesia.

With sedative/anxiolytic for standing chemical restraint.

Presentation: 10 mL multidose bottle, 0.3 mg/mL for injection.

Dose: 0.005–0.02 mg/kg IV/IM. Lower doses can be used when combined with α_2 agonists for sedation/restraint. Beware increased locomotor activity at the highest dose.

Notes:
- Analgesia lasts around 6–8 hours.
- As a partial μ opioid receptor agonist, buprenorphine is not as efficacious as the full μ opioid receptor agonists, morphine and methadone. Nevertheless, buprenorphine should provide better analgesia, of longer-duration, than butorphanol.
- As a Schedule 3 controlled drug, it should be stored in a locked receptacle.
- Relatively recently licensed for use in horses in UK so further information will become available with time.

Side effects:
Increased locomotor activity occurs if the highest doses are given to non-painful animals.

Contraindications:
Few absolute contraindications.

As with all opioids, relatively contraindicated in head-trauma patients with already raised intracranial pressure.

METHADONE
No licensed product is available for equine use in the UK CD (S-II).

Indications:
- Relief of severe pain.
- Useful with sedative/anxiolytic for standing chemical restraint.

Presentation: Methadone hydrochloride, 1 mL ampoule (10 mg/mL).

Dose: 0.1–0.5 mg/kg IM/IV.

Notes:
- Duration of action 2–4 hours.
- May be administered epidurally (0.1–0.2 mg/kg), in combination with morphine (0.1–0.2 mg/kg) for provision of analgesia with a duration of at least 12 hours. The preservative-free preparations are preferred for this route of administration.

Side effects:
Can cause some increased locomotor activity, e.g. box walking.

Contraindications:
As with all opioids, relatively contraindicated in patients with head trauma and already raised intracranial pressure.

Must be kept in a locked receptacle and purchase and dispensing registered in a bound record book.

MORPHINE SULPHATE
No licensed product is available for equine use in the UK CD (S-II).

Indications:

- Relief of severe pain.
- Useful in combination with a sedative/anxiolytic for standing chemical restraint.
- Can be administered by the epidural or intra-articular routes for the relief of pain without loss of motor nerve function (NB preservative-free preparations are preferred). Often combined with methadone for epidural analgesia (see below).

Presentations:

Morphine hydrochloride, single-dose vial – 10 mg/mL or 60 mg/2 mL.

Preservative-free formulation is variably available in single-dose vials containing 10 mg/mL, 2 mg/mL and 2.5 mg/5 mL.

Dose: 0.1–0.2 mg/kg IM/IV; 0.1–0.2 mg/kg for epidural or intra-articular administration.

Epidural doses:

- 0.1 mg/kg made up to final volume 10 mL for 500 kg horse (with, e.g. sterile 0.9% NaCl; analgesia at least to L1, 0.2 mg/kg analgesia up to Th9). Onset of analgesia may take up to 4 hours. Analgesia duration is usually at least 12 hours and sometimes may extend up to 24 hours. When combined with preservative-free methadone (0.1 mg/kg), the methadone provides analgesia within 30 minutes, but this lasts only 2–3 hours; so methadone's effects are waning at the time when morphine's effects are becoming apparent. The mixture is an excellent mixture for providing long-duration epidural analgesia.
- Other combinations have been reported, e.g. morphine 0.05–0.1 mg/kg + detomidine 30 μg/kg. The addition of the α_2 agonist ensures quick-onset analgesia without the danger of motor block, similar to the use of methadone. However, α_2 agonists are rapidly absorbed systemically from the epidural site so the animal may become obviously sedated.

Notes:

Duration of action 2–4 hours following systemic administration.

- Very good analgesia.
- Preservative-free presentation should be used for epidural and intra-articular administration.
- Box walking may be apparent in normal, pain-free horses if high doses are administered.
- Although morphine has been described as a cause of postoperative ileus, recent studies showed NO proof of this fact and its analgesic and sedative properties outweigh this risk by far.

Must be kept in a locked receptacle and purchase and dispensing registered in a bound record book.

PETHIDINE
POM V/CD (S-II)

Indications:

- Relief of musculoskeletal and gastroenteric pain.
- Effective spasmolytic.
- Useful in combination with a sedative or anxiolytic for standing chemical restraint.

Presentation:

Pethidine hydrochloride.

50 mg/mL.

Dose: 3.5–10 mg/kg IM (35–100 mL/500 kg).

Notes:
- Onset of action within 5–10 minutes
- Duration of action 30 minutes.
- Do not administer IV: causes histamine release!
- Analgesia is dose-dependent.

Must be kept in a locked receptacle and purchase and dispensing registered in a bound record book.

α_2 *Agonists*
POM V

Indications:

- Sedative and analgesic with muscle-relaxant effects.
- Premedication prior to ketamine (or thiopental) anaesthetic induction.
- Useful in recovery stages of anaesthesia if horse is excited/distressed.
- Sedative of choice for hepatoencephalopathy.
- Can be used for epidural analgesia without danger of motor paralysis (in combination with morphine).

   See above for individual agents (detomidine, romifidine and xylazine).

(c) Anaesthetic Agents

1. Volatile/gaseous agents

- Agents in current use include the vapour nitrous oxide (N_2O) and the volatile liquid agents isoflurane, sevoflurane and desflurane. Only isoflurane is licensed for use in horses in the UK at present. Halothane is no longer available. Nitrous oxide's use in horses remains controversial as it can partition into spaces already occupied by even lower solubility gases (such as nitrogen, hydrogen and methane) faster than these other gases can partition out of these spaces and so distension of the gastrointestinal tract is possible. However, this has never been documented to have caused colic.

- To define a dose for an inhalational agent the term MAC is used: this is the Minimal Alveolar Concentration necessary to prevent 50% of the population moving (with gross purposeful movement) in response to a supramaximal noxious stimulus (skin incision, for example).

- Apart from nitrous oxide, inhalational agents have NO ANALGESIC PROPERTIES – so other analgesic drugs need to be added to the protocol.

ISOFLURANE
POM V

Indications: Maintenance of anaesthesia. Induction of anaesthesia in foals.

Presentation: Colourless, volatile liquid with pungent, unpleasant smell.

Dose: MAC 1.3%. Expect to deliver, into a circle system, somewhere between 2% and 3% during anaesthetic maintenance, depending on the other sedative, anaesthetic and analgesic drugs used. If you can monitor inspired and end-tidal isoflurane concentrations, then the end-tidal value is a guide to the alveolar concentration, so you can tell how near MAC the horse is receiving. Most patients will require between MAC and 1.5× MAC in order to remain adequately anaesthetised during noxious stimulation.

Notes:
- Cardiovascular effects: causes dose-dependent cardiovascular depression, mainly in the form of vasodilation and thereby hypotension is common.
- Respiratory effects: dose-dependent respiratory depression. Isoflurane is a particularly pungent agent and can cause breath-holding when used for inhalation induction in foals. Although a cuffed endotracheal tube should bypass the sensory olfactory mucosa, some people believe there are 'pungent receptors' in the lungs too, which might explain the reluctance of most isoflurane-anaesthetised horses to breathe!
- Low solubility gives relatively rapid induction and recovery from anaesthesia (useful for performing inhalation anaesthetic induction in foals).

SEVOFLURANE
Not licensed for equine use.

Indications: Maintenance of anaesthesia.

Induction of anaesthesia in foals.

Presentation: Colourless, volatile liquid with pungent smell (but more tolerable than isoflurane) in a plastic bottle.

Dose: MAC 2.3%. Expect to deliver, into a circle system, somewhere between 2% and 4% during anaesthetic maintenance, depending on the other sedative, anaesthetic and analgesic drugs used. If you can monitor inspired and end-tidal sevoflurane concentrations, then the end-tidal value is a guide to the alveolar concentration, so you can tell how near MAC the horse is receiving. Most patients will require between MAC and 1.5× MAC in order to remain adequately anaesthetised during noxious stimulation.

Notes:

- Cardiovascular effects: causes dose-dependent cardiovascular depression mainly via causing vasodilation and, thereby, hypotension.

- Respiratory effects: causes dose-dependent respiratory depression but because it's reportedly less pungent than isoflurane, theoretically sevoflurane should produce less respiratory depression than anaesthesia at an equivalent depth with isoflurane. In practice, however, respiratory depression with both isoflurane and sevoflurane can be marked at equivalent anaesthetic depths! That said, however, foals do tend to breath-hold less during anaesthetic induction with sevoflurane than with isoflurane, so this is one potential advantage.

- Low solubility gives relatively rapid induction and recovery from anaesthesia. Useful for performing inhalation anaesthetic induction in foals and, due to its lower solubility in blood than isoflurane, the induction of anaesthesia may be slightly quicker.

- Recovery is much the same as following isoflurane anaesthesia. Its lower blood solubility should offer a slightly faster recovery but, for most anaesthetics lasting at least an hour, its greater fat solubility offsets its lower blood solubility and negates any potential advantage. Rapid recoveries aren't necessarily better recoveries though!

- At the moment more expensive than isoflurane.

DESFLURANE
Not licensed for equine use.

Indication: Maintenance of anaesthesia.

Presentation: Colourless, volatile liquid in a plastic-reinforced glass bottle, very pungent smell. Requires special, heated vaporizer to blend pure desflurane vapour into the fresh gas stream to the desired output concentration.

Dose: MAC 6–9%. Expect to deliver, into a circle system, somewhere between 8% and 9% during anaesthetic maintenance, depending on the other sedative, anaesthetic and analgesic drugs used. If you can monitor inspired and end-tidal desflurane concentrations, then the end-tidal value is a guide to the alveolar concentration and you can tell how near MAC the horse is receiving. Most patients will require between MAC and 1.5× MAC in order to remain adequately anaesthetized during noxious stimulation.

Notes:

● Cardiovascular effects: dose-dependent cardiovascular depression, similar to isoflurane and sevoflurane. Occasionally, at light planes of anaesthesia, sympathetic stimulation may occur.

● Respiratory effects: dose-dependent respiratory depression but also very pungent such that intermittent positive pressure ventilation is usually required. Not suitable for induction of anaesthesia.

● Very low solubility – rapid change of anaesthetic depth and recovery from anaesthesia can, therefore, be expected. Special vaporiser allows refilling while turned on because of this!

● Due to its physical properties, desflurane needs a special vaporiser (very expensive).

NITROUS OXIDE
POM *V*

Indications:

● Adjunct during induction and maintenance of general anaesthesia with volatile agents.

● Weak analgesic.

Presentation: Colourless, sweet-smelling vapour in cylinders (BLUE). Full cylinders contain compressed liquid nitrous oxide, above which is a saturated vapour. Beware because the cylinder contents gauge will show no reduction until all the liquid has been evaporated and only vapour remains.

Dose: Where gas monitoring is not available, *never exceed* 50% mixture with oxygen in rebreathing systems to ensure that a hypoxic gas mixture isn't delivered to the patient. Where gas monitoring is not available, another precaution against delivering hypoxic gas mixtures to the patient is to use relatively high-flow, semi-closed rebreathing systems (circle systems or To and Fro systems).

Notes:

- Use with care in heavy horses in dorsal recumbency which are particularly prone to becoming hypoxaemic. In these cases, where high inspired oxygen concentrations will be required to help offset the hypoxaemia, there is often no 'room' left for nitrous oxide.

- Ideally and especially when using nitrous oxide, the patient's oxygenation status should be monitored using arterial blood gas analysis or, at the very least, pulse oximetry. This will help to guide any necessary interventions.

- Second gas effect theoretically useful during induction of anaesthesia or during transition from intravenous induction to inhalation maintenance.

- Diffusion hypoxia is suggested as a hazard at the end of anaesthesia if oxygen isn't supplemented after nitrous oxide is first discontinued. This effect has also been suggested to occur in young delivered by Caesarean section such that nitrous oxide is not favoured in these cases.

- Do not use in colic or any other situation where closed gas-filled spaces may exist (see above). Some people don't use it in healthy horses because of the worry of causing distension/displacement colic.

- Nitrous oxide has been linked to bone marrow depression in people and so extra care must be taken for human safety (i.e. good scavenging). Pregnant women should not come into contact with it because of the suggested risks of teratogenesis, abortion and infertility.

- Greenhouse gas!

- The role of nitrous oxide use in equine anaesthesia is questionable, as its benefits do not outweigh the problems occurring with the use of this gas.

2. Intravenous anaesthetic drugs

KETAMINE
POM *V*

Indication: Short duration general anaesthesia with xylazine, romifidine or detomidine.

Presentation: 10 or 50 mL multidose vials, 100 mg/mL.

Dose: 2–2.5 mg/kg IV.

Notes:
- Ensure adequate sedation with an α_2 agonist before administration of ketamine.
- Once administered, it can take 60–120 seconds for anaesthetic induction to be complete.
- Very wide therapeutic index.
- Minimal cardiorespiratory depression.
- Useful for anaesthetic maintenance for procedures of <1 hour duration in-field (in combination with guaiphenesin and an α_2 agonist).
- Analgesia an advantage. Useful during anaesthesia if administered as an infusion at sub-anaesthetic dose for additional systemic analgesia (doses 0.5–1.5 mg/kg/hour).
- **NEVER administer ketamine alone or first!** (Ensure pre-filled syringes are clearly labelled).

PROPOFOL
Not licensed for equine use in UK. POM *V*

Indication: Induction of anaesthesia in foals/small ponies. (Induction quality can be poor in horses so it's often not recommended.)

Presentations: White emulsion (10 mg/mL), single-use 20 mL vials, multidose 20 mL vials with preservative (benzyl alcohol).

Dose: 2–5 mg/kg IV; doses towards the lower end of this dose range following premedication with an α_2 agonist.

Notes:
- Only efficacious when administered IV, so IV catheter advised. Not irritant if extravascular deposition occurs.
- Mild cardiorespiratory depression. Large, rapid boluses may cause apnoea.
- Rapidly metabolised, short-acting. Has been used as part of an anaesthetic maintenance technique, but high infusion rates may cause sufficient respiratory depression to warrant intermittent positive pressure ventilation; therefore, often not used as the sole maintenance agent.
- Expensive.
- Useful for small ponies/young foals as induction agent/short procedures (e.g. entropion).
- Discard single-use bottle 24 hours after opening. (Product with preservative has shelf-life of 28 days following first use.)

ALFAXALONE
Not licensed for equine use in UK. POM V

Indications: Anaesthetic induction; possibly useful for maintenance as it is rapidly metabolised.

Presentation: Clear solution of alfaxalone solubilised in 2-hydroxypropyl-β-cyclodextrin in 10 mL multidose vials; 10 mg/mL.

Dose: Following premedication, 1–3 mg/kg IV.

Notes:
- Large volume of injectate required and relatively expensive, so may be more useful in foals and small ponies.
- Minimal cardiovascular depression. Some respiratory depression, especially with higher doses given rapidly IV.
- Rapid metabolism should enable relatively quick recovery from anaesthesia, especially following short field procedures. Recovery quality similar to that following ketamine-based anaesthetic protocols.
- Still a relatively new agent so more details of its use in horses and ponies should emerge with time.

THIOPENTAL (THIOPENTONE) SODIUM
Licensed product no longer available in the UK but can be imported under Special Treatment Certificate from Australia. POM V

Indication: Anaesthetic induction for short-duration procedures.

Presentation: Dry powder reconstituted to 2.5%, 5% or 10% solution – sterile water diluent provided.

Dose: 10–15 mg/kg (1–1.5 g/100 kg) following *light* premedication.

5–10 mg/kg (0.5–1 g/100 kg) following *heavy* premedication.

Notes:
- Do not reconstitute with Hartman solution or Ringer's lactate solution.
- Extremely alkaline – very irritating extravascularly, use of IV catheter obligatory. Immediate action if extravascular injection suspected (using copious amounts of saline ± lidocaine [lignocaine] HCl).
- Preferably, use solutions of <10%.

GUAIPHENESIN
Not licensed for equine use in the UK but can be imported under SIC from The Netherlands. POM V

Indications: Not an anaesthetic agent but a centrally acting muscle relaxant with some sedative effects that may be used in conjunction with thiopental or ketamine for anaesthetic induction; and in combination with ketamine and an α_2 agonist for maintenance of short-term intravenous anaesthesia.

Presentation: Plastic bottle containing 500 mL of a 10% solution (100 mg/mL) of guaiphenesin.

Dose: 20–120 mg/kg IV (often only 20–50 mg/kg when used as co-induction agent following α_2 agonist premedication). Irritant to vascular endothelium and, if extravascular deposition occurs, IV catheter must be used. Beware doses >150 mg/kg which may be associated with prolonged, ataxic recoveries; higher doses still are associated with toxicity (cardiac arrhythmias, respiratory depression).

Administration: By infusion; either for induction of anaesthesia where its infusion usually precedes a bolus of thiopental or ketamine; or for maintenance of anaesthesia (previously induced usually with ketamine following an α_2 agonist), in combination with ketamine and an α_2 agonist (triple drip). A typical recipe for such a 'triple drip' would be: into 500 mL of 10% guaiphenesin, add 1000 mg of ketamine and 500 mg of xylazine (i.e. eventual concentrations are: 100 mg/mL guaiphenesin; 2 mg/mL ketamine and 1 mg/mL xylazine). The infusion rate is around 1 mL/kg/hour which, for a 20 drops/mL giving set, would be about 3 drops/second for a 500 kg horse.

(d) Muscle Relaxants

Atracurium

Not licensed for equine use in UK.

Indications: Peripherally acting skeletal muscle relaxant; useful for better surgical access in some procedures, eye surgery (eyeball stays in centre of orbit and does not move).

Presentation: 10 mg/mL, 2.5 mL, 5 mL, 25 mL.

Dose:

- First dose: 0.1–0.25 mg/kg IV.
- Top up doses: ¼–½ initial dose IV.

Notes:

- Because atracurium affects all muscles – IPPV MUST BE PERFORMED! Only consider using this drug if special equipment is available to provide ventilation and also, ideally, to monitor the degree of neuromuscular blockade (e.g. requiring a peripheral nerve stimulator).

- Undergoes spontaneous chemodegradation in the plasma at normal body temperature and pH by 'Hofmann elimination'.

- Reverse with, ideally, edrophonium 0.1 mg/kg IV or, if not available, with neostigmine 0.04 mg/kg and atropine 0.01 mg/kg, both IV.

- 'Depth' of muscle relaxation can be monitored using either a 'train-of-four' or 'double burst' pattern of peripheral nerve stimulation. Superficial motor nerves commonly used for such stimulation include branches of the facial nerve (if you have access to the head), stimulation of which causes a muzzle twitch or the superficial peroneal nerve, stimulation of which causes a foot flick.

Dantrolene sodium
POM V

Indications:

- Direct-acting skeletal muscle relaxant.
- Prevention or treatment of malignant hyperthermia-associated myopathy exertional rhabdomyolysis.

Presentation: 100 mg caps for ORAL use.

Dose: 10 mg/kg po loading dose, 3–5 mg/kg po q 1 h.

As prophylactic – full loading dose 60 minutes before surgery.

Use cautiously before surgery (not fully evaluated).

Very expensive and very short half-life, therefore rarely stocked.

Guaiphenesin/glyceryl guaiacolate ether BP (GGE)
POM V

Indications: Spinally acting muscle relaxant. Use for anaesthetic induction in combination with anaesthetic agent (ketamine, thiopental) or for anaesthetic maintenance as 'Triple-drip' (GGE+ketamine+α_2 agonist as rate-adjustable, continuous infusion). See also above.

Presentation: White crystalline powder.

Homemade – dissolve 50 g powder in 500 mL 5% dextrose or saline solution to make a 10% solution. Very difficult to dissolve. Helps to warm solution.

Available from The Netherlands, Gujatal® is a 10% solution.

Dose: For co-induction of anaesthesia 20–120 mg/kg IV slowly until desired effect is attained. Following α_2 agonist premedication, dose required is often lower, i.e. 20–50 mg/kg (i.e. approx. half bodyweight [kg] in millilitres of 10% solution, as a guide).

Notes:

- May precipitate out of solution, if very cold.
- Best to make up fresh. Make up any 'triple drip' solutions fresh and use that day.
- Very irritating – if suspected, infiltrate with large volumes of saline solution.
- **DO NOT USE ALONE FOR CASTRATION** – this drug has no analgesic/anaesthetic properties!
- It is also reported to be a useful expectorant (po) (doubtful efficacy).

Methocarbamol
POM V

Indication: Central muscle relaxant, reduces muscle spasm in musculoskeletal conditions.

Presentations: Solution for injection (100 mg/mL). Tablets 500 and 750 mg.

Dose: 4.4–55 mg/kg slow IV q 6h (use higher doses for severe conditions.

Oral 50–100 mg/kg q 12–24 h

> **Note:**
> ● Use in tetanus controversial.

Suxamethonium

Not licensed for equine use.

Indications: Depolarising muscle relaxant. Can be useful adjunct to injectable euthanasia. Classically used as part of anaesthetic induction technique.

Presentation: White, water-soluble powder reconstituted for injection.

Dose: 0.1–0.2 mg/kg IV.

> **Notes:**
> ● Muscle fasciculation occurs before paralysis ensues. Inactive in alkaline solution.
> ● DO NOT mix with barbiturates in syringe!
> ● Additive to thiopental for euthanasia in difficult circumstances (followed by large-volume pentobarbitone – 200 mg/mL).

(e) Opioid Antagonists

Naloxone

Not licensed for veterinary use. CD (S-II)

Indication: Respiratory depression associated with potent opioids.

> Antidote against inadvertent human self-administration of potent opioids.

Presentations: Single-dose (1 mL) vials 0.4 mg/mL for injection.

Dose:

For antagonism of opioid overdose or unwanted side effects (pure μ-agonists) in animals: 0.04–1.0 mg/kg.

(f) Parasympathomimetics

Neostigmine

Not licensed for veterinary use.

Indications:

● Non-depolarising neuromuscular blocker antagonist: through its action as an anti-cholinesterase it increases acetylcholine presence at neuromuscular junctions. The increased concentration of acetylcholine can compete with the neuromuscular blocker for effects on the muscle's motor end plate.

- Stimulates motility (but not necessarily co-ordinated motility) and tone of the GI tract.
- Miotic effects on iris.
- Atropine poisoning/toxicity.

Presentation: 2.5 mg/mL (1:500) aqueous injection in 1 mL vials.

Dose: 0.02–0.04 mg/kg IV/SC.

Dosing intervals determined by response.

> **Note:**
> - May need to give 0.01 mg/kg atropine slow to effect in horses to counteract neostigmine's muscarinic effects (NB: monitor ECG closely). Magnesium may inhibit the efficacy of anticholinesterase therapy in antagonising neuromuscular blockade by reducing post-synaptic calcium ingress and calcium-mediated muscle contraction.

Edrophonium
Not licensed for veterinary use.

Indication: Non-depolarising neuromuscular blocker antagonist.

Presentation: 1 mL vials; 10 mg/mL.

Dose: 0.1–0.5 mg/kg IV/SC.

Dosing intervals determined by response.

> **Note:**
> - Can use edrophonium alone in horses to reverse atracurium. It has minimal muscarinic effects and, therefore, an anticholinergic, such as atropine, is rarely required.

Bethanecol
POM V

Indications: Oesophagitis, gastroduodenal ulcers, incontinence, gastrointestinal motility stimulant.

Presentation: 25 mg tablets.

Dose: 0.025–0.030 mg/kg every 4 hours for 24 hours SC, 0.35–0.45 mg/kg orally every 6–8 hours.

> **Note:**
> - At higher doses diarrhoea and colic may occur.

Physostigmine
POM V

Indication: Diagnosis of narcolepsy.

Dose: 0.06–0.08 mg/kg slow IV.

> **Note:**
> ● This will precipitate a narcoleptic attack within 3–10 minutes after administration. Atropine sulphate 0.04–0.08 mg/kg reduces severity of attacks and can prevent them reoccurring.

(g) Parasympatholytics

Atropine
POM V

Indications: Parasympatholytic (anticholinergic, mydriatic, cycloplegic). Relief of smooth muscle spasm, antidote to parasympathomimetic drugs (including organophosphate). For intraoperative bradydysrhythmias. In cardiopulmonary resuscitation. Bronchodilation. Glaucoma, relief of iris spasm.

Presentations: Clear aqueous solution, 10 mg/mL, 50 mL multidose vials, also 1 mL vials; 0.6 mg/mL.

Dose: 0.01–0.04 mg/kg IV/IM/SC.

0.015 mg/kg IV/IM/SC as treatment for acute bronchoconstriction.

> **Notes:**
> ● Side effects (may be prolonged) and include:
>   1. Sinus tachycardia, ectopic complexes.
>   2. Vision disturbances (mydriasis (may cause panic - use darkened room), photophobia, cycloplegia, possible but not marked increases in intra-ocular pressure).
>   3. Abdominal distension, ileus.
>   4. Urinary retention.
> ● Ophthalmic ointment or drops (1/2%) can cause systemic effects on gut motility in particular. Ophthalmic effects include reduction in intra-ocular pressure in glaucoma due to high unconventional (uveoscleral) drainage of aqueous in horses (beware of cause of glaucoma).

Glycopyrrolate
No licensed veterinary product available.

Indication: Counteract vagal reflex in emergency resuscitation.

Presentation: 1 and 3 mL vials; 300 µg/mL.

Dose: 2 µg/kg IV.

Notes:
- Onset of action slower than atropine (1–3 minutes), therefore, less useful in an emergency. Duration of action is also longer (2–3 hours cardiovascular effects).
- More gastrointestinal side effects than atropine.

Hyoscine butylbromide
POM *V*

Indication: Anti-spasmodic. Relief of spasmodic colic; facilitation of rectal examination in horses that strain during the procedure.

Presentations: 1 mL ampoules, 20 mg/mL and 50 mL multidose bottles, 20 mg/mL. With metamizole (as Buscopan compositum) 100 mL multidose glass bottle; each mL contains 4 mg butylscopolamine bromide and 500 mg metamizole.

Dose: 0.3 mg/kg hyoscine; 0.2 mg/kg hyoscine with 25 mg/kg metamizole IV.

Notes:
- May cause a transient increase in heart rate post-administration.
- Metamizole is a non-steroidal anti-inflammatory and administration of further anti-inflammatory drugs should only be done with caution.

(h) Sympathomimetics
Dobutamine
No specific veterinary licensed product. POM *V*

Indications: Hypotension, particularly during general anaesthesia. It is a positive inotropic agent (β_1 agonist) indicated for short-term cardiovascular support in patients with poor cardiac performance due to decreased contractility. Overall effects on vascular resistance are believed to be minimal. At normal doses, cardiac rates are also not significantly affected, but rates may increase at higher dosages.

Presentations: Dry powder 250 mg/bottle or 250 mg solution for dilution.

Dose: Reconstitute with 1 L 5% glucose or 0.9% saline to yield a solution having a concentration of 250 µg/mL.

Administer IV at 1–5 µg/kg/minute, which, for a 500 kg horse, means starting at about 1 drop per second of a 250 µg/mL solution; but administer and titrate to effect.

Notes:
- ECG monitoring for tachyarrhythmias and, rarer, bradyarrhythmias, is essential.
- Drug interactions: oxytocic drugs may cause a severe hypertension when used with dobutamine. Dobutamine may be ineffective if β-blocking drugs, e.g. propanolol have recently been given.

Dopamine

No specific veterinary licensed product. POM *V*

Indications: Correction of haemodynamic imbalances in shock.

Oliguric pre-renal renal failure.

Presentations: To prepare solution: add 250 mg to 1 L of normal saline or Hartman solution to give concentration of 250 µg/mL. 5 mL ampoules containing either 40 or 160 mg/mL.

Dose: Variable according to effect desired (2–10 µg/kg/minute by continuous IV infusion).

<2.5 µg/kg/minute dopaminergic effects said to predominate, including splanchnic vasodilation and possibly increased urine output.

2.5–5 µg/kg/minute for β_1 effect.

>5–10 µg/kg/minute causes α effects in addition to β and dopaminergic effects; arrhythmias may occur at these infusion rates.

Notes:
- Only used in intensive care (especially neonates).
- Severe necrosis/sloughing if accidental extravascular deposition occurs (if suspected, infiltrate site with 5–10 mg phentolamine in 10–15 mL normal saline).
- Monitor urine flow, cardiac rate/rhythm/blood pressure.
- Cease if severe arrhythmias, such as premature ventricular contractions (PVCs), develop.
- Half-life in circulation 5–9 minutes.

Ephedrine sulphate

No specific veterinary licensed product. POM *V*

Indications: An ino-constrictor with direct and indirect pressor effects. May be given as a bolus to help support arterial blood pressure in anaesthetised horses. Depth of anaesthesia and intravascular volume status should also be assessed when treatment of hypotension is undertaken.

Presentation: Aqueous solution for injection (30 mg/mL) 1 mL vials.

Dose: 0.03–0.2 mg/kg IV.

Notes:
- Besides an increase in arterial blood pressure, heart rate may also increase.
- Re-dosing is less successful as tachyphylaxis is displayed.

Epinephrine/adrenaline

No specific veterinary licensed product. POM *V*

Indications:

- Adrenergic effects (α and β).
- Bronchodilator.
- Increases systolic blood pressure.
- First-line drug in cardiac resuscitation.
- Prolongs effect of local anaesthetics because of vasoconstriction localising the agents to the site of administration and delaying systemic absorption.
- Capillary haemostasis (local), e.g. in eyes/iris – see Ophthalmic drugs.

Presentation: Clear, aqueous solution for injection. 1 mg/mL (1 in 1000) as adrenaline acid tartrate BP.

Doses: 0.1–0.2 mL/50 kg by IV/IC injection. 0.01–0.02 mg/kg IV.

For anaphylaxis: 0.2–0.4 mL/50 kg by IM or SC injection (2–4 mL/500 kg horse).

Notes:

- Use care with dose calculation. Best to dilute to 1 in 10 000 using water for injection.
- Ophthalmic drops (1%) are available but can have systemic effects.
- This solution can be diluted to create a 0.5% solution for use in the equine dysautonomia (grass sickness) test.

Isoprenaline

No specific veterinary licensed product available. POM V

Indications:

- Non-specific β receptor agonist
- Emergency relief of bronchospasm
- Has been used as positive inotrope but has positive chronotropic actions, too.

Presentation: Injectable 1 in 5000 (0.2 mg/mL) 1 mL vial.

Dose: Best used as IV infusion administered to effect.

Note:

- Causes dangerous tachycardia and arrhythmias especially under halothane anaesthesia. Superseded by new specific β_1 agonist drugs.

Noradrenaline (norepinephrine)

No specific veterinary licensed product available. POM V

Indications: Predominantly α adrenergic effects (slight β effects).

For hypotension associated with anaesthesia or shock.

Presentation: 4 mg in 4 mL ampoule.

Dose: Dissolve 4 mg in 1 L saline solution.

Administer as IV drip. Very short acting – administer according to effect.

> **Notes:**
> - Potent vasoconstrictor.
> - May cause decreased organ perfusion and increased myocardial work. Avoid prolonged infusions.
> - Very short shelf-life – dispose of after use.

Phenylephrine

No specific veterinary licensed product available. POM *V*

Indications: α_1-adrenergic agonist. Useful in phenothiazine-induced hypotension. May be used during general anaesthesia but must treat other causes of hypotension (e.g. excessive anaesthetic depth; hypovolaemia).

Valuable adjunct to therapy of some cases of nephrosplenic ligament entrapment (entrapment of the left colon in the nephrosplenic space).

Presentation: 1 mL ampoule 10 mg/mL.

Dose: 5–8 µg/kg IV (up to 0.01 mg/kg) bolus will increase blood pressure in anaesthetised horses. Heart rate will usually decrease in response to a baroreceptor reflex.

Most frequently used as an infusion and administered to effect (0.1–0.2 µg/kg/ minute).

Dose for treatment of nephrosplenic ligament entrapment: 20–80 µg/kg dissolved in 500 mL 0.9% NaCl and given IV over 15 minutes, ideally during lunging. (Note that the heart rate must be carefully monitored during infusion.) This treatment relies upon categoric diagnosis and should not be used in suspected (i.e. unproven) cases.

> **Note:**
> - High dose can increase myocardial work and decrease organ perfusion. Do not use in cases of myocardial failure.

(i) Sympatholytics

Propanolol

No specific veterinary licensed product available. POM *V*

Indications: β-adrenoreceptor blocker (correction of supraventricular tachyarrhythmias).

Presentation: Aqueous injection (1 mg/mL), 1 mL glass vial.

Dose: 0.03–0.15 mg/kg IV slowly.

Note:
- Usually begin at low dose and titrate to effect. Can be used to correct serious tachydysrhythmias produced by β_1 agonist. Can be used to treat some cases of atrial fibrillation, either as a total treatment or as an adjunct to other methods.

  NB: This drug is, by definition, a negative inotrope. Use with caution. A shorter acting β-blocker is Esmolol, dose 0.05–0.15 mg/kg IV.

(j) Anticonvulsants

The management of seizures in horses is critical both for safety of personnel and for the patient. Inevitably, there are problems with the drug protocols that are used and so it is important to follow established guidelines.

Protocol for anticonvulsive therapy in horses

(After Mayhew IG, 1989, Large Animal Neurology, Lea and Febiger, London.)

- Select one drug only.
- Institute at recommended dose. Adjust until no untoward effects present.
- Administer oral drugs at least 1–2 hours before feeding (empty stomach).
- If side effects (e.g. drowsiness/collapse) without control of convulsions, reduce drug and add second at recommended dose.
- If seizures are controlled, gradually taper dose of first drug (to discontinue after 1–2 weeks) provided no seizures develop.
- If seizures return as first drug is withdrawn, return to controlling dose and continue for 3 months.
- Do not alter drugs until animal has been seizure-free for 4 weeks at least.
- Do not suddenly withdraw drugs – severe seizures may follow.
- Monitor blood concentrations of drugs if seizures are difficult to control. Aim for seizure control by maintaining blood levels of pentobarbital of 5–15 μg/mL. Tolerance is a serious/difficult problem.
- If routine drugs fail to control seizures, use other drugs with caution – more drugs make coordination more difficult and may induce severe seizures.
- Horses with convulsions are dangerous to themselves/peers and handlers.
- If convulsions are controlled for 3 months try to reduce doses – if seizures return discuss outlook with owner. The need for long-term therapy makes prognosis very guarded (dangers and welfare).
- Beware of drug interactions (e.g. chloramphenicol/tetracycline prolong the effects of phenytoin; ketamine is seizurogenic anyway)!
- Low blood proteins may increase effect of protein-bound drugs at standard doses.
- Ivermectin is always contraindicated in convulsive horses (severe seizures may be seen within days).

Carbamazepine
POM V

Indication: Anticonvulsant with sodium channel-blocking effects. Used mainly for treatment and diagnostic confirmation of trigeminal neuralgia (headshaking syndrome). Little anticonvulsant effect due to short half-life.

Presentation: 400 mg tablets.

Dose: Initially 10 mg/kg q 6 h. Dose increased to 20 mg/kg q 12 h and then to 40 mg/kg q 24 h. All efficacy tests to be performed within 2 hours of a dose.

Notes:
- The drug is expensive and has more value in differentiating trigeminal neuralgia cases (part of headshaking syndrome) from post-herpetic neuralgia and other forms of the headshaking syndrome.
- Major difficulty with this drug is short half-life in horses (2 hours) compared with humans (27 hours).

Diazepam
POM V/CD (S-IV)

Indications: Anticonvulsant, sedative, muscle relaxant.

Useful sedative/muscle relaxant and premedicant in foals.

Presentation: Solution for injection 5 mg/mL in 2 mL single-dose vials.

Dose: Pre-anaesthetic (foals): 0.05–0.5 mg/kg IV (average 0.25 mg/kg).

Status epilepticus: up to 1 mg/kg (slow IV).

Notes:
- Unacceptable ataxia if given alone to adult horses.
- Use slow IV injection (<10 mg/minute).
- Diazepam solubilised in propylene glycol may cause thrombophlebitis.
- Minimal cardiorespiratory effects.
- Do not dilute or mix with other agents (may be mixed with ketamine provided used immediately).
- May replace GGE in anaesthetic induction protocols (especially foals).

Midazolam
POM V/CD (S-IV)

Indications: As for diazepam (anticonvulsant activities).

Presentation: 10 mg in 2 mL vials, i.e. 5 mg/mL.

Dose: As for diazepam. IV dose titrated against the response.

Notes:
- Short-acting benzodiazepine. Not yet fully evaluated in foals but appears similar to diazepam for premedication.
- Can be mixed with other agents. Does not cause thrombophlebitis.

Phenobarbital
POM V

Indication: Anticonvulsive therapy.

Presentations: Aqueous solution for IV injection 60 and 200 mg/mL.

15, 30, 60 and 100 mg tablets for oral dosing.

Dose: Convulsing foals: 5–20 mg/kg IV (diluted in 30 mL saline and given slowly over 30 minutes).

Adults: 12–20 mg/kg initial dose (diluted in saline and given over 30 minutes), followed by 1–9 mg/kg for maintenance.

Oral: 2–12 mg/kg q 12–24 h (aim to maintain blood drug levels at a concentration of 15–45 µg/mL).

Note:
- Reduce dosage according to effect. Prolonged high doses may cause hepatic failure.

Phenytoin
POM V

Indication: Anticonvulsive therapy in foals.

Presentations: Aqueous solution for IV injection 50 mg/mL.

25 and 100 mg capsules for oral dosing.

Dose: 5–10 mg/kg initial dose followed by 1–5 mg/kg q 2–4 h (reducing after 12 hours to q 6–12 h IV/po pnr).

Note:
- Reduce dosage according to effect. Prolonged high doses may cause hepatic failure.

Primidone
POM V

Indication: Anticonvulsive therapy in foals.

Presentation: 250 mg tablet for oral dosing.

Dose: 2 g po for 50 kg foal as loading dose, then 1 g q 12 h.

Note:
- Long-term use may result in tolerance and/or hepatopathy.

Section 2
Drugs acting on the cardiovascular system

(a) Angiotensin Converting Enzyme (ACE) Inhibitors
Enalapril
POM *V*

Indications: Mitral regurgitation, congestive heart failure (CHF), other conditions associated with cardiac enlargement.

Dose: 0.5 mg/kg q 24 h.

Note:
- Very poor oral bioavailability; effective doses have not been established.

Quinapril
POM *V*

Indications: See Enalapril above.

Dose: 120 mg/horse po q 24 h.

Note:
- Demonstrated to increase stroke volume and cardiac output in cases of mitral regurgitation.

(b) Anti-arrhythmic Drugs
Bretylium
POM *V*

Indication: Refractory ventricular tachycardia.

Presentations: 50 mg/mL injection; 10 mL bottle.

Dose: 3–5 mg/kg IV.

Digoxin
POM *V*

Indications: Atrial fibrillation, congestive heart failure, supraventricular arrhythmias.

See 'Cardiac glycosides'.

Flecainide

Indications: Class IC antiarrhythmic agent – blocks fast sodium channels. Used in an experimental atrial fibrillation model.

Dose: Oral dose 4 mg/kg.

Note:
- Ineffective IV and can induce serious ventricular dysrhythmias in some horses. Collapse and sudden death have also been associated with its oral use.

Glycopyrrolate
POM V

Indication: Vagal-induced bradycardia.

See 'Anticholinergics'.

Hyoscine
POM V

Indication: Vagal-induced bradycardia.

See 'Anticholinergics'.

Lidocaine (lignocaine)
POM V

Indications: Class IB antidysrhythmic agent. Ventricular tachycardia.

Presentations: 1 and 2 mg/mL in glucose intravenous infusion.

Dose: 0.25–0.5 mg/kg IV q 5 minutes. 2–4 mg/kg total maximum dose *OR* 20–50 µg/kg/minute IV infusion.

Side effects: Excitement reactions common in conscious horses. Control neurologic reactions with diazepam.

Notes:
- Drug of choice to control ventricular tachycardia during anaesthesia.
- NOT effective for supraventricular tachycardia.

Magnesium sulphate

Indications: *Torsades des pointes*, refractory ventricular tachycardia.

Dose: 2–5 mg/kg diluted in saline over 20 minutes; 50 mg/kg maximum total dose.

Note:
- NOT effective for supraventricular tachycardia.

Phenytoin

(See also Anticonvulsants in Drugs Acting on the Nervous System.) POM V

Indications: Ventricular tachycardia induced by digoxin.

Dose: 7.5 mg/kg IV or 20 mg/kg po q 12 h loading dose, then reduce to 10–12 mg/kg q 12 h.

Note:
- Similar cardiovascular effects to lidocaine (lignocaine).

Procainamide

POM V

Indications: Class IA antidysrhythmic agent. Ventricular tachycardia and atrial fibrillation.

Presentations: Tablets 250 mg; injection 100 mg/mL; 10 mL.

Dose: 1 mg/kg/minute IV; 20 mg/kg maximum total dose. Oral dose 22–35 mg/kg q 8h.

Note:
- Not vagolytic, hypotension less of a problem than with quinidine, compatible with digoxin.

Propafenone

POM V

Indication: Ventricular tachycardia.

Dose: 0.5–1 mg/kg IV in 5% dextrose over 5 minutes.

Note:
- Little known about effects and pharmacokinetics in horses as yet.

Propranolol

POM V

Indications: β-adrenoreceptor blocker. Has been suggested for control of supraventricular and ventricular tachydysrhythmias and digoxin-induced dysrhythmias.

Presentation: Aqueous injection (1 mg/mL) 1 mL glass vial.

Dose: 0.03–0.15 mg/kg IV slowly (over 2–4 minutes).

0.38–0.78 mg/kg po q 8h.

Note:
- Usually begin at low dose and titrate to effect. Can be used to correct serious tachydysrhythmias produced by β_1 agonist drugs.

Side effects: May cause bronchial smooth muscle constriction. Hepatic impairment increases the $t_{1/2}$, therefore decrease dosing frequency.

Quinidine gluconate

Indications: Class IA antidysrhythmic agent. Acute onset atrial fibrillation, ventricular tachycardia.

Dose: 0.5–2.2 mg/kg IV q 10 min; maximum total dose 12 mg/kg.

Side effects: Hypotension, increased serum concentrations of both drugs when used with digoxin.

> **Note:**
> ● Limited availability. Not available in UK.

Quinidine sulphate

No applicable category.

Indications: Treatment of supraventricular cardiac arrhythmias (*atrial fibrillation*, supraventricular tachycardia).

Negative inotrope (systemic hypotension). Increases ventricular rate.

Presentation: Powder for oral administration.

Dose: 22 mg/kg po q 2 h until effects seen or a total of 132 mg/kg. If fail to convert, continue at 22 mg/kg po q 6 h. Some cases take over 350 g to convert.

Normal regime for 500 kg horse:

● *Day 1*: test dose for idiosyncratic reaction (Note: many cardiologists do not consider this to be necessary): 5 g (by stomach tube in solution). If safe, proceed to:

● *Day 2*: 10 g doses (po) at 2-hour intervals.

● Careful cardiac monitoring by clinical appraisal and continuous ECG (Holter monitors or telemetry).

● Continue until conversion or up to 6th dose (i.e. total 60 g).

● If not converted, several different options have been suggested:

  (a) 24 hours without therapy then repeat regime as before.

  (b) Continue with quinidine sulphate at 22 mg/kg every 6 hours.

  (c) 24 hours without therapy then repeat regime and additional digoxin (0.011 mg/kg orally q 12 h) until conversion.

After conversion:

● Rest for 4–5 weeks – check ECG.

● Gentle work 4–5 weeks – check ECG.

If failure to convert:

● Assay serum levels of drug to ensure a serum concentration of 2–5 μg/mL. Estimations of $t_{1/2}$ are helpful to identify required individual dosing intervals.

- Horses, which persistently fail to convert, are likely to never do so. Long history of atrial fibrillation or other cardiac disease (e.g. valvular regurgitation and atrial enlargement) increases risk of non-conversion and toxicity.

Notes:
- TEST DOSE of 5 mg/kg (5 g) given to detect untoward effects (nasal congestion, laryngeal and pulmonary oedema, urticaria, laminitis, colic, diarrhoea, cardiac arrhythmia).
- Early indications of toxicity by >25% lengthening of QRS complex.
- Always test electrolyte status before conversion (especially K+).
- If decreased myocardial function present digitalise first (qv). **Otherwise DO NOT digitalise unless needed during conversion.**

ABSORBED THROUGH HUMAN SKIN! (GLOVES + AVOID CONTACT).

(c) Cardiac Glycosides
Digoxin
POM *V*

Indications: Positive inotrope (calcium influx), negative chronotrope (increased refractory period, decrease in conductivity through the myocardium, autonomic nervous system effects).

Parasympathomimetic (slowing of sino-atrial node, delayed conduction of AV node). Congestive heart failure, atrial fibrillation/flutter, supraventricular arrhythmias.

Presentations: Oral: 62.5, 125 and 250 µg tablets; IV: 250 µg/mL injection in 2 mL single-dose vials.

Dose: 11 µg/kg po q 12 h or 2.2 µg/kg IV.

Note:
- Horses with atrial fibrillation and concurrent CHF and/or tachycardia should be digitalised before administration of quinidine sulphate (but those with no CHF should NOT). In theory, the two drugs should not be given simultaneously, but evidence suggests that low doses of digoxin may stabilise the ventricular activity during administration of quinidine sulphate for conversion. Decrease dose in renal disease.

Side effects: Include sudden death, A-V block, arrhythmias, anorexia, diarrhoea and depression. Blood levels should be monitored carefully, particularly if no effects seen. Serious toxicity has been reported. ALWAYS DIGITALISE WITH EXTREME CARE – use regular ECG and auscultation monitoring of cardiac activity.

(d) Anticholinergics

Atropine
POM *V*

Indications: Parasympatholytic (anticholinergic, mydriatic, cycloplegic). Relief of smooth muscle spasm, antidote to parasympathomimetic drugs (including organophosphate). For intraoperative bradydysrhythmias. In cardiopulmonary resuscitation. Bronchodilation. Glaucoma, relief of iris spasm.

Presentations: Clear aqueous solution, 10 mg/mL, 50 mL multidose vials, also 1 mL vials; 0.6 mg/mL.

Dose: Cardiac effects: 0.01–0.4 mg/kg IV or SQ.

0.015 mg/kg IV/IM/SC as treatment for acute bronchoconstriction.

Organophosphate poisoning: 1 mg/kg (to effect mydriasis and cessation of salivation) q 2–6 h as needed.

Notes:
- Side effects (may be prolonged) include:
  1. Sinus tachycardia, ectopic complexes.
  2. Vision disturbances (mydriasis, photophobia, cycloplegia, possible but not marked increases in intra-ocular pressure) (mydriasis may cause panic – use darkened room).
  3. Abdominal distension, ileus.
  4. Urinary retention.
- Ophthalmic ointment or drops (1/2%) can cause systemic effects on gut motility in particular. Ophthalmic effects include reduction in intra-ocular pressure in glaucoma due to high unconventional (uveoscleral) drainage of aqueous in horses (beware of cause of glaucoma).

Glycopyrrolate
No licensed veterinary product available.

Indications: Anticholinergic (anti-muscarinic) actions similar to atropine but does not cross into CNS (fewer side effects). Treatment of bradydysrhythmias due to increased parasympathetic tone. During head and neck or ocular surgery to block vagal responses.

Presentation: 1 and 3 mL vials; 300 µg/mL.

Dose: 2 µg/kg IV.

Bronchodilator effects: 2–3 mg IM q 12 h (450 kg horse).

Notes:

- Onset of action slower than atropine (1–3 minutes), therefore, less useful in an emergency. Duration of action is also longer (2–3 hours cardiovascular effects).

- More gastrointestinal side effects than atropine.

- More expensive than atropine. Supposedly more potent antisialagogue with fewer arrhythmogenic tendencies.

- Advantage over atropine in the horse not proven but does decrease CNS effects.

- Incompatible with chloramphenicol, dexamethasone, diazepam, thiopentone (thiopental).

(e) Vasodilators
Sildenafil
POM V

Indication: Treatment of pulmonary hypertension in foals.

Presentation: 25, 50 and 100 mg tablets.

Dose: 0.5–2.5 mg/kg po up to q 4 h.

Side effects: Systemic hypotension at high doses.

(f) Shock Treatments
Adrenaline/epinephrine
POM V

Indications: Adrenergic (α and β) effects.

Bronchodilator. Increases systolic blood pressure.

First-line drug in cardiac resuscitation.

Anaphylaxis.

Prolongs effect of local analgesics when given in combination.

Local capillary haemostasis.

Presentation: Clear, aqueous solution for injection, 1 mg/mL (1 in 1000).

Dose: 0.01–0.02 mg/kg IV.

Notes:

- Use care with dose calculation.

- Ophthalmic drops available and can have systemic effects.

Side effects: Anxiety, restlessness, tachycardia, ventricular arrhythmias.

Noradrenaline/norepinephrine
POM V

Indications: α_1 and β_1 activity, with variable β_2 activity. Potent vasopressor; also inotropic and chronotropic effects.

Dose: 0.2–2 µg/kg/minute.

Dobutamine
POM V

Indications: Synthetic catecholamine with principal activity as a positive inotropic agent via action as a β_1-adrenergic agonist (some activity also at β_2 and α_1 receptors). Short-term support of hypotension (particularly during general anaesthesia) due to decreased myocardial contraction. Tachycardia can develop in some individuals at clinically applicable doses.

Presentations: Dry powder, 250 mg/bottle or 250 mg solution for dilution.

Dose: Reconstitute with 1 L 5% glucose or 0.9% saline to yield a solution having a concentration of 250 µg/mL. Administer IV at 1–5 µg/kg/minute. Can increase rate above this but at high infusion rates (10–20 µg/kg/minute) β_2 and α_1 receptor-mediated effects may be seen and tachyarrhythmias are more likely.

Notes:
- ECG monitoring for tachyarrhythmias essential.
- Drug interactions: oxytocic drugs may cause a severe hypertension when used with dobutamine.
- Dobutamine may be ineffective if β-blocking drugs (e.g. propanolol) have recently been given.

Dopamine
POM V

Indications: Correction of haemodynamic imbalances in shock. Oliguric renal failure. Agonist at dopamine, β_1, β_2 and α_1 receptors, activity is somewhat dose dependant.

Presentations: To prepare solution: add 250 mg to 1 L of normal saline or Hartman solution to give concentration of 250 µg/mL.

Dose: Variable according to desired effect:

<2.5 µg/kg/minute – dopaminergic effects predominate resulting in vasodilation (especially in renal and splanchnic beds), reduced afterload and increased cardiac output.

2.5–5 µg/kg/minute – β_1 effects predominate producing positive inotropic effects (may see positive chronotropy as well).

>5 µg/kg/minute – α_1 effects become evident causing increasing systemic vascular resistance (vasoconstriction).

Notes:
- Only used in intensive care (especially neonates).
- Severe necrosis/sloughing if extravascular injection occurs. Monitor urine flow, cardiac rate/rhythm/blood pressure. In case of severe arrhythmias (e.g. ventricular premature contractions) discontinue administration.
- Half-life: 5–9 minutes.

Vasopressin (antidiuretic hormone)
POM V

Indications: Increases mean arterial pressure, systemic vascular resistance and urinary output in patients with septic shock unresponsive to catecholamines.

Also used for treatment of diabetes insipidus.

Dose: 0.1–2 mU/kg/minute IV.

Treatment of diabetes insipidus, 60 IU/500 kg IV q 6 h.

Section 3
Drugs acting on the respiratory system

(a) Bronchodilators

1. Sympathomimetics – receptor agonists:

   Specific and non-specific agents (β_1 and β_2 receptors).

   Specific β_2 agonists prevent side effects associated with β_1 stimulation.

   Very effective bronchodilators.

   Decreased release of inflammatory mediators.

   Enhanced ciliary activity and less viscous secretions.

   Aerosolised preparations offer decreased systemic effects.

2. Parasympatholytics:

   Antagonism of the parasympathetic muscarinic receptors on airway smooth muscle.

   Systemic preparations not used in respiratory disease due to potential for severe side effects (e.g. ileus). Aerosolised preparations offer decreased systemic effects.

3. Xanthine derivatives:

   Bronchodilation via inhibition of phosphodiesterase and other mechanisms.

   May increase tidal volume by stimulation of the medulla.

   Less effective than β receptor agonists in chronic respiratory disease (action affected by airway remodelling).

   CNS and myocardial stimulants and diuretics.

Aminophylline
POM V

Indications: Xanthine derivative (see above 'xanthine derivatives' for actions). Bronchodilator, but it also increases mucociliary clearance and acts as a respiratory stimulant.

Presentations: 25 mg/mL injectable solution.

100 and 200 mg tablets for oral administration.

Dose: 2–5 mg/kg IV q 8–12 h (slow).

5–10 mg/kg po q 12 h.

Side effects: Excitability, tachycardia, sweating, muscular tremors.

113

Clenbuterol
POM *V*

Indications: Specific β_2 agonist with sympathomimetic effects. Bronchodilation and increased mucociliary clearance. Acute and long-term therapy of recurrent airway obstruction (RAO, 'heaves') and inflammatory airway disease (IAD). Also used to induce uterine relaxation during parturition or to prevent early placental separation and delay or reduce uterine contraction during obstetric manipulations.

Presentations:
Granules for oral feed administration 0.016 mg/g (1 level measure/200 kg q 12 h).

Syrup for oral dosing/in feed 72.5 µg/mL (available in 100, 330 and 460 mL bottles).

Aqueous solution for injection 30 µg/mL (2.7 mL/100 kg q 12 h by slow IV injection).

Dose: 0.8 µg/kg po/IV q 12 h.

Notes:
- Intravenous dose useful for immediate relief of bronchospasm (effective for 12 hours, follow by oral preparation q 12 hours). Most used bronchodilator for long-term therapy of RAO; must be combined with strict environmental dust control and corticosteroid administration (systemic – short term/inhaled – long term).
- Rapid desensitisation and down regulation of β_2 receptors occurs after administration of clenbuterol. This can be prevented by corticosteroid administration.

Side effects: Sweating, tachycardia, transient muscle tremors and restlessness are more common with intravenous administration. Minimised by slow administration. Antagonises effects of $PGF_2\alpha$ and oxytocin.

Contraindications: High doses may reduce uterine contractions, therefore, discontinue use in pregnant mares at expected delivery time. Withdrawal periods. Do not use in horses intended for human consumption.

Etamiphylline camsylate
POM *V*

Indications: Xanthine derivative (see above 'xanthine derivatives' for actions). Respiratory disease (relief of bronchospasm and pulmonary oedema). Cardiovascular collapse (myocardial stimulation and relief of pulmonary oedema). Respiratory stimulation of neonates (see 'Respiratory stimulants').

Presentation:
Aqueous solution 140 mg/mL for injection IM/SC.

Dose: 3 mg/kg IM/SC/po q 8 h.

Notes:
- Can be given IV slow/diluted. Used as bronchodilator, mostly superseded by specific β_2 agonists.
- Oral administration failed to improved pulmonary function in horses with RAO.

Side effects: No data in pregnant animals, CNS stimulation that is readily countered if necessary by the use of a suitable hypnotic.

In overdoses, hypokalaemia and convulsions may occur. Treat with intravenous infusion of potassium chloride and intravenous diazepam, respectively.

Ipratropium bromide
POM *V*

Indications: Parasympatholytic. Conditions in which bronchospasm is a problem (RAO; IAD).

Presentations: Metered dose inhaler, $17\,\mu g$/actuation.

Nebuliser solution: $250\,\mu g$ in $1\,mL$ or $500\,\mu g$ in $2\,mL$

Dose: $2–4\,\mu g/kg$ q 12 h maximum; inhaled.

Notes:
- Not effective if extensive airway remodelling has occurred.
- Minimal systemic absorption following inhalation.
- No adverse effect on mucociliary clearance. Effects are short lived.

Pentoxyfylline
POM V

Indication: Methylxanthine derivate. Bronchodilator with some anti-inflammatory effects.

Presentations: $20\,mg/mL$ injectable solution (for nebulization).

$400\,mg$ tablets.

Dose: $8–10\,mg/kg$ po q 12 h.

Notes:
- Higher doses ($16\,mg/kg$ q 12 h) were as beneficial as atropine to relieve airway obstruction.
- Limited oral absorption.

Salbutamol (Albuterol)
POM *V*

Indications: Short-acting specific β_2 agonist.

Acute exacerbations of recurrent airway obstructive disease (RAO) and short-term therapy of IAD.

Lung function testing to assess reversibility of the condition.

Presentations: Metered dose inhaler $100\,\mu g$/actuation.

Combination salbutamol/ipratropium in a MDI commercially available.

Dose: 1–2 µg/kg inhaled q 12 h.

Notes:
- Rapid onset of action. Short duration of effect (30–60 minutes).
- Not suitable for long-term treatment of RAO on its own (short-acting).
- Regular use of β_2 agonists in the absence of anti-inflammatory medication (corticosteroids) may mask progression of the disease (particularly, further airway obstruction with mucus).

Side effects: Low incidence, excessive use (or in sensitive individuals) may result in systemic effects of trembling, anxiety and cardiac arrhythmias. Sometimes transient paradoxical bronchoconstriction occurs.

Salmeterol
POM V

Indications: Long-acting β_2 agonist.

Long-term therapy of RAO.

Dose: 210 µg q 12–24 h inhaled.

Notes:
- Slow onset of action – not suitable for acute crisis.
- Duration of action normally 6–8 hours.
- May have other beneficial effects in management of RAO (inhibition of smooth muscle proliferation; increased force of contraction of the diaphragm and intercostal muscles; mild anti-inflammatory action on neutrophils; epithelial protective agent and improved mucociliary function).
- Regular use of β_2 agonists in the absence of anti-inflammatory medication may mask progression of the disease.
- Long-term therapy of RAO requires concurrent environmental management and corticosteroid therapy.

Side effects: Few side effects reported.

Excessive use (or in sensitive individuals) may result in systemic effects of trembling, anxiety and cardiac arrhythmias.

Terbutaline sulphate
POM V/CD (S-IV)

Indications: β_2-receptor agonist – more-or-less specific for respiratory/bronchial receptors. Has largely been replaced by more specific and effective clenbuterol. May be useful in acute respiratory distress as nebulised preparation.

Dose: 0.02–0.06 mg/kg IV or inhaled.

Presentation: 1 mg/mL solution for injection.

Notes:
- Not licensed for animal use.
- Very short half-life.

Side effects: Higher doses may stimulate β_1 receptors.

Major side effects limit use in horses.

Sweating and CNS signs can develop.

Cardiac dysrhythmias may need treatment with β-blockers (e.g. propanolol).

Theophyline
Indications: Xanthine derivative. Bronchodilation, mild diuretic, CNS stimulant. Supportive therapy for RAO, IAD and congestive heart failure (with pulmonary oedema).

Dose: 12 mg/kg IV initial dose then 6 mg/kg IV q 12 h.

5 mg/kg po q 12 h.

Note:
- IV solutions should be diluted in >100 mL of water/isotonic saline for injection. Administer very slowly. Not IM. Diuretic effect is weak, therefore, rarely used alone as diuretics.

Side effects: Narrow therapeutic index!

Excitement, tremors and visual disturbances may be induced.

Antagonistic effect with β-blockers (e.g. propanolol).

Contraindications: Pregnancy; myocardial disease.

(b) Antihistamines
Definition: In the true sense, these are chemicals that block the action of histamine at receptor sites. They may also stabilise mast cells and have antiserotonin properties. Many mediators other than histamine are responsible for hypersensitivity reactions. Antihistamines have limited use only.

Cetirizine
Indications: Second generation antihistamine. Conflicting reports on its efficacy, research showed no evidence supporting its use for insect bite hypersensitivity.

Presentation: 10 mg tablets.

Dose: 0.2–0.4 mg/kg q 12 h.

Chlorpheniramine (chlorphenamine) maleate
Indications: Histamine 1 receptor antagonist. Premedication for drugs that may induce anaphylactic reactions; pruritus in allergic skin disorders; compulsive scratching. Unlikely to be useful in respiratory disease in horses.

Presentations: Tablets 4 mg; syrup 400 μg/mL.

Dose: 0.25–0.5 mg/kg q 12 h po.

Note:
● Limited success in horses.

Side effects: Minimal. Light sedation or behavioural changes.

Cyproheptadine hydrochloride
Indications: Serotonin antagonist with anticholinergic and antihistaminic effects. Pituitary pars intermedia dysfunction (PPID/equine Cushing's disease syndrome).

Photic headshaking.

Dose:
PPID: adjunct to pergolide; if no response to pergolide and endocrinological tests remain abnormal, addition of 0.3–0.5 mg/kg of cyproheptadine may improve the clinical status.

Headshaking: 0.3 mg/kg q 12 h for 1 week. If no response, increase by 0.1 mg/kg every week thereafter for a further 3 weeks.

Note:
● Rarely used alone for PPID. Limited success in headshaking.

Side effects: Few reported adverse effects in horses; occasional drowsiness and even stupor at high doses. These are usually transient and are worst following the first administration. In humans, drowsiness, nausea, ataxia and anorexia are reported.

Diphenhydramine
POM V

Indications: First generation antihistamine. Also used for fluphenazine toxicity.

Presentations: 50 mg/mL solution for injection, 25 mg tablets.

Dose: 0.6 mg/kg IV q 24–48 h.

0.5–1 mg/kg po.

Side effects: Mild sedation possible.

Doxepin hydrochloride
Indications: Tricyclic antidepressant with antihistamine properties used for its anxiolytic properties for the treatment of psychogenic pruritus in cases of atopic dermatitis or insect bite hypersensitivity.

Presentation: 10, 25 and 50 mg tablets.

Dose: 0.5–0.75 mg/kg po q 12 h.

Hydroxyzine hydrochloride
POM V

Indications: First generation antihistamine. Allergic dermatitis (insect hypersensitivity). May be useful in some cases of headshaking if an allergic trigger factor is present.

Presentation: 25 mg tablets.

Dose:
Dermatitis: 0.5–1.5 mg/kg q 8 h IM or po.
Headshaking: 1.4 mg/kg q 12 h po.

> **Note:**
> ● Very useful antihistamine for insect hypersensitivity (sweet itch) and other pruritic dermatosis. Less effective than corticosteroids in allergic dermatitis but fewer side effects. Treatment of urticaria is usually disappointing; remission in 3–4 days if going to be useful. Very few cases of headshaking will respond. Can be combined with carbamazepine in treatment of headshaking.

Side effects: Some sedative effects can be seen early in the treatment course. Usually this subsides.

Sodium cromoglycate (sodium cromoglicate)
POM V

Indications: Mast cell inhibitor (stabilises membranes, blocks degranulation and decreases amount of histamine in mast cells). Prophylaxis and control of respiratory tract allergic conditions (RAO; summer pasture associated obstructive pulmonary disease [SPAOPD]).

Dose: 80 mg q 24 h via nebuliser for 1–4 days.

> **Note:**
> ● Most extensively used and studied mast cell inhibitor in horses to date. Single course (4 days) expected to provide prophylaxis for 3–20 days. (Not predictable.) MUST be accompanied by full range of management/supportive measures. THIS IS NOT A TREATMENT FOR RAO/SPAOPD – it is a prophylactic compound and is not effective in acute attack. Sometimes resented by horses (possibly bad taste).

Nedocromil sodium
Has been used in horses. Longer duration of action and possibly more potent than the above.

Dose: Suggested dose is 17.5 mg q 12–24 h.

Presentation: Nebuliser solution.

Side effects: May cause cough.

Contraindications: Manufacturer recommends that it is not administered in first trimester of pregnancy.

(c) Antitussives

Coughing is a protective mechanism and aids in elimination of excessive bronchial secretions. Antitussives should not be used if the cough is productive. They are rarely used as therapy in horses but may be useful to aid diagnostic respiratory tract procedures (e.g. bronchoalveolar lavage [BAL]).

Butorphanol tartrate
POM V/CD (S-IV)

Indications: Mixed opioid agonist–antagonist.

Effective antitussive, useful for control of coughing during diagnostic procedures of the respiratory tract (e.g. bronchoalveolar lavage).

Analgesia and sedation (see 'Opioids' and 'Drugs acting on the Central Nervous System').

Codeine phosphate BP
POM V/CD (S-V)

Indications: Opioid analgesic. Diarrhoea. Suppression of non-productive cough.

Presentation: Codeine phosphate (non-proprietary): tablets 60 mg.

Dose: 1–3 mg/kg q 12–24 h.

> **Note:**
> ● Little analgesic activity. Symptomatic treatment only.

Side effects: Constipation.

Contraindications: Known hepatic disease; respiratory conditions with excess secretion; CNS depression.

(d) Mucolytics

Mucolytics reduce mucus viscosity and allow more effective mucociliary clearance.

Acetylcysteine

Indications: Mucolytic used for control and treatment of respiratory conditions associated with excess mucus (e.g. of RAO), IAD, sinusitis.

Presentations: Acetylcysteine (non-proprietary) – oral powder (10 mg/g); aqueous solution for injection (3 mg/mL).

Dose: 0.1–0.3 mg/kg oral daily for up to 5 days or longer.

1.5 mg/kg IM/IV q 12 h.

Enema: for meconium impaction in foals (4% solution); 8 g acetylcysteine, 20 g baking soda ($NaHCO_3$), 200 mL water.

> **Note:**
> ● Parenteral dose may be useful initially followed by oral use. May safely be administered over prolonged courses.

Bromhexine HCl
POM V

Indications: Assists control and treatment of respiratory tract infections and hypersensitivity conditions where there is excess mucus (e.g. sinusitis, bronchitis).

Presentation: Oral powder (10 mg/g).

Dose: 200–400 µg/kg oral once daily.

> **Note:**
> ● May safely be administered over prolonged courses. May be mixed with sulphonamides/potentiated sulphonamides for oral use.

Contraindications: Minimal. Do not use in horses for human consumption.

Dembrexine
POM V

Indications: Assists control and treatment of respiratory tract infections and hypersensitivity conditions where there is excess mucus (e.g. sinusitis, bronchitis).

Presentation: Powder 5 mg/g active ingredient. Multidose 420 g tub.

Dose: 0.3 mg/kg in feed q 12 h for 12–14 days.

> **Note:**
> ● Very safe. Useful adjunct to management of upper and lower respiratory tract infections – hastens return to normal function. Do not exceed 28 days' treatment (reassess diagnosis and management). Concurrent antibiotics may be indicated. May be mixed with sulphonamides/potentiated sulphonamides and/or clenbuterol for oral use.

Contraindications: No data in pregnant mares.

(e) Respiratory Stimulants

These are primarily used to stimulate apnoeic neonates. They may be used with caution to reverse respiratory depression associated with general anaesthesia, sedative or hypnotic drugs – but they can paradoxically worsen hypoxia or induce seizures. Ensure adequate airway and ventilation first.

Caffeine
POM V

Indication: Respiratory stimulant in neonatal foals.

Presentation: 10 mg/mL oral solution.

Dose: 10 mg/kg loading dose, then 2.5 mg/kg po or per rectum for maintenance.

> **Note:**
> ● Conflicting reports regarding its efficacy.

Doxapram hydrochloride
POM *V*

Indications: Respiratory stimulation in newborn animals. Stimulation of respiration following anaesthesia, sedatives or hypnotic drugs.

Presentations: Drops for sublingual use; vials for topical sublingual or parenteral use.

Dose:

Neonates: 0.5–1.0 mg/kg IV/SC/IM (or sublingual 40–100 mg). As a CRI, 0.5 mg/kg loading dose followed by 0.03/0.08 mg/kg/minute.

Adults: 0.5–1.0 mg/kg IV.

> **Notes:**
> - Recent studies have shown that this drug decreases blood flow to the brain and it is no longer recommended in foals.
> - Increases respiratory drive but this may in turn increase oxygen consumption, potentially worsening the hypoxaemia.

(f) Corticosteroids

Most effective therapy for control of RAO. Decrease smooth muscle contraction and epithelial damage, inhibit inflammatory cells and their mediators, potentiate bronchodilatory effect of catecholamines, decrease mucus production. Maximum clinical effect is seen within 2–7 days. Combine with bronchodilators to provide symptomatic relief (especially in the acute crisis). Inhaled and systemic preparations used. Inhaled forms achieve high local concentrations and minimise systemic side effects. Prolonged use of high doses of systemic drugs should be avoided. Remember, the more potent the anti-inflammatory effect the greater potential for side effects. The preparations commonly used in RAO are outlined below. For information regarding side effects and further indications see 'Hormones/steroids' (p. 147) and 'NSAIDS – Adrenal corticoids' (p. 152).

Systemic

1. *Dexamethasone*: Most commonly used corticosteroid for RAO. 0.05–0.1 mg/kg IV q 24 h followed by decremental doses and alternate day doses IM. Suggested maximum of 3–5 days to avoid systemic effects. **Check formulation before injection – confirm route compatibility.**

2. *Isoflupredone*: Same efficacy as dexamethasone in RAO. 0.03 mg/kg IM once a day for 5 days then alternate days and taper to low dose over 10–20 days.

3. *Triamcinolone acetate*: Long acting (at least 5 weeks clinical efficacy). Do not use unless short-acting preparations are absolutely not an option due to potential for side effects.

4. *Prednisolone*: Less potent/less side effects. Useful for longer-term management if inhaled preparations not an option. 1 mg/kg q 24 h in feed in the morning – decremental doses over 4–6 weeks to minimum effective dose.

> **Note:**
> - Prednisone has no clinical efficacy in horses (it is poorly absorbed from the equine gut).

Inhaled

Drugs of choice for long-term therapy. Concurrent use of a bronchodilator may enhance delivery and will provide symptomatic relief:

1. *Beclomethasone (beclometasone) dipropionate*: Available as a metered dose inhaler (MDI). Improvement seen in 3–4 days. 500–3500 µg/horse q 12 h (µg/actuation depends on formulation).

2. *Fluticasone propionate*: Available as an MDI. 1000–2500 µg/horse q 12 h (µg/actuation depends on formulation). Less systemic effects and shorter withdrawal time than beclomethasone.

Aerosolised steroid drugs

Aerosols are finely suspended solid or liquid particles in a gas. At present, corticosteroids and bronchodilators are used clinically in aerosol form in the horse. For all aerosolised drugs the delivered pulmonary concentration depends on the formulation of the product, the delivery device, correct operator use, patient co-operation and the disease process (degree of airway obstruction). Aerosols are available in three forms:

1. *Dry powder inhalants*: Pulmonary drug delivery decreased in conditions of high relative humidity (>95%). Compatible delivery devices are:

   - 'Equi poudre' (Agritronics Int).
   - 'Equine Aeromask' with adaptor (Trudell Medical International).

2. *Metered dose inhalers (MDI)*: Drug in prepared canister designed to release a specific dose on each activation. Main advantage of consistent dose release. Most now propelled by hydrofluroalkane-134a (HFA) an environmentally friendly product which has largely replaced the old CFC-driven preparations. The delivered dose of each drug depends on its propellant type (check manufacturer's instructions). Compatible delivery devices are:

   - 'Equine haler' (Equine Healthcare APS), spacer device, hand held, fits over one nostril, use with MDIs only, drug wastage at external nares, most likely to be well tolerated.

   - 'Equine Aeromask' (Trudell Medical International) – versatile (MDIs, nebulisers and dry powders), fits over the entire muzzle, drug wastage at external nares and upper respiratory tract, compliance may be poor in some horses.

   - 'Aerohippus' (Trudell Medical International) spacer device, hand held, fits over one nostril, use with MDIs only, most likely to be well tolerated.

Note:
- Careful technique is required with all the devices to minimise drug wastage.

3. *Nebuliser solutions*: Less widely used than the other two forms. Require special nebuliser unit (for example, Flexineb Equine Nebuliser, Nortev) or can be used with 'Equine Aeromask'. Disadvantage of potential for environmental contamination of delivered solution.

(g) Antimicrobials

Table 3.3 The rationale for antibiotic selection in pulmonary infection in horses

Condition	Predisposing factors	Commonly involved organisms	Suggested empirical antibiotic therapy	Samples for culture and sensitivity
Bacterial pneumonia	Stress, viral infection, transport	Gram +ve: Strep. zooepidemicus (opportunistic, most commonly involved in early stages, prolonged condition may have involvement of Gram –ve organisms and anaerobes as for pleuropneumonia)	Benzyl sodium penicillin and gentamicin. Third-generation cephalosporin good alternative. (Anaerobic infection should be suspected if there is brown nasal discharge and foul odour – include metronidazole in therapy.)	Tracheal aspirate
Pleuropneumonia	General anaesthesia, head held in upright position for prolonged periods, long-distance travel, thoracic trauma	Gram +ve: Strep. zooepidemicus; Gram –ve: E. coli; Klebsiella; Pasteurella, anaerobes (e.g. Bacteroides)	Benzyl sodium penicillin, gentamicin and metronidazole	Pleural fluid and tracheal aspirate. (Sample fluid from both sides of the chest as bacterial populations may differ.)

INDEX OF DRUGS USED IN EQUINE MEDICINE

Section 4
Drugs acting on the urinary tract

(a) Diuretics

Increase urinary excretion of Na^+ and water. Classified according to their site of action in the renal nephron. *Carbonic anhydrase (CA) inhibitors*, *osmotic agents* and *xanthines* act on the proximal convoluted tubule. *Loop diuretics* act on the ascending Henle's loop. *Thiazides* act on the early distal convoluted tubule. *K^+ sparing diuretics* act on the late distal convoluted tubule and collecting duct.

Acetazolamide
POM V

Actions: Carbonic anhydrase inhibitor.

Indications: Modest diuretic. Mainly used in the management of HYPP. Also used in the treatment of glaucoma.

Presentations: 500 mg vial for injection; 250 mg tablets.

Dose: 2.2–4.4 mg/kg po q 12 h for HYPP.

Furosemide (frusemide)
POM *V*

Actions: Loop diuretic. Increased venous capacitance.

Indications: Oedematous conditions, congestive heart failure, oliguric renal failure, cerebral oedema, exercise-induced pulmonary haemorrhage.

Presentations: Aqueous 5% solution for injection (50 mg/mL), 10 mL multidose vial.

Dose: 0.5–2 mg/kg IV q 12–24 h pnr.

Note:
- Potent diuretic. Rapid onset (increased Na^+/water excretion without significant loss of K^+ over short courses). Majority of drug excreted unchanged in the urine within 4 hours. Monitor electrolytes over treatment course. Effects on exercise-induced pulmonary haemorrhage limited/equivocal (1–2 hours pre-racing, permissible in certain countries/states only). Oliguric renal failure – use if horse remains oliguric after 12–24 hours of appropriate fluid and electrolyte replacement, administer at 1 mg/kg IV q 2 h. If urine is not voided after the second dose mannitol (1 mg/kg as a 10–20% solution) can be added.

Side effects: Prolonged use may cause significant hypokalaemia – arrhythmia, increased susceptibility to cardiac glycoside toxicity – and hypochloraemia. Consider potassium supplementation during use, especially if concurrent anorexia. Hypovolaemia (in excessive use). Electrolyte alterations in the endolymph of the inner ear may exacerbate effects of ototoxic drugs (e.g. aminoglycoside antibiotics).

Contraindications: Glomerulonephritis, urinary obstruction, electrolyte deficiency syndromes.

Mannitol
POM V

Actions: Osmotic diuretic (unabsorbed solute in proximal tubule causes diuresis). Saluretic effect low (ability to promote Na^+ and Cl^- loss). Increased renal medullary blood flow.

Indications: Reduction of intracranial (CSF) and intra-ocular pressure. Adjunct to furosemide (frusemide) in oliguric renal failure (see above).

Presentation: 20% solution (200 mg/mL) in 500 mL single-dose bottle.

Dose: 0.25–2.0 g/kg slow IV (drip) as 20% solution (never stronger).

> **Note:**
> - Check for crystals (warm solution) – always use in-line filter. Monitor electrolytes throughout usage, especially in oliguric renal failure.

Side effects: Extravascular injection causes thrombophlebitis.

Contraindications: Congestive heart failure, pulmonary oedema. (Initial expansion of ECF because minimal Na^+/Cl^- loss accompanies water loss. Oedema may be exacerbated leading to decompensation.) Do NOT mix with other electrolyte solutions unless very diluted (precipitates)!

(b) Other Drugs
Ammonium chloride

Indications: Urinary acidification in attempt to dissolve urinary calculi especially of the sabulous types. Enhances renal excretion of some drugs and effect of urinary antiseptics and antibiotics which work better in acid solution (e.g. tetracycline and penicillin G) (c.f. aminoglycosides work best in alkaline solution).

Dose: 0.3–0.6 g/kg q 24 h po.

> **Note:**
> - Do not use commercially available enteric-coated tablets (unchanged in gut!). Palatability is questionable (smell of ammonia not liked!). Monitor electrolytes.

Contraindications: Hepatic failure/compromise, renal failure.

Ascorbic acid (vitamin C)
Indication: Urinary acidification.
Dose: 0.5–2 g/kg q 12/24 h po.

> **Note:**
> ● More efficacious than ammonium chloride in acidifying the urine of horses.

Bethanecol chloride
POM V

Actions: Synthetic cholinergic agonist with predominantly muscarinic effects.

Indications: Primarily used to stimulate bladder contractions in paralytic bladder syndromes (e.g. sorghum poisoning, idiopathic bladder paralysis).

Also used as oesophageal and intestinal prokinetic.

Presentations: Tablets 10 and 25 mg.

Dose: 0.25–0.75 mg/kg po q 8–12 h.

Contraindications: Urinary obstruction.

(c) Antimicrobials

General principles of antimicrobial use for urinary tract infection (UTI):

● *Lower UTI*: Continue therapy for at least 1 week.

● *Upper UTI*: Continue therapy for at least 2–6 weeks.

● Collect midstream urine sample for culture/sensitivity before initiation of therapy; 2–4 days into treatment and 1–2 weeks after treatment has been discontinued.

● If the UTI recurs and the same organism is isolated, suspect primary underlying disorder as focus of infection (e.g. urolithiasis).

Table 3.4 Antibiotic selection for use in urinary tract infections

Trimethoprim/sulphonamide	Usually good efficacy Consider the metabolism of the sulphonamide For example, *Sulphadiazine [sulfadiazine]*: is excreted largely unchanged in the urine, therefore, is a good choice
Penicillin and ampicillin	Upper or lower urinary tract infections caused by susceptible *Corynebacterium* spp., *Streptococcus* spp. and *Staphylococcus* spp. Ampicillin is highly concentrated in urine and, therefore, may be effective even if *in vitro* resistance reported. In horses with severely compromised renal function, potentiated penicillins (e.g. ticarcillin) may be an alternative to aminoglycosides
Gentamicin/amikacin	Nephrotoxic Reserve for highly resistant organisms or acute life-threatening Gram −ve infections
Cephalosporins	Concentrated in urine Broad-spectrum
Fluoroquinolones	Enrofloxacin useful in resistant cases

INDEX OF DRUGS USED IN EQUINE MEDICINE

Section 5
Drugs acting on the gastrointestinal tract

(a) Antacids/Anti-ulcer Drugs

Cimetidine
POM V

Actions and indications: Used to treat/prevent gastric and duodenal ulcers in adults and foals. Histamine (H_2) receptor antagonist (competitively inhibits histamine thus reducing acid output from stomach).

Interesting immunomodulation effect (reverses suppressor T-cell mediated immune suppression) – used for treatment of melanoma.

Weak anti-androgenic activity.

Presentations: Tablet for oral use, 200, 400 or 800 mg.

Syrup for oral use, 40 mg/mL.

Injection, 100 mg/mL (2 mL vials).

Dose: 6.6 mg/kg IV q 6–8 h.

20–25 mg/kg po q 6–8 h.

> **Note:**
> - Poor gut absorption, so higher oral doses are required. Reduced hepatic clearance of warfarin, β-blockers, quinidine sulphate, metronidazole, diazepam. Important to appreciate parietal cells can secrete acid via other mechanisms, so histamine inhibition not gold standard.

Side effects: Rare; diarrhoea and/or dizziness reported in humans.

Omeprazole
POM V

Actions and indications: Omeprazole is a substituted benzimidazole, acting as a proton pump inhibitor resulting in complete suppression of gastric acid secretion by specific inhibition of the H^+/K^+ ATPase enzyme system at the secretory surface of the parietal cells.

Gold standard for treatment of equine gastric ulceration syndromes (adults and foals).

Presentation: Oral capsules, 10, 20, 40 mg.

Oral paste in syringes, 400 mg/unit.

Dose: 4 mg/kg q 24 h po healing dose.

2 mg/kg q 24 h po maintenance/prevention dose.

Note:
- Expensive. Dosing required daily. Capsules are difficult to handle – need to be broken open before administration (by drench) – inconvenient. Paste formulation easy to use. IV preparation available in some countries (0.5 mg/kg).

Side effects: May delay the elimination of warfarin, no other interactions reported in the horse. Avoid direct contact with human skin and eyes as may cause hypersensitivity. Zero days withdrawal period.

Contraindications: Not recommended in pregnant or lactating mares.

Ranitidine
POM V

Actions and indications: As for *cimetidine* (above) but no proven effect on melanoma. Reported to be more potent than cimetidine (more reliable oral absorption), but omeprazole recognised as gold standard.

Presentations: Tablet oral, 75, 150 mg.

Syrup for oral use, 15 mg/mL.

Solution for injection, 25 mg/mL.

Dose: 6.6 mg/kg po q 8 h.

1–2 mg/kg IV q 8 h.

Note:
- More expensive than cimetidine – less frequent dosing necessary.

Side effects: Rare; allergic reactions reported in humans.

Sucralfate
POM V

Actions and indications: Complex of aluminium hydroxide and sulphated sucrose. In acid medium forms non-absorbable ion (binds to protein exudate creating 'bandage' over ulcers). Stimulates increased prostaglandin E1 synthesis and mucus secretion. Gastrointestinal ulceration.

Presentation: Suspension, oral 200 mg/mL.

Tablet, oral, 1 g.

Dose:

Adults: 20–40 mg/kg po q 8 h.

Foals: 20–80 mg/kg po q 6 h.

Note:
- Should be given on empty stomach (>1 hour before feed). Most effective if used in conjunction with other antacids particularly for the treatment of glandular ulcers.

Side effects: Rare; allergic reactions reported in humans.

Contraindications: Large quantities required for effective treatment of adults, questionable choice of treatment in the face of ready availability of omeprazole.

(b) Intestinal Stimulants

Bethanecol chloride
POM V

Actions: Synthetic cholinergic agonist with predominantly muscarinic effects.

Indications: Primarily used to stimulate bladder contractions in paralytic bladder syndromes (e.g. sorghum poisoning, idiopathic bladder paralysis).

Also used as oesophageal and intestinal prokinetic. Increases contractions in caecum and ventral colon but its efficacy in the small intestine has not been determined.

Presentations: Tablets 10 and 25 mg.

Dose: 0.25–0.75 mg/kg po q 8–12 h.

Contraindications: Urinary or intestinal obstruction.

Cisapride
POM V

Actions and indications: Cisapride is a substituted benzamide acting as an indirect cholinergic agent to enhance release of acetylcholine leading to increased calcium flux and enhanced gastroduodenal coordination. Prophylaxis/treatment of ileus. Treatment of certain types of grass sickness (only selected chronic cases).

Presentations: Cisapride has been withdrawn from the market in Europe and USA because of infrequent cardiac side effects in humans.

Dose: 0.1 mg/kg IM q 8 h (continue until motility returns).

0.8 mg/kg po q 8 h.

Contraindications: Oral preparation contraindicated in horses in postoperative ileus producing positive volumes of reflux.

Erythromycin lactobionate
POM V

Actions and indications: Erythromycin is a macrolide antibiotic, which, at lower levels, acts as a motilin agonist, mimicking the effects of endogenous motilin. Erythromycin also acts via 5-HT receptors to release acetylcholine and promote gastroduodenal coordination. Used for prophylaxis/treatment of ileus.

Presentations: 500 mg and 1 g vials for preparation as IV infusion.

Dose: 1–2 mg/kg IV (as infusion in 1 L saline given over 1 hour) q 6 h, until motility returns. Higher doses can disrupt propulsive activity.

Note:
- Cases treated with this drug as an antibacterial agent may develop diarrhoea which is presumed to be due to the prokinetic effects.

Side effects: Abdominal pain, antibiotic-induced diarrhoea.

Lidocaine (lignocaine) hydrochloride
POM V

Actions and indications: Suppresses activity of afferent neurones in the bowel wall, in turn suppressing sympathetic reflex inhibition of gut motility. Anti-inflammatory properties also can directly stimulate enteric smooth muscle. Analgesic effects may play a role in anecdotal clinical improvement in equines. Prophylaxis/treatment of ileus. Prokinetic.

Presentations: Solution for injection 1% w/v, 2% w/v. Also 0.2% solution in 5% glucose (500 mL) available.

Dose: 1.3 mg/kg IV infusion in polyionic fluids over 15 minutes as a loading dose. 0.05 mg/kg/minute IV infusion in polyionic fluids as continuous infusion until motility returns.

Note:
- Lidocaine (lignocaine) has been shown to shorten the duration of ileus in humans. However, the efficacy in equines is still uncertain. Anecdotally one of the more promising prokinetic agents.

Side effects: Muscle fasciculations, ataxia and possibly seizures. These signs are more likely if the initial bolus is administered too rapidly.

Contraindications: Lidocaine (lignocaine) should not be used simultaneously with cimetidine or metronidazole. Available commercial combinations of lidocaine with adrenaline are not suitable for this purpose.

Metoclopramide
POM V

Actions and indications: Metoclopramide is a substituted benzamide that acts as a dopamine receptor antagonist, adrenergic blocker and a 5-HT4 agonist. Prophylaxis/treatment of ileus. Prokinetic drug.

Presentations: Solution for injection 5 mg/mL, 2 mL glass ampoule.

10 mg tablets of metoclopramide hydrochloride BP.

Dose: 0.25 mg/kg/hour over 1 hour only, q 6 h (dilute in 500 mL saline).

0.04 mg/kg/hour continuous infusion.

Note:
- GI prokinetic with central and peripheral anti-dopaminic effects as well as direct and indirect stimulatory effects on cholinergic receptors. May cause transient reversible excitement at higher doses.

Side effects: Excitement (this can be profound), restlessness, sweating, colic.

Neostigmine
POM V

Indications: Acetyl-cholinesterase inhibitor. Promotes caecal and colonic contractile activity.

Presentation: Solution for injection 0.5 and 2.5 mg/mL.

Dose: 0.011–0.033 mg/kg SQ q 4 h.

Can be given IV but is associated with signs of abdominal discomfort.

Contraindications: Should be avoided in horses with impaction or intestinal distension.

(c) Intestinal Sedatives/Antispasmodics

Butorphanol tartrate
POM V/CD (S-IV)

Actions and indications: Butorphanol is a mixed agonist–antagonist that provides superior visceral analgesia compared with NSAIDs. Relief of musculoskeletal and visceral pain (colic).

With sedative/tranquilliser for standing sedation/restraint. Effective antitussive, useful for control of coughing due to respiratory tract procedures (e.g. bronchoalveolar lavage).

Presentation: 10/50 mL multidose bottle, 10 mg/mL for injection.

Dose: 0.05–0.2 mg/kg IV/IM/SC. Lower doses are used when combined with α_2 agonists for sedation/restraint.

> **Note:**
> - Unlikely to cause excitement after intravenous injection, but to minimise this risk the drug is best used in conjunction with α_2 adrenergic agonists. Should provide up to 4 hours of intestinal sedation/analgesia unless pain is very severe.

Side effects: Minimal, CNS excitation, decreased GI motility.

Hyoscine butylbromide
POM V

Actions and indications: Intestinal antispasmodic and *also analgesic* as a result of dipyrone component. Used for treatment of spasmodic colic and obstructive colic and as an aid to rectal examination by reducing straining. Aids relief of oesophageal intraluminal obstructions (choke).

Presentation: Sterile aqueous solution for injection, 1 mL vials and 50 mL multidose bottles containing 20 mg/mL hyoscine.

100 mL multidose vials (combination of 4 mg/mL hyoscine + 500 mg/mL of the NSAID dipyrone, also known as metamizole).

Dose: 0.3 mg/kg IV.

Combination product (hyoscine + dipyrone): 5 mL/100 kg.

Note:

- Dipyrone is a non-steroidal analgesic. Failure of colic to respond may indicate more severe problems (investigate further). **NOT FOR IM injection (marked local reaction).** Extravascular injection may cause thrombophlebitis.

Side effects: May cause transient increase in heart rate post-administration.

Contraindications: Repeated doses are not indicated! Dipyrone is a non-steroidal anti-inflammatory and administration of further anti-inflammatory drugs should only be done with caution.

Morphine sulphate
CD (S-II)

Actions and indications: Morphine is a pure opioid agonist. Provides relief of severe pain (see opioid section in analgesics).

Presentation: Morphine hydrochloride, single-dose vial, 10 mg/mL or 60 mg/2 mL.

Preservative-free formulation is variably available in single-dose vials containing 10 mg/mL, 2 mg/mL and 2.5 mg/5 mL.

Dose: 0.02–0.1 mg/kg IM/IV.

Notes:

- Excitement/box walking normal in pain-free horses.
- Very good analgesia of 2–4 hours following systemic administration.
- Must be kept in a separate, locked receptacle and purchase and dispensing registered in a bound record book.

Side effects: Excitement/box walking is common in pain-free horses. Has also been implicated in impaction colic as a result of reduced GI motility.

Contraindications: As an analgesic in colic, due to the side effects.

Pethidine
POM V/CD (S-II)

Actions and indications: Relief of musculoskeletal and gastroenteric pain.

Effective spasmolytic.

Presentation: Multidose vial, 50 mg/mL for injection.

Dose: 3.5–10 mg/kg IM.

Note:

- Do not administer IV: causes histamine release with profuse sweating/excitement.

Side effects: See above.

Contraindications: See above regarding IV injection. Overdose may also cause CNS stimulation and/or convulsions. Do not use where there may be renal impairment or in combination with detomidine. Do not use in pregnant mares or in animals intended for human consumption.

Xylazine
POM V

Actions and indications: α_2 agonist with sedative, analgesic and muscle relaxant effects. Premedication prior to general anaesthesia with ketamine/thiopentone (thiopental), etc. Often used in combination with butorphanol to enhance analgesia (see p. 80).

Presentation: 20 mg/mL (20 mL multidose vial) for injection.

100 mg/mL (10 mL multidose vial) for injection.

500 mg dry powder (10 mL single-dose vial)+diluent.

Dose: 0.25–1.1 mg/kg IV (slow).

Notes:

- Peak effect 3 minutes after IV administration.
- Duration of action somewhat dose-dependent but commonly 10–20 minutes.
- Marked local reaction/unreliable effect if administered IM (2–3× IV dose).
- Bradycardia with first- and second-degree heart block is common following administration.
- Ataxia more marked at higher doses and may be more pronounced when combined with an opioid.
- Diuresis and sweating are commonly observed.
- Not licensed for use in pregnant mares as no safety data. However, no good evidence exists for any teratogenic or ecbolic effects.

Side effects: Bradycardia, cardiac arrhythmias, polyuria, hypotension.

Contraindications: Do not use during last month of pregnancy due to risk of inducing parturition. Use with caution during the first trimester. Not to be used in horses intended for human consumption.

(d) Laxatives/Cathartics
Acetylcysteine
No applicable category.

Actions and indications: Strongly mucolytic at pH >7.5. Management of retained meconium/meconium impaction (primary or secondary).

Presentations: Pure powder.

Acetylcysteine enema (4%).
The required 4% solution can be made up as follows:

- 8 g acetylcysteine.
- 20 g baking soda ($NaHCO_3$).
- 200 mL water.

Dose: Single 200 mL dose administered intrarectally repeated after 60 minutes as required.

Notes:

- This is a highly effective procedure that should be used wherever the condition exists.
- The solution is administered slowly UNDER GRAVITY FLOW at room temperature or 37 °C, via a Foley catheter into rectum and the procedure is repeated after 1 hour. The procedure is very effective and is especially useful in the colt foals with secondary 'high meconium impaction in the terminal rectum due to a congenital narrowing of the pelvic inlet'.[1]

Dioctyl sodium sulfosuccinate (DSS)
AVM-GSL

Indications: Intestinal impaction. DSS acts as a surfactant and facilitates the movement of water into desiccated ingesta.

Presentation: Water- and oil-based solution for oral use only.

Dose: 10–20 mg/kg by stomach tube as a 5% solution q 48 h.

Note:

- Surfactant laxative. Not recommended for use with liquid paraffin.

Lactulose BP
AVM-GSL

Actions and indications: Mainly used in the management of hepatic encephalopathy to reduce production and absorption of ammonia from the gastrointestinal tract.

Presentation: Oral suspension (3.35 g/5 mL).

Dose: 0.2 mL/kg po q 12 h.

Liquid paraffin BP
AVM-GSL

---

[1]Madigan JE, Goetzman BW (1990). Use of acetylcysteine solution enema for meconium retention in the neonatal foal. Proceedings of the American Association of Equine Practitioners, pp. 117–118.

Actions and indications: Liquid paraffin acts as a faecal softener and lubricant. Indicated for impaction of the intestines, particularly pelvic flexure impaction, meconium impaction in foals.

Presentation: Oily liquid.

Dose: 2–6 L by stomach tube/pump q 12–24 hours to effect.

   100–150 mL foals q 24 h.

Notes:
- Administration facilitated by mixing with warm water, to a total volume of 6–8 L for a 500 kg horse.
- **NOT practical to dose effective amounts by drenching; nasogastric tube essential to avoid inhalation (often fatal).** If the liquid paraffin has appeared at the anus without significant volumes of faeces, fluid therapy may be indicated.

Contraindications: Do not use in horses with positive volumes of reflux on passing a nasogastric tube. Do not use if surgical colic suspected!

Magnesium sulphate BP (Epsom salt)
AVM-GSL

Actions and indications: Magnesium sulphate acts as an ionic cathartic to actively draw water into the bowel lumen. Used as treatment for intestinal impaction.

Presentation: Crystals/powder (100%).

Dose: 1 g/kg via nasogastric tube q 12–24 hours to effect.

Notes:
- Osmotic laxative. Effects often severe.
- Do not administer for more than 3 days because of severe enteritis and possible magnesium intoxication.

Side effects: Magnesium toxicity rare but possible with repeated administration.

Sodium phosphate/biphosphate
POM V

Indications: Meconium retention, small colon/rectal impaction.

Presentation: Suppositories or plastic packs with extension nozzle.

Dose: pnr.

Note:
- Safe, reliable, effective. Multiple enemas (of any type) may cause mucosal irritation/oedema. Recommended for treatment of meconium impaction in foals. Not big enough for adults.

Sodium sulphate BP (Glauber's salt)
GSL

Indications: Intestinal impaction, purgation.

Presentations: Crystals/powder.

Dose: 1 g/kg by stomach tube or in feed (palatable) q 12 h.

Note:
- Very safe – severe diarrhoea sometimes results.

Psyllium hydrophilic mucilloid
GSL

Action and indications: Psyllium is a bulk-forming laxative which causes the fluid and ion content of the faeces to increase by absorbing water. It is considered to be particularly useful for treating sand impactions.

Presentations: Flakes/powder.

Dose: 1 g/kg po q 8–24 h.

Psyllium can be administered long term at 1 g/kg q 24 h.

Note:
- The efficacy of psyllium hydrophilic mucilloid in treating sand impactions has been questioned.

(e) Antidiarrhoeals
Bismuth subsalicylate

Indication: Diarrhoea.

Presentation: Oral suspension (17.5 mg/mL).

Dose:
Foals: 30 mL every 2–4 hours.
Adults: 500 mL every 4 hours.

Note:
- Generally safe.

Codeine phosphate BP
POM V/CD (S-V)

Indications: Diarrhoea, cough suppression.

Presentation: Tablets oral 60 mg.

Dose: 0.2–2 g/day.

> **Note:**
> - Symptomatic treatment only and very few doses usually required. Overuse can cause impaction!

Kaolin (light)
No applicable category.

Indications: Intestinal absorbent – symptomatic treatment of diarrhoea. Useful as lining agent (with liquid paraffin) for intestinal inflammation (not affected by gastric secretions).

Presentation: Mixture of kaolin.

Dose: 50–200 g/day pnr.

> **Notes:**
> - Symptomatic treatment only.
> - Only useful for foals – do not attempt to control diarrhoea in adult horses with this – very messy and poor efficacy.

Section 6
Hormones/steroids and non-steroidal anti-inflammatory drugs

(a) Sex Steroids (Drugs Used to Manipulate Equine Reproduction)

Oestrogens
Prepare the female reproductive tract for fertilisation and the developing of the secretory tissue of the mammary gland. Causes behavioural signs of oestrus. Anabolic activity.

Oestradiol (estradiol)
Banned for use in food-producing animals in the EU.

In the UK, oestradiol 17β can only be used under the CASCADE if animals are signed out of the human food chain.

Progestogens
These drugs are used to prepare and maintain the female reproductive tract for implantation and pregnancy. They inhibit oestrous behaviour.

Altrenogest
POM *V*

Indications:

- Inductions of cyclic ovarian activity in mares with some follicular activity, either early in the season or in response to poor cyclicity at other stages.
- Treatment of lactation anoestrus in absence of corpus luteum. Suppression of oestrus and oestrus behaviour in normally cycling mares. Management and manipulation of oestrus cycle.

Presentation: Regumate Equine: Clear/light yellow oily solution for oral use 2.2 mg/mL. Available as 250 mL or 1 L multidose containers with built-in dose-regulating cup (1 L only, 1 mL/50 kg bodyweight).

Actions: Synthetic progestogen.

Dose: 0.044 mg/kg po.

Courses of 15 days or more used to suppress/regulate oestrus.

Meat withdrawal period: 9 days.

> **Note:**
> ● **DO NOT use in pregnant mares/stallions or mares where uterine infections have been identified.** Mixing with feed should be immediately before administration. May alter behaviour – possibly useful in some cases of headshaking. **Women of child-bearing age should not handle the product. Protective measures (gloves, sleeves, etc.) should be used when handling concentrate or feed.**

Androgens
Responsible for physical and psychological male sexual characteristics.

Testosterone
Banned for use in food-producing animals in the EU.

Gonadotrophins

HUMAN CHORIONIC GONADOTROPHIN (LUTEINISING HORMONE/LH)
POM V

Indications: Glycoprotein excreted in the urine of pregnant women.

Stimulation of ovulation and formation of corpus luteum (predicted timing of ovulation).

Suboestrus (follicles >2 cm), post-partum lactation failure, nymphomania, prolonged oestrus. Used as part of test for cryptorchidism (see cryptorchidism test, p. 52).

Poor libido in stallions.

Actions: Similar effect to LH.

Presentation: Single-dose vials, 1500 IU, white soluble powder+solvent.

Dose: 1500–3000 IU IV or IM injection 24 hours before mating or AI.

> **Notes:**
> ● IM/SC injections may be associated with abscess formation or clostridial myositis.
> ● Rare anaphylaxis after IV.
> ● When used for lactational failure, oxytocin should be given simultaneously.

Buserelin
POM V

Indications: Infertility of ovarian origin. Improvement of conception rates.

Presentation: Aqueous solution for injection 0.004 mg/mL.

Dose: To induce ovulation of a mature follicle; 10 mL total dose single IM (IV or SC injection may be used). Administered on first day of maximum follicle size, 6 hours before service. Repeat 24 hours if ovulation has not taken place.

Note:
- Synthetic GnRH analogue.

Deslorelin
POM *V*

Indications: Infertility of hypothalamic origin.

Induction of ovulation within 48 hours in oestrus mares with follicle diameter >30 mm.

Presentation: Subcutaneous biocompatible, cylindrical implant (2.3 mm diameter × 3.6 mm) containing 2.1 mg deslorelin acetate in preloaded plastic syringe.

Note:
- Synthetic nonapeptide analogue of GnRH. 100× more potent than GnRH.

Posterior pituitary hormones

OXYTOCIN
POM *V*

Indications: Stimulation of smooth muscle in uterus and mammary gland. Induction of parturition. Treatment of retained placenta. Post-partum haemorrhage and increased speed of uterine involution.

Uterine prolapse.

Stimulation of lactation.

Presentation: Sterile aqueous solution for injection 10 IU/mL, multidose 25 mL bottle.

Dose:

25–100 IU SC/IM/IV.

50 IU in 500 mL saline as IV infusion over 30 minutes for placental retention.

2–10 IU (total dose) in 5–10 mL saline by slow IV injection for parturition induction (parturition in 30–90 minutes).

2–10 IU by slow intravenous injection for uterine prolapse.

Notes:
- Sweating, colic may be seen.
- Not to be used in obstructive dystocia.
- ONLY to be used for induction of parturition when milk calcium concentration ≥10 mmol/L.

Prostaglandins

These drugs are either analogues or synthetic forms of prostaglandin F2α. They cause regression of the corpus luteum (CL). The CL is refractory to prostaglandins for up to 5 days post-ovulation in mares. Used to destroy persistent corpora lutea (treatment of prolonged dioestrus), induce oestrus for therapy or diagnostic purposes, return to oestrus early for covering and induction of abortion (before 35 days).

Notes:
- Absorbed through human skin. Should not be handled by women of child-bearing age/pregnant women. Accidental skin contact should be washed immediately with cold water. May also cause bronchospasm.

DO NOT USE WITH NON-STEROIDAL ANTI-INFLAMMATORY DRUGS.

ALFAPROSTOL
POM *V*

Indications: Luteolytic control of oestrous cycle including termination of persistent dioestrus, control of sub-oestrus and induction of abortion.

Presentation: Sterile aqueous solution for injection, 40 mL vials; 2 mg/mL.

Dose: 2–10 mg *total dose IM.*

Note:
- Sweating, colic, tachycardia, polypnoea. Spontaneous resolution after 5–10 minutes.

CLOPROSTENOL
POM *V*

Indications: Luteolytic control of oestrous cycle including termination of persistent dioestrus, control of sub-oestrus and induction of abortion.

Presentations: Sterile aqueous solution for injection, 10 or 20 mL multidose vials, 0.25 mg/mL.

Dose:

Horses: 250–500 µg *total dose IM.*

Ponies and donkeys: 125–250 µg *total dose IM.*

Note:
- Sweating, colic, tachycardia, polypnoea. Spontaneous resolution after 5–10 minutes.

DINOPROST PROMETHAMINE
POM *V*

Indications: Luteolytic control of oestrous cycle, treatment of sub-oestrous, abortion induction (before 35 days), termination of persistent dioestrus.

Presentation: Aqueous solution for injection 5 mg/mL, 10 mL and 30 mL multidose vials.

Dose: 5 mg *total dose IM*.

> **Note:**
> - Side effects include sweating, colic (usually disappear spontaneously after 10–15 minutes).

Myometrial relaxants

Clenbuterol
(see p. 117)

Spasmolytics: Hyoscine-n-butyl bromide
(see p. 139)

(b) Anabolic Steroids

Synthetic derivatives of testosterone. They promote nitrogen retention in metabolic disease. Retention of sodium, calcium, potassium, chloride, sulphate and phosphate also occur with most. Other effects include stimulation of appetite, increased erythrocyte production, increased skeletal muscle mass, retention of intracellular water, premature closure of growth plates and increased skin thickness. Some androgenic activity is present in most of these drugs and so hormonal effects on both male, neutered male and female horses can be expected.

Nandrolone phenylpropionate
POM V

Indications: Anabolic stimulation, metabolic enhancement, metabolic and endocrine-related anaemia, supportive management of chronic renal failure.

Actions: Clinical efficacy of anabolic steroids is unproven. In anaemia, effects due partly to increased erythropoietin production and partly from direct stimulation of bone marrow.

Presentations: None licensed for use in horses. Various forms available (e.g. oily solution for IM injection). 25 mg/mL, 10 mL vial.

Dose: 1 mg/kg IM. Repeated at 2–3 week intervals.

> **Notes:**
> - Administration to geldings at full dose may induce severe virilisation with behavioural problems (use half doses at 10-day intervals). Most horses respond after two to three injections. Contraindicated in all neoplastic conditions.
> - Use in competition horses not allowed in many countries!

(c) Adrenal Corticoids

Corticosteroids are reported to be potentially dangerous in inducing or exacerbating laminitis and are, therefore, specifically CONTRAINDICATED IN THE TREATMENT OF LAMINITIS and related conditions.

> The clinician is warned that due deliberation should be given before any horse is subjected to systemic or oral corticosteroid therapy.

However, the therapeutic value of these compounds in the treatment of disease is undisputed and the assessed risk to a particular horse should be carefully weighed. Many clinicians consider that the risk of corticosteroids is much lower than is commonly appreciated and that it is only those animals with a marked tendency towards laminitis and those with disease conditions which might predispose to laminitis on whom the drugs should not be used without extreme care and careful discussion of the potential effects with the owner.

Aside from the contraindications associated with laminitis and the general suppression of immune responses (and consequent effects on infectious processes) one of the strongest contraindications is in corneal ulceration.

- Corneal ulceration should never be treated with corticosteroids of any nature.
- Where anti-inflammatory effects are required in the presence of corneal ulceration, alternative non-steroidal anti-inflammatory drugs may be indicated.

However, as soon as corneal epithelium has definitely covered the corneal defect, corticosteroids have a dramatic effect in reducing the extent of subsequent fibrosis and scar/leukoma formation.

General properties of corticosteroids

1. Duration and relative potency of common corticosteroid drugs.

Table 3.5 The duration of action and the relative potency of corticosteroid drugs used in equine practice

Drug	Equivalent anti-inflammatory dose (mg)	Anti-inflammatory potency (relative)	Mineralo-corticoid potency (relative)	Approx. half-life *in vivo* (minutes)	Duration of effect (IV/po)
Hydrocortisone	20	1	2	60	<12 hours
Betamethasone	0.6	25	0	>300	>48 hours
Dexamethasone	0.75	30	0	120	>48 hours
Methylprednisolone	4	5	0	100	12–24 hours
Prednisolone	5	4	1	120	12–24 hours
Prednisone	5	4	1	60	12–24 hours
Triamcinolone	4	5	0		12–24[a]

[a]Lasts for weeks if given IM.

2. General physiological properties
   - Cardiovascular system:
     Reduces capillary permeability; enhances vasoconstriction (hence value in shock) but needs very high doses.
   - Nervous system:
     Lowers seizure threshold; reduces response to pyrogens; stimulates appetite.
   - Endocrine system:
     Suppresses ACTH/TSH/FSH/prolactin/LH release from pituitary.
     Reduces conversion of T_3 to T_4.
     Reduces ADH production – diuresis.
   - Musculoskeletal system:
     Inhibits osteoblast function (endocrine function).
     Muscular weakness, atrophy, osteoporosis.
     Inhibited bone growth.
     Increased Ca excretion and inhibition of vitamin D absorption.
   - Metabolic effects: Stimulates gluconeogenesis; mobilisation of fats (increased triglycerides and cholesterol).

- Immune system (high dose only): Suppression of T-lymphocytes, lymphokines, acute phase proteins. Reduced neutrophil chemotaxis. Decreased mast cell degranulation.
- Haematopoietic system: Increases circulating platelets, neutrophils and RBCs. Platelet aggregation inhibited. Reduced lymphocytes, eosinophils, monocytes.
- Gastrointestinal system: Increased secretion of gastric acid/pepsin/trypsin; decreased mucosal cell proliferation/repair; increased absorption of iron/ calcium but decreased fat absorption.
- Integumentary system: Thinning of skin and hair loss.

Beclomethasone (beclometasone) dipropionate
POM V

Indications: Maintenance therapy of non-infectious airway inflammatory diseases including IAD and recurrent obstructive airway disease (RAO/ COPD) and summer pasture associated airway obstructive disease (SPAOPD), nasal hypersensitivity and headshaking syndromes associated with nasal irritations.

Actions: Inhaled corticosteroid, with longer duration of action and less systemic absorption. Inhibits the production of inflammatory mediators, decreases goblet cell hyperplasia and decreases airway hyper-reactivity. Approximate onset of action 24 hours.

Presentations: MDI, HFA formulation, μg/actuation depends on formulation, administration by suitable inhaler.

Dose: 500–3500 μg/horse (of HFA formulation) by inhaler q 12–24 h.

Note:
- Maintenance inhaled corticosteroids essential for successful management of RAO. Expensive. Systemic corticosteroids may be needed in an acute attack in conjunction with bronchodilators. Do not use beclomethasone (beclometasone) parenterally! Interactions/precautions as for dexamethasone (below). Horses receiving other steroids by other routes may require lower dose. Older chlorofluorocarbon (CFC) formulation MDI largely replaced by hydrofluoroalkane (HFA). The HFA formulation produces finer drug particles resulting in a 2× to 10× increase in pulmonary drug deposition compared to the CFC preparations.

Dexamethasone
POM V

Indications: Treatment of inflammatory/hypersensitivity/allergic conditions including acute airway obstruction, insect-induced hypersensitivity (sweet itch), urticaria, insect stings and zootoxicosis reactions.

Specific treatment of purpura haemorrhagica/immune-mediated vasculitis and other immune-mediated conditions such as immune-mediated thrombocytopenia/anaemia and autoimmune skin conditions of the pemphigus and lupus groups.

Presentations: Many preparations for oral and systemic use (e.g. solution containing dexamethasone sodium phosphate 2 mg/mL and benzyl alcohol as preservative), for IV or IM injection, 50 mL multidose vial.

Dose: 0.05–0.2 mg/kg IV/IM/po (higher doses for shock and hypersensitivity conditions, lower dose range for inflammatory conditions).

Notes:
- Single dose usually well tolerated, but severe side effects may be seen in long-term use. Symptoms of Cushing's disease with significant alterations in carbohydrate, fat, protein and mineral metabolism may be seen. Hypothalamic–pituitary–adrenal suppression occurs during therapy – withdraw treatment gradually.

- Do not administer to pregnant animals.

- Delayed wound healing and increased susceptibility to infection – use antibiotic cover if risk of or pre-existing infection.

- Viral infections may be exacerbated.

- Contraindicated as part of topical or systemic therapy where infectious agent involved, laminitis and where corneal ulcers are present.

CHECK FORMULATION BEFORE INJECTION – CONFIRM ROUTE COMPATIBILITY.

Fluticasone propionate
POM V

Indications: Maintenance therapy of IAD, recurrent airway obstructive disease (RAO/COPD), summer pasture associated airway obstruction (SPAOPD), nasal hypersensitivity and headshaking syndromes associated with nasal irritations.

Actions: As for beclomethasone (beclometasone).

Presentations: MDI µg/actuation depends on formulation. Administration by suitable inhaler.

Dose: 1000–2500 µg/horse q 12–24 h.

Note:
- Most potent inhaled corticosteroid with longest pulmonary residence time and least adrenal suppression.

Methylprednisolone
POM V

Indications: Shock, anti-inflammatory therapy (joints and bursae), inflammatory and immune-mediated conditions.

Presentation: Suspension for injection containing methylprednisolone acetate 4.0%, 5 mL vials.

Dose: 0.2–0.7 mg/kg IM.

Intra-articular: 80–120 mg joint. Use care when injecting multiple joints, as dose is cumulative.

Notes:
- Side effects as for dexamethasone.
- Some formulations available for IV for rapid effect (shock, head trauma: *controversial!*).
- Duration of effect variable – average 3–4 weeks.
- Effect in treatment of sweet itch and small airway disease dubious.
- Few applications for this drug other than intra-articular or bursal injections. Has high risk of infection when given into synovial cavities or into bursae, so strict asepsis must be observed during the procedure.

Prednisolone
POM *V*

Indications:

Anti-inflammatory, anti-allergic therapy.

Immune-mediated conditions.

Temporary treatment of malabsorption/intestinal lymphosarcoma.

Presentation: 5 and 25 mg tablets.

Dose: 0.5–2 mg/kg po q 12 h taper dose according to effect.

Note:
- Interactions and side effects as for dexamethasone. Short duration of effect, therefore, decreased potential for side effects and most suitable for maintenance therapy.

Triamcinolone
POM *V*

Indications: Dermatoses, inflammatory conditions.

Useful as intralesional injection (very small doses) in allergic collagen necrosis disorder of the skin (collagen granuloma).

Commonly used as intra-articular steroid.

Presentation: Solution for injection 10 mg/mL.

Dose: 0.02–0.05 mg/kg IM.

Intrarticular 5–10 mg/joint up to a maximum dose of 18–20 mg.

Notes:
- Interactions and side effects as for dexamethasone above.

POTENTIAL RISK OF LAMINITIS – probably the most risky corticosteroid. Recent research suggests, however, that this risk may be overstated; as yet, there is no definitive advice. In general, it should probably be avoided except in low doses in defined conditions.

(d) Non-steroidal Anti-inflammatory Drugs

None licensed for animals less than 6–10 weeks of age, all carry contraindications in pregnancy, in animals suffering from cardiac, hepatic or renal disease or where there is a possibility of gastrointestinal ulceration or bleeding, dehydrated, hypovolaemic or hypotensive animals. Use of more than 1 NSAID concurrently or within 24 hours of a different NSAID is contraindicated.

Acetaminophen (paracetamol)
POM V

Indications: Analgesic and anti-pyretic, poor anti-inflammatory. Treatment of pyrexia associated with respiratory disease in pigs. Analgesia for acute traumatic pain in dogs.

Presentation: 200 mg/g powder, 200 mg/mL solution licensed in pigs for administration in drinking water.

400 mg tablets in combination with 9 mg codeine phosphate licensed in dogs (note legal category VFA-VPS).

500 mg tablets.

120, 250 mg/5 mL oral suspension.

10 mg/mL solution for IV injection.

Dose: Not licensed in horses but use reported at 20 mg/kg po q 12 hours.

Note:
- Good oral bioavailability in horses.

Acetylsalicylic acid
POM V

Indications: Anti-pyretic, analgesic, anti-inflammatory.

Presentations: Aspirin – 325 mg tablet, white powder, gel for topical application (in combination with heparin and levomenthol).

Dose: Very short half-life in horses limits its use as a systemic anti-inflammatory, anti-pyretic and analgesic agent. Very high doses are needed (10–100 mg/kg po q 8–24 hours). Much more potent as an antithrombotic agent where duration of effect is dose dependant. Single IV doses of 4 and 12 mg/kg shown to significantly prolong bleeding time for 4 and 48 hours, respectively. Prolonged effect due to irreversible acetylation of active sites on COX enzyme with platelets being unable to synthesise new enzymes.

Topical application: maximum of 50 g gel per day applied directly to affected area.

Notes:
- Only the topical preparation in combination with heparin and levomenthol is currently licensed in UK for use in horses for treatment of localised musculoskeletal inflammation.
- Powdered form licensed for use in cattle and pigs for treatment of pyrexia associated with acute respiratory disease and inflammation.

Carprofen
POM V

Indications: Prostaglandin sparing anti-pyretic, analgesic, non-steroidal anti-inflammatory drug. Musculoskeletal pain, laminitis and soft tissue injury. Reduction/control of postoperative pain and inflammation.

Presentations: Solution for IV injection (50 mg/mL).

White granules for oral use (8.7% w/w).

Dose: 0.7 mg/kg IV or po q 24 h for up to 10 days.

Notes:
- Analgesia with weak anti-inflammatory action and long half-life in the horse.
- 'Prostaglandin sparing' NSAID. Mechanism of action not clearly defined, appears to produce minimal inhibition of COX; therefore, may work via non-COX mechanisms, contributing to favourable side effect profile and wide therapeutic index.
- COX-2 selectivity demonstrated in dog and cat has not been shown to be the case in the horse.

Dimethyl sulphoxide (dimethyl sulfoxide)
POM V

Indications: Topical/IV anti-inflammatory. Decreases intracranial pressure.

Used as a carrier – aids skin penetration of other drugs (e.g. corticosteroids).

Presentations: 90% (900 mg/mL) solution in non-sterile analytical reagent bottles. Premixed in bottles with steroids for topical application to skin (applicator or paint brush supplied).

Dose: 0.25–1.0 g/kg very slow IV as diluted (20%) solution in normal saline. High doses are used to control intracranial pressure (110 mL of concentrate in 1 L saline as drip for 500 kg horse).

Topical: apply three to four times daily to shaved area.

Notes:
- Handle with care. Rapid skin penetration. Wear gloves – skin penetration is suggested by a strong taste in the mouth shortly after contact.
- May show diuretic effect when given IV.
- If given fast, IV may cause significant haemolysis.

Dipyrone (metamizole)
POM V

Indications: Pyrazolone analgesic, anti-pyretic, anti-inflammatory.

Presentation: Only available in combination with butylscopolamine (hyoscine) currently in the UK.

Dose: 25 mg/kg IV.

> **Notes:**
> - Localised tissue reaction if given extravascularly or IM.
> - Do *NOT* use with phenothiazine ataractics (hypothermia). May cause blood dyscrasia, hepatitis, nephropathy, colic, diarrhoea.
> - Good anti-pyretic and antithrombotic, poor anti-inflammatory.

Eltenac
POM V

Indications: Postoperative swelling. Anti-inflammatory, anti-pyretic, anti-oedematous activity.

Presentations: Clear, colourless solution for injection containing 50 mg eltenac, 1 mg sodium bisulphite and 150 mg propylene glycol per mL.

Dose: 0.5 mg/kg IV q 24 h for up to 5 days.

> **Note:**
> - **Do not give IM.** Do not use for horses intended for human consumption or animals less than 6 weeks of age.

Firocoxib
POM V

Indications: Treatment of lameness due to inflammation associated with osteoarthritis.

Presentation:

Paste (7.32 g) containing 60 mg (8.2 mg/g) firocoxib for oral dosing.

Solution for injection (20 mg/mL), 25 mL multidose vials

Dose:

0.1 mg/kg po q 24 hours.

0.09 mg/kg IV q 24 hours

Manufacturer states treatment should not exceed 14 days.

Flunixin meglumine
POM V

Indications: Analgesia, anti-pyresis, anti-inflammatory. Visceral pain associated with colic.

Presentations:

Solution for injection (50 mg/mL), 50 and 100 mL multidose vials.

Granules sachets (10 g) containing 250 mg flunixin for oral administration.

Paste (10 g) containing 500 mg flunixin for oral dosing.

Dose: 1.1 mg/kg IV/IM/po q 24 hours up to 5 days.

0.25 mg/kg q 6–8 h for endotoxaemia/septic shock.

> **Note:**
> - Use with great care in colic, masks cardiovascular effects of endotoxaemia.

Isopyrin (ramifenazone)
POM V

Indications: Analgesia, anti-pyresis, anti-inflammatory effect.

Presentation: Solution for injection each mL containing 240 mg isopyrin (ramifenazone)+121.4 mg phenylbutazone.

Dose: 4.2 mg/kg phenylbutazone and 7.8 mg/kg isopyrin (3.5 mL/100 kg) IV q 24 h.

> **Notes:**
> - Administer slow IV (over at least 1 minute).
> - UK preparation discontinued.

Ketoprofen
POM V

Indications: Analgesia, anti-pyresis and anti-inflammatory action. Visceral pain associated with colic.

Presentations: Aqueous 1% and 10% solutions (multidose vials), 5 and 20 mg tablets. Only the 10% solution is licensed for use in the horse. A 10% oral solution for administration in drinking water is available but only licensed for use in pigs.

Dose: 2.2 mg/kg of the 10% solution IV q 24 h, for up to 5 days for musculoskeletal pain. 2.2 mg/kg of the 10% solution IV as a single dose for analgesia in cases of abdominal pain.

> **Notes:**
> - Do not administer concurrently with phenylbutazone or flunixin meglumine.
> - Only licensed postoperatively.
> - Poor oral bioavailability in horses.
> - Analgesic, anti-inflammatory and anti-endotoxic effects similar to flunixin meglumine.

Meclofenamic acid
POM V

Indications: Anti-inflammatory, analgesic, anti-pyretic.

Presentation: 10 g sachets white granules for oral use in feed.

Dose: 2.2 mg/kg q 24 h po for up to 7 days.

> **Notes: Variable bioavailability following oral administration**
> - Manufacturers advise maximum of 7 days treatment.
> - Slow onset of action, requiring 36–96 hours of treatment before evidence of clinical efficacy.

Meloxicam
POM V

Uses: Non-steroidal, anti-inflammatory drug used for alleviation of inflammation and pain relief in acute and chronic soft tissue and orthopaedic disorders and pain associated with colic.

Dose and formulation: 0.6 mg/kg IV/po or mixed in feed.

Oral suspension containing 15 mg/mL q 24 h for maximum of 14 days (dosing syringe with weight calibration supplied).

Solution for intravenous injection containing 20 mg/mL (50 and 100 mL multidose bottles). Licensed for single injection only (treatment can be continued using oral formulation).

> **Note:**
> - Transient, self-limiting swelling may occur at injection site. Urticaria and diarrhoea are occasional side effects.

Naproxen
POM V

Indications: Relief of inflammation and pain associated with muscle and soft tissues. Marked analgesic and anti-pyretic effects (prostaglandin inhibitor).

Presentation: Single-dose sachets (4 g active substance in granule form) for oral use.

Dose: 10 mg/kg po q 12 h in feed for 14 days (pnr).

> **Notes:**
> - Structurally similar to ibuprofen and ketoprofen. Poor oral bioavailability (50%).
> - Slow onset of action, requiring 48–96 hours of treatment before evidence of clinical efficacy.
> **NOT to be used in pregnancy.** Safe under other circumstances.

Paracetamol (see Acetaminophen, p. 151)

Phenylbutazone
POM V

Indications: Analgesia, anti-pyresis and anti-inflammatory activity. Pain associated with musculoskeletal disorders and reduction in post surgical soft tissue reaction.

Presentations: Sachets of white powder for oral administration containing 1 g phenylbutazone.

Oral paste 32 mL syringe containing 6 g phenylbutazone in dose graduated (kg) syringe.

Solution for intravenous injection containing 200 mg/mL.

200 mg tablets.

Dose: Solution: 4.4 mg/kg IV for up to 5 consecutive days.

Oral (granules or paste).

Day 1: 4.4 mg/kg q 12 h.

Days 2–5: 2.2 mg/kg q 12 h.

Then: 2.2 mg/kg q 24 h or q 48 h.

Notes:
- Extensive hepatic metabolism produces primary active metabolite oxyphenbutazone as well as inactive metabolites. Oral absorption can be delayed by certain feeds and can result in a second peak of absorption from the colon.
- Narrow therapeutic index in horses but long-term administration at low doses appears to be generally safe in normal horses.
- European law bans the use of phenylbutazone in horses intended for human consumption.

Ramifenazone (see Isopyrin, p. 154)

Suxibuzone
POM V

Indications: Pain and inflammation associated with musculoskeletal conditions and soft tissue inflammation.

Presentations: Yellow granules supplied in 10 g sachets containing 1.5 g suxibuzone for oral administration.

Dose: Horses: Days 1–2: 6.25 mg/kg q 12 hours.

Days 3–5: 3.1 mg/kg q 12 hours.

3.1 mg/kg q 24 hours or eod, reducing to minimum clinically effective dose.

Ponies: Administer at half the recommended horse dose, i.e.:

Days 1–2: 6.25 mg/kg q 24 hours.

Days 3–5: 3.1 mg/kg q 24 hours for 3 days or 6.25 mg/kg eod, reducing to minimum clinically effective dose.

> **Note:**
> ● Derivative of phenylbutazone. Reduced incidence of gastrointestinal ulceration vs PBZ.

Vedaprofen
POM V

Indications: Anti-inflammatory and analgesic for musculoskeletal pain, soft tissue injury of both traumatic and surgical origin. Can be used pre- and postoperatively.

Presentation: Oral gel 100 mg/mL vedaprofen with 130 mg/mL propylene glycol.

Solution for injection 50 mg/mL, 100 mL multidose vials. Licensed for single injection only (treatment can be continued using oral formulation).

Dose:

Injectable 2 mg/kg IV.

Oral.

Day 1: 2 mg/kg q 12 hours.

Days 2–5: 1 mg/kg q 12 hours for up to 14 consecutive days.

> **Notes:**
> ● The only NSAID licensed for pre-operative administration.
> ● Not to be used in animals less than 6 months of age.
> ● Manufacturer states can be used during pregnancy.

(e) Pituitary Suppression Drugs
Used for the treatment of PPID (equine Cushing's disease). In PPID, abnormal pars *intermedia* cells produce excessive amounts of proopiomelanocortin (POMC) and other POMC-derived peptides in addition to adrenocorticotropic hormone (ACTH). Debate continues as to the pathogenesis of PPID. It may be that abnormality of the pars *intermedia* occurs as a spontaneous pituitary disease or that there is loss of dopaminergic innervation (i.e. a primary hypothalamic disorder). (Aminergic neurones arising in the hypothalamus regulate melanotrophs in the pars intermedia. Dopamine is the primary neurotransmitter of these secretory neurones and it tonically inhibits release of hormones from melanotrophs.)

Cyproheptadine
POM *V*

Indications: Treatment of PPID. Limited efficacy as a monotherapeutic agent, normally given in combination with pergolide when maximal doses of pergolide alone are insufficient to resolve the clinical signs.

May be useful in some cases of idiopathic headshaking (trigeminal-summation or post herpetic neuralgia) (in conjunction with carbamazepine).

Actions: Serotonin antagonist with additional anticholinergic and antihistaminic effects. (Serotonin has been shown to be a potent secretagogue of ACTH in isolated rat pars *intermedia* tissue.)

Presentation: 4 mg tablets.

Dose:

Week 1: 0.3 mg/kg q 12–24 h.

Week 2: 0.4 mg/kg q 12–24 h.

Week 3–4: 0.5 mg/kg q 12–24 h.

Week 5–6: 0.6 mg/kg q 12–24 h.

Notes:
- Temporary and equivocal response. 6–8 weeks before clinical improvement (reduced polydipsia/hair coat restoration).

Not to be used in animals with inflammatory airway disease (IAD/RAO). May cause sedation and ataxia at higher doses.

Pergolide mesylate
POM V

Indication: Treatment of PPID.

Action: Dopamine agonist.

Presentation: 1 mg tablets for oral administration.

Dose: Suggested protocol is 0.002 mg/kg (1 mg/500 kg), po, q 24 h. If no improvement noted within 4–8 weeks, increase daily dose by 0.001–0.002 mg/kg (0.5–1 mg/500 kg) monthly up to a total dose of 0.01 mg/kg. Alternatively, if unsatisfactory response to 0.004–0.006 mg/kg pergolide and endocrine tests remain abnormal, 0.3–0.5 mg/kg of cyproheptadine can be added to pergolide therapy.

Notes:
- Appears to be most effective treatment at present. Improvement of clinical signs best measure of response, as normalisation of endocrine tests may be slow.
- Side effects of anorexia (and secondary hyperlipaemia), diarrhoea and colic may be seen with higher doses.
- Pergolide is an ergot alkaloid and may have some vasoconstrictive effects, which has led to concerns over exacerbation of laminitis – no confirmed problems.

Trilostane

Indications: Trials suggest efficacy in treatment of PPID.

Actions: Specific adrenal gland suppression. Competitive 3-β-hydroxysteroid dehydrogenase inhibitor (enzyme required for synthesis of cortisol from cholesterol in the adrenal medulla).

Presentation: Hard gelatin capsules 60, 120 mg – no reports of use with this preparation in horses. Licensed for dogs.

Dose: 1 mg/kg suggested dose po q 24 h.

> **Notes:**
> - Clinical improvement reported in lethargy, laminitis, polyuria/polydipsia and weight distribution while having little effect on hirsutism. Approximately 3 months for full clinical effect. Monitor with DST/TRH endocrine test. No reported side effects. Further trials are necessary.
> - Not licensed for equine use.

(f) Others

Adrenocorticotrophic hormone (ACTH)
POM *V*

Indications: Stimulation of adrenal activity in premature/dysmature foals. Diagnosis of pituitary–adrenal axis disorders.

Actions: ACTH causes release of cortisol from the adrenal cortex. Endogenous ACTH released from the anterior pituitary. Negative feedback by cortisol.

Presentations: Aqueous solution: 250 μg/mL, 1 mL single-use vials.

Dose: 100–250 μg total dose for 50 kg foal IM single dose.

Insulin
POM *V*

Indications: Specific therapy for insulin-responsive diabetes mellitus. Treatment of hyperlipaemia in ponies. Diagnosis of certain endocrine conditions (combined glucose insulin test).

Actions: *Hyperlipaemia* – Insulin helps prevent development of hyperlipaemia by inhibiting tissue hormone-sensitive lipase (enzyme causing lipolysis of adipose tissue). Also stimulates gluconeogenesis in the liver and activates lipoprotein lipase (enzyme causing uptake of fatty acid from very low density lipopolysaccharides [VLDL] in the blood by adipose tissue).

Presentations: Regular insulin 100 units/mL, 10 mL vial.

Protamine zinc insulin (long-acting insulin) 100 units/mL, 10 mL vial.

Dose: Titration in diabetes mellitus.

Hyperlipaemia: insulin zinc: 0.15 IU/kg subcutaneous q 12 h, can be increased
    in increments of 0.05 IU/kg if hyperglycaemia occurs (monitor blood glucose
    levels carefully).

CRI regular insulin (combined with glucose infusion!): 0.07 IU/kg/hour (monitor
    blood glucose levels carefully).

Notes:
- Hyperlipaemia: Treatment of lipaemia/hyperlipaemia should be carried out in
  conjunction with oral (or IV) glucose therapy at 0.25 g/kg po q 12 h.
- May have poor efficacy due to relative insulin insensitivity.
- Diabetes mellitus: Few, if any, horses showing clinical signs of diabetes
  mellitus such as hyperglycaemia, glycosuria, PU-PD, weight loss, etc.,
  are true diabetics – almost all will be PPID cases and some may be
  hyperlipaemia cases.

Misoprostol
POM V

Indications: Prostaglandin E₁ analog, used for the treatment of right dorsal colitis.

Presentation: 100 and 200 µg tablets.

Dose: 1.5–5 µg/kg po q 8 h.

Note:
- The higher doses have been associated with sweating, colic and diarrhoea.

Thyroxine (levothyroxine)
POM V

Indications: Hypothyroidism (rare in horses). Used in the management of Equine
    Metabolic Syndrome as a way to aid weight loss.

Presentations: 0.1, 0.2, 0.3, 0.4, 0.5, 0.6, 0.7, 0.8, 1 mg tablets.

Dose: 0.1 mg/kg po q 24 h.

INDEX OF DRUGS USED IN EQUINE MEDICINE

Section 7
Anti-infective drugs

(a) Antiviral Drugs

Idoxuridine

Indications: Superficial herpes viral keratitis.

Presentation: 0.1% or 0.5% eye ointment.

Dose: Apply every 2–4 hours until epithelial defect closed, then every 4–6 hours for further 3–4 days.

> **Note:**
> - Epitheliotoxic, may retard closure of epithelial defects. Do not use in pregnant mares.

Acyclovir
POM V

Indications: Superficial herpes viral keratitis, EHV-1 myeloencephalopathy, EHV-5 multinodular pulmonary fibrosis.

Presentation: Eye ointment, acyclovir 3%; 4.5 g.

200, 400 and 800 mg tablets.

Solution for injection 50 mg/mL.

Dose: For herpetic keratitis apply every 3–4 hours.

20 mg/kg po q 8 h.

10 mg/kg IV q 12 h.

> **Notes:**
> - Unpredictable efficacy but generally effective for herpetic keratitis.
> - Very poor oral bioavailability in horses.
> - Questionable efficacy for EHV-1 myeloencephalopathy.

Ganciclovir
POM V

Indications: Acute herpetic keratitis. EHV-1 myeloencephalopathy, EHV-5 multinodular pulmonary fibrosis.

Presentation: Eye drops, 0.15% in gel basis.

Solution for injection: 10 mg/mL.

Dose: Apply every 2–4 hours until epithelial defects closed, then every 4–6 hours for further 4–7 days. Usual duration of treatment is 14–21 days.

2.5 mg/kg IV q 8–12 h.

> **Notes:**
> - May cause ocular irritation and secondary punctuate ulceration (check status of cornea before medication).
> - Believed to be more efficacious than Acyclovir for EHV-1 infection.

Trifluridine

Indications: Superficial herpes viral keratitis.

Presentation: Eye drops 1%.

Dose: Apply every 2–4 hours until epithelial defect closed, then every 4–6 hours for further 3–4 days.

> **Note:**
> - Only available in UK on request from Moorfields Eye Hospital, 162 City Road, London, EC1V 2PD.

Valacyclovir

Indications: EHV-1 myeloencephalopathy, EHV-5 multinodular pulmonary fibrosis.

Presentation: Eye ointment 3%.

Dose: Apply every 3 hours until epithelial defect closed, then every 12 hours for 7 days (human).

> **Note:**
> - Human drug, efficacy in horses not known, anecdotally good.

Vidarabine

Indications: Superficial viral keratitis due to equine herpes virus infection.

Presentation: 500 and 1000 mg tablets.

Dose: 18–40 mg/kg po q 8–12 h.

> **Note:**
> - Expensive but better bioavailability and efficacy over acyclovir.

Interferon α_2A

Indications: Prevention or alleviation of viral respiratory disease.

Presentation: Different number of preparations available for injection (3, 6, 9, 18 and 36 million units), but can be given orally in horses.

Dose: 1000 IU/horse po q 24 h.

Notes:
- Human drug, equivocal results in horses.
- Can be applied topically for treatment of herpetic keratitis.

(b) Antibacterials

Notes:
- Every precaution should be taken to ensure the use of swabs, cultures and sensitivity testing of bacteria. Resistance *in vitro* does not always mean that the compound is of no value but due note must be taken of such results. Sensitivity *in vivo*, likewise may not result in sensitivity *in vitro*. Tissue availability of the compound may alter the effects significantly. Doses should be accurately calculated from the bodyweight of the patient and courses should be completed to avoid resistance as far as possible.
- Commercial preparations containing more than one antibiotic agent may require dosage adjustment for one or other of the drugs included. It may be impossible to give the correct dosage of both or all the agents.

Antibacterial resistance

Antibacterial selection in horses is different than that in many other species for a number of reasons. The sensitivity of hindgut fermenters, such as horses, to antibacterial-induced colitis means that a significant proportion of antibacterials available for use in animals cannot be used safely in horses. Limited markets and lengthy and costly development periods further limit the development of equine-specific preparations by drug companies. Furthermore, extrapolated doses of human antibiotic preparations applied to horses is often prohibitively expensive, inappropriate and sometimes dangerous (e.g. risk of colitis). Licensing laws, which regard the horse as a food-producing animal in some parts of Europe, make using these human products potentially illegal.

Further, antibacterial resistance is an increasing problem facing all medical practice. This is not a new problem; veterinarians frequently encounter resistant organisms and are trained to select the most appropriate antibiotic type as necessary. Recent interest in public awareness and concern over antibacterial resistance, for example, methicillin-resistant strains of S. *aureus* (MRSA) outbreaks in human hospitals are becoming major issues to equine practitioners. Although the highly resistant organisms encountered in human hospitals are not thought to be a problem in veterinary hospitals, MRSA has already been reported in a number of outbreaks. The irresponsible use of antibacterials by veterinarians is perceived by the medical profession as a source of public concern. Clearly, social and political pressures on the veterinary profession have resulted in some changes. However, great care should be taken to demonstrate that the profession does have a responsible attitude to antibacterial use. This not only safeguards the immediate welfare of animals, but, perhaps more importantly, safeguards the future use and effectiveness of veterinary antibiotics.

Choice of antibacterial
Before selecting an antibacterial the clinician MUST first consider two factors:

1. *The specific needs of the patient*. For example, neonatal foals have different pharmacodynamics than adults in many respects and some of the drugs have known toxicity to one or other organ/system. Also, for example, enrofloxacine has specific harmful effects on growth plates that make this drug contraindicated in foals. Tetracycline may cause flexor laxity in foals or diarrhoea in adults and so due attention should be paid to the case itself. Likewise, hepatic failure may have a profound effect on metabolism of drugs in all ages of horse. Known individual allergies to antibacterials should mean that those drugs are specifically contraindicated. Most current antibacterials in equine practice have a relatively wide margin between therapeutic and toxic effects and so toxicity is not usually regarded as a significant factor in most cases. However, there are individual drugs that have significant toxicity.

2. *The likely organism*. This has a profound influence on the choice of drug! There are many reports of 'common organisms' in the various disease processes and their likely sensitivities and so these data should be used to guide selection. The final choice will usually, in theory at least, be determined by specific culture and sensitivity. Unfortunately, these are all too seldom performed.

Antibacterial policy
Polices should be directed at 'best practice'. This will result in minimal opportunities for resistance and toxicity and maximal return in efficacy. In general:

- viral infections should not be treated with antibiotics
- samples should be taken to establish the nature and sensitivity of the bacteria involved
- doses should be carefully calculated according to the weight (or surface area) of the patient and should be maintained at the correct interval for a suitable duration. Inadequate doses predispose resistance and in some infections a higher than normal dose may be indicated – but this may result in significant toxicity
- the route of administration is also important and must be considered carefully
- lack of response should trigger a complete reassessment of the case to establish if this is due to an error of diagnosis, an error of selection of drug or development of a resistance complication.

(1) β-Lactams

Table 3.6 Suggested antibiotic drugs for use in horses

Drug	Route	Dose (mg/kg)	Interval (hours)	Comments
Amikacin	IM/IV/SC	15–25 (25 mg/kg in foals)	24	Therapeutic concentration monitoring ideal
Amoxicillin (amoxycillin) ($3H_2O$)	IM/SC po po/IM	Injectable 5–12 Oral 30–50 Foals 10–30	12 8–12 12	Reactions sometimes severe NOT LA forms
Ampicillin	IV/IM	10–80	6–8	Useful pleural cavity irrigation Not LA forms
Ampicillin	IV/IM	10–80	6–8	Useful pleural cavity irrigation Not LA forms
Ceftiofur	IV	2	12–24	EXPENSIVE BUT GOOD ACTIVITY/ PENETRATION
Chloramphenicol (succinate)	IV	25	12	Resistance problems, risk of aplastic anaemia, etc.?
Enrofloxacin	po po IV	7.5 4 5	24 12 24	Contraindicated in horses less than 3 years of age (high risk of cartilage disorders)
Gentamicin sulphate	IV/IM*	6.6 (11 mg/ kg in foals less than 7 days old)	24	Nephrotoxicity Therapeutic concentration monitoring ideal, especially in foals
Kanamycin sulphate	IM	10	12	No veterinary formulation – availability?
Neomycin	IM	5	24	With penicillin IV forms not available in UK

Continued

Table 3.6 Suggested antibiotic drugs for use in horses—cont'd

Drug	Route	Dose (mg/kg)	Interval (hours)	Comments
Oxytetracycline	IV (slow)	5–7	12	Diarrhoea risk Not LA forms or IM
Penicillin-Na G	IV/IM	15–25 000 IU	6	K salts not to be given IV
Procaine penicillin G	IM	20 000 IU	24	Useful routine antibiotic cover
Streptomycin sulphate	IM/IV	8–12	4	Probably useless in horses!
Ticarcillin/ clavulanate	IV	50–75	6	Expensive Very effective for foals (septicaemia)
Ticarcillin	IV	50–75	6	Expensive Effective for foals (septicaemia)
Trimethoprim-sulphadoxine	IV/IM*po	15–20 (total)	12	Oral forms useful Broad-spectrum effects Minimal toxicity

Note: The list is not complete but covers some of the more common drugs available in the UK.
*Not recommended.

Ampicillin

POM V

Indications: β-lactam infections due to Gram +ve organisms (except penicillinase producers) and most Gram –ve organisms (poor for *E. coli*).

Not for Mycobacteria, *Proteus* (except *P. mirabilis*), *Pseudomonas*, *Rickettsia*, *Mycoplasma*.

Presentations: 500 mg, 2 g powder for reconstitution single-dose vials; 150 mg/mL suspension IM injection, 50/100 mL multidose vials.

Dose: 20 mg/kg sodium salt (IV/IM) q 6–8 h.

20 mg/kg trihydrate salt (IM) q 12 h.

20 mg/kg trihydrate salt (po) q 8 h.

Notes:

- Soluble salt only stable for 1–2 hours after reconstitution.
- Low oral bioavailability in adults.
- Useful adjunct to metronidazole for pleural irrigation in infective pleuritis.

Long-acting forms are contraindicated (**SEVERE LOCAL REACTIONS/ANAPHYLAXIS**).

Penicillin (G-K, G-Na, G-procaine)
POM V

Indications: β-lactam infections due to penicillin-sensitive Gram +ve bacteria.

Presentations: Na-Penicillin 3 g (5 meg units) powder-vials.

Procaine penicillin: 300 mg/mL solution, 100/30 mL multidose bottles.

Dose: See Table 3.7 below.

Table 3.7 Dose, route and interval for penicillin in horses

Name	Route	Dose (mg/kg)	Dose (IU/kg)	Interval (hours)
Na benzyl-	IV	10–17	22 000–25 000	6–8
Procaine-	IM	10–17	22 000–25 000	12

Notes:

- Intravenous Na$^+$ or K$^+$ benzathine penicillin occasionally is associated with sudden death and/or abrupt cardiac arrhythmias. These drugs should not be administered *during anaesthesia or in combination with other drugs likely to affect cardiac rhythm*.
- Na$^+$ salts are absorbed more slowly when given IM. **Avoid concurrent bacteriostatic agents.**
- Always check formulation for suitable route of administration.
- **DO NOT mix with other drugs.**
- Allergies possible (anaphylactic reactions – if these are encountered DO NOT use cephalosporin either).
- Anaphylactic shock requires emergency treatment with adrenaline (epinephrine).
- There are no effective oral preparations for horses.

Warning: Check contents/permitted route before use (many products are cocktails of drugs). Mixtures of different drugs may make accurate dosage of all components difficult!

Ticarcillin
POM V

Indications: β-lactam broad-spectrum, bactericidal. Particularly active against J-haemolytic Streptococci and *Pseudomonas aeruginosa*, *Staphylococcus aureus*, *Klebsiella pneumoniae*, *Bacteroides fragilis*.

Intrauterine flush, joint infections and neonatal septicaemia.

Presentation: 1 g, 5 g dry powder for reconstitution. Combinations with clavulanic acid available.

Dose: 50 mg/kg q 6 h IM/SC/IV.

Uterine flush: 6 g dissolved in 100–500 mL saline q 24 h×3 (during oestrus).

Note:
- Expensive. No veterinary product licensed in UK. Good tissue penetration. Potentiation with clavulanic acid is effective but rapid resistance can develop to either form. Some good reports of use in septicaemia in foals but some disappointing.

(2) Cephalosporins

Cefalexin
POM V

Indications: First-generation cephalosporin. Indicated for Gram +ve bacteria; less activity against Gram –ve than second, third and fourth generation cephalosporins.

Presentation: 125, 250 and 500 mg capsules.

Dose: 25–30 mg/kg po q 6–8 h.

Cefazolin
POM V

Indications: First-generation cephalosporin. Indicated for Gram +ve bacteria; less activity against Gram –ve than second, third and fourth generation cephalosporins.

Presentation: 500 mg, 1 g and 2 g.

Dose: 11–20 mg/kg IV or IM q 6–8 h.

Note:
- Poor oral bioavailability in adult horses. For foals only.

Cefepime
POM V

Indications: Fourth-generation cephalosporin.

Presentation: Solution for injection equivalent to 250 mg, 500 mg, 1 g and 2 g per vial.

Dose: 11 mg/kg IV q 8 h for foals.

2.2 mg/kg IV q 8 h for adult horses.

> **Note:**
> ● No veterinary preparations available. When used orally can cause colic.

Cefquinome
POM V

Indications: Fourth-generation cephalosporin, licensed in horses for IV and IM use.

Presentation: 30 mL vial (1.35 g) and 100 mL vial (4.5 g).

Dose: 1–2 mg/kg IV or IM q 24 h.

Foals: Dose can be increased up to 4.5 mg/kg q 6–12 h.

> **Notes:**
> ● Licensed in adult horses for respiratory disease.
> ● Licensed in foals for severe bacterial infections with a high risk of septicaemia.

Ceftiofur
POM V

Indications: Broad-spectrum, bactericidal, third-generation cephalosporin antibiotic. CNS, joint, eye, urinary and peritoneal infections. Good effect in respiratory disease, especially *Streptococcus equi/zooepidemicus* and *Pasteurella* infections showing penicillin resistance. Limited spectrum against Gram +ve and extended spectrum against Gram −ve.

Presentations:
1 g vial containing powder (+20 mL diluent).

4 g vial containing powder (+80 mL diluent).

Dose: 1–5 mg/kg IV q 6 h, 1–5 mg/kg IM q 24 h.

Usual adult dose: 2.2 mg/kg q 12 h IV or IM.

Usual foal dose: 5 mg/kg q 6 h, can give up to 10 mg/kg, IV or IM.

> **Notes:**
> ● Good tissue penetration with rapid metabolism (metabolites are still active) – concentrates in tissue compartments. Excreted via urine and faeces. 10-day courses are usually required.
> ● If given IM, maximum of 10 mL should be placed in any one site.
> ● Diarrhoea has occurred after IV injections of long courses at high doses.
> ● Not licensed for IV use.

Ceftriaxone
POM V

Indications: Third-generation cephalosporin. Broad-spectrum, Gram +ve, Gram –ve, some anaerobes. Excellent penetration into most body tissues, pleural fluid, peritoneal fluid, bile, bronchial mucosa, bone, myometrium, inflamed and healthy blood CSF barrier. Relatively non-toxic.

Presentations: 125, 250, 500, 1000 and 2000 mg vials for injection.

Dose: 25–50 mg/kg IV or IM q 12 h.

> **Notes:**
> - Human drug.
> - Quite expensive (foals only?).

(3) Aminoglycosides

Amikacin
POM V

Indications: Aminoglycoside infections due to Gram +ve organisms (except penicillinase producers) and most Gram –ve organisms, especially if gentamicin resistance.

Presentation: 50/250 mg amikacin base/mL solution for IM injection.

Dose: 10–15 mg/kg q 24 h slow IV or IM.

Foals: 20–25 mg/kg q 24 h slow IV/IM.

Subconjunctival 75–100 mg.

Intra-articular 250–750 mg/joint.

Regional limb perfusion: 2–5 mg/kg.

Intrauterine: 2 g in 200 mL normal saline q 72 h×3.

> **Notes:**
> - This class of antibiotic exhibits concentration-dependent bactericidal activity and a postantibiotic effect. The longer interval between dosing provides a drug-free period, which allows reversal of adaptive resistance.
> - No formulation in UK licensed for horses. Higher dosage regimens for respiratory infections.
> - Very useful for septicaemic foals where higher dose rates are due to a larger volume of distribution.
> - Also useful for intrauterine use in mares (no significant systemic absorption from uterus).
> - Useful for intra-articular use (probable antibiotic of choice for most infective joint disorders).
> - Foals' blood concentrations should be monitored.
> - Nephrotoxicity problems similar to other aminoglycosides.

Gentamicin
POM *V*

Indications: Infections due to most Gram −ve and some Gram +ve organisms. Particularly *Ps. aeruginosa*, *R. equi*. Bactericidal. Intrauterine infections (use infusion).

Presentation: 20/40/80 mg/mL single-dose (2 mL) vials.

50 mg/mL; 50 mL.

Ophthalmic preparations.

Dose: Adults 6.6 mg/kg IV q 24 h.

Foals up to 7 days old, 11 mg/kg sid.

Notes:
- Foals and dehydrated animals may show severe nephrotoxicity. Monitor renal function before and during therapy.

DO NOT USE WITH OTHER NEPHROTOXIC DRUGS.

- Poor oral absorption. Rapid resistance.
- Therapeutic concentration monitoring ideal, especially in foals. Do not use with loop diuretics.

Neomycin
POM *V*

Indications: Aminoglycoside used to reduce ammonia-producing organisms in large intestine in cases of hepatic encephalopathy. Gram −ve infections (especially enteric organisms). Decreases microbes in colon prior to colon surgery.

Ophthalmic infections.

Presentations: 500 mg tablets.

Ophthalmic preparation.

Dose: For hepatic encephalopathy 5–15 mg/kg orally once daily.

Note:
- No products licensed in UK for use in horses. Toxic effects as for gentamicin. Not as effective as other aminoglycosides against *Pseudomonas*, *Klebsiella* and *E. coli*.

(4) Chloramphenicol and derivates

Chloramphenicol
POM *V*

Indications: Broad-spectrum, bacteriostatic. Suspected/confirmed chloramphenicol-sensitive salmonellosis (plasmid-borne resistance widespread). Active against rickettsial and chlamydial infections, most anaerobes, most Gram +ve aerobes, non-enteric aerobes. CNS infections (because it readily crosses lipid barriers). Corneal ulceration (topical).

Presentations:

Chloramphenicol palmitate 25 mg/mL oral suspension. Capsules 250 mg, 500 mg and 1 g.

500 mg and 1 g as sodium succinate powder for reconstitution.

Ophthalmic preparation.

Dose: 25–50 mg/kg q 6–12 h.

> **Notes:**
> - Not licensed for equine use or food-producing animals. Rapid metabolism in horses.
> - Prolonged courses may result in reversible aplastic anaemia in horses, although has been used for many years in safety. Significant interactions with penicillin and rifampicin. Possibly over-rated as antibiotic for corneal/conjunctival infections (consider gentamicin first) but does penetrate into anterior chamber.
>
> **Use with extreme caution – avoid skin contact. Risk of aplastic anaemia in 1 in 30,000 people approximately.**

Florfenicol
POM *V*

Indications: Broad-spectrum, bacteriostatic. Good penetration because it readily crosses lipid barriers.

Presentation: Solution for injection 300 mg/mL.

Dose: 20 mg/kg IM q 48 h.

> **Notes:**
> - Not licensed for equine use.
> - Foals only, serious risk of colitis in adults.

(5) Potentiated sulphonamides

Sulphadiazine + trimethoprim
POM *V*

Indications: Broad-spectrum antibacterial (most Gram –ve, some Gram +ve).

Presentations:

Sulphadiazine 200/400 mg/mL + trimethoprim 40/80 mg/mL solution for injection; 50 and 100 mL multidose vials.

Single-dose oral sachets (37.5) with 12.5 g sulphadiazine and 2.5 g trimethoprim.

Dose: 30 mg/kg combined ingredients (25 mg sulphadiazine + 5 mg trimethoprim) q 12–24 h orally.

24–30 mg/kg by slow IV q 12–24 h.

Notes:
- Dose of 30 mg/kg po q 12 h is commonly found to be more effective. **USE CARE GIVING IV INJECTIONS – MUST BE VERY SLOW.** Increased pulmonary penetration when used in combination with clenbuterol. Takes time to be effective; therefore, no significant benefit parenteral versus oral administration and latter much safer. Consider injection route in cases of choke lasting more than 24 hours.

- *Ps. aeruginosa* resistant. Oral courses effective over long periods without apparent toxic effects. Check formulation and permitted route before administration. Better absorption after starvation (possibly best administered on empty stomach – difficult to manage).

- Do not administer detomidine, xylazine, romifidine or halothane to horses receiving potentiated sulphonamide medication (risk of death from heart failure).

(6) Tetracyclines

Doxycycline
POM *V*

Indications: Bacteriostatic tetracycline. Broad-spectrum, not *Pseudomonas*, *Enterobacter* or *Enterococcus*.

Used for treatment of *Neorickettsia risticii* (Potomac horse fever) and other equine *Neorickettsia* (oxytetracycline is the first-line treatment for this condition). Mycoplasmal respiratory infections, *Ehrlichial* infections, *Lawsonia intracellularis* and *Borrelia*.

Anti-MMP effect, useful in keratomalacia and immune-mediated keratopathies. Appropriate concentration in tear film following oral administration.

Presentations: 100 mg tablet/capsule.

Oral solution 100 mg/mL.

Dose: 10 mg/kg po q 12 h or 20 mg/kg q 24 h.

Notes:
- NOT for parenteral use – fatal cardiac arrhythmias, collapse, death. Rapid absorption and longer effect than oxytetracycline.

- Ophthalmic solutions have a useful anti-collagenase activity in addition, but are not generally available. Concentrations are critical (weak solutions must be used!) but are not yet established for horses.

Oxytetracycline
POM *V*

Indications: Broad-spectrum bacteriostatic tetracycline. Urinary and respiratory tract bacterial infections.

Useful effect in the treatment of contracted tendon syndromes in young foals. First-line treatment of *Neorickettsia* infections (e.g. *Neorickettsia risticii*/Potomac horse fever), *Ehrlichial* infections, *Lawsonia intracellularis* and *Borrelia*.

Presentation: 5%, 10% and 20% solution for injection for SLOW IV administration.

Dose: 6.6 mg/kg IV slow q 12 h.

> **Notes:**
> **Tetracyclines have been associated with some fatal cases of diarrhoea especially in adults – this risk may be small but it does exist and due note should be taken before embarking on this drug in adult horses.** The drug is actually used widely and there are very few reports of any problems. Long-acting solutions should not be used in horses under any conditions:
>
> - IM injection may cause large local reactions (which may abscessate).
> - Contraindicated in stressed animals (e.g. surgery, trauma, anaesthesia) – dysbacteriosis of large colon and diarrhoea.
> - The drug is well tolerated by foals. Septicaemia and joint infections are treatable.
> - Some evidence that foals with contracted tendons can improve following administration of a single (or two) large doses of the drug (2.5–3 g diluted in 1 L saline q 24 h). Risk of nephropathy with this dose!
> - Antagonistic effect with bactericidal drugs.

(7) Fluoroquinolones

Enrofloxacin
POM *V*

Indications: Bactericidal, broad-spectrum quinolone includes Gram –ve aerobes and staphylococci, but no activity against anaerobes; hence, antibiotic-associated diarrhoea rare. Used for pleuropneumonia due to aerobes and first-line choice for salmonellosis.

Presentations: 25 mg/mL solution for SLOW IV injection.

2.5% and 10% oral solution.

Dose: 5 mg/kg IV q 24 h.

7.5 mg/kg orally q 24 h.

> **Note:**
> - Not licensed for equine use. Contraindicated in horses less than 3 years of age (high risk of cartilage disorders).

Marbofloxacin
POM *V*

Indications: Bactericidal, broad-spectrum quinolone.

Presentations: 2% and 10% solution for IV injection.

5, 20 and 80 mg tablets.

Dose: 2 mg/kg IV q 24 h.

3.5–4 mg/kg orally q 24 h.

> **Note:**
> - Risk of cartilage disorders in young horses.

(8) Macrolides

Azithromycin
POM *V*

Indications: Macrolide antibiotic, similar properties and spectrum of activity to erythromycin. Effective for Gram +ve organisms, *Chlamydia*, *Mycoplasma*, *Listeria*, *Rhodococcus*, *Corynebacterium*. Rapid development of resistance so always use in combination with another drug (usually rifampin).

Presentations: Capsules containing azithromycin dihydrate 250 mg, 500 mg and 1 g. 500 mg vials for injection.

Dose: 10 mg/kg po q 24 h, after 5 days, q 48 h.

> **Notes:**
> - Can cause hyperthermia in foals and fatal colitis in adults. DO NOT USE IN ADULT HORSES.
> - Only practical for use in foals with *Rhodococcus equi* infection.

Clarithromycin
POM *V*

Indications: Macrolide antibiotic, similar properties and spectrum of activity to erythromycin. Effective for Gram +ve organisms, *Chlamydia*, *Mycoplasma*, *Listeria*, *Rhodococcus*, *Corynebacterium*. Rapid development of resistance so always use in combination with another drug (usually rifampin).

Presentations: 250 and 500 mg tablets.

Dose: 7.5 mg/kg po q 12 h.

> **Notes:**
> - Can cause hyperthermia in foals and fatal colitis in adults. DO NOT USE IN ADULT HORSES.
> - Used in foals with *Rhodococcus equi* infection in combination with rifampin.

Erythromycin
POM *V*

Indications: Macrolide-static or -cidal activity according to dose rate/susceptibility. Effective for Gram +ve organisms, *Chlamydia*, *Mycoplasma*, *Listeria*, *Rhodococcus*, *Corynebacterium*. Rapid development of resistance so always use in combination with another drug (usually rifampin).

Presentations: 250 and 500 mg tablets.

500 mg and 1 g vials and 100 mg/mL solution for injection.

Dose: 25 mg/kg po q 6–8 h.

> **Notes:**
> - Avoid if hepatic function not normal.
> - Can cause hyperthermia in foals and fatal colitis in adults. DO NOT USE IN ADULT HORSES.
> - Used in foals with *Rhodococcus equi* infection in combination with rifampin.
> - Erythromycin acts as intestinal prokinetic.
>
> **AVOID PARENTERAL FORMS (human preparations) – severe local reactions, especially IM.**

(9) Miscellaneous antibacterials

Imipenem–cilastatin sodium
POM *V*

Indications: A carbepenem. Very broad-spectrum. Almost all Gram+ve and Gram –ve, including *Pseudomonas*, *Listeria*, *Enterococcus*. Not anaerobes. Good penetration except CNS. Toxic effects can include hepatocellular jaundice, auto-immune-mediated haemolytic anaemia, diarrhoea, fits, nausea, pruritis, rash, pseudomembranous colitis (all in humans).

Presentation: Powder for reconstitution and injection. To store, make up with 1% lignocaine (lidocaine) solution; lasts 4 hours at room temperature, 24 hours in refrigerator.

Dose: 10 mg/kg IM q 8–12 h.

> **Notes:**
> - Human drug.
> - Expensive (foals only?).

Metronidazole
POM *V*

Indications: Nitroimidazole specifically for treatment of anaerobes, narrow spectrum including protozoa and Gram +ve and Gram –ve anaerobes. May have intestinal anti-inflammatory activity. Used for clostridial enteritis, peritonitis. Soaked swabs may control local anaerobic infections (e.g. feet/wounds).

80% oral systemic availability.

Presentations: 200/250/400/500 mg tablets. 5 mg/mL solution for injection.

Powder for reconstitution and oral paste also available.

Dose: 15 mg/kg IV loading dose then 7.5 mg/kg IV q 6 h, inject over 1 hour.

15 mg/kg q 8 h orally.

30–60 mg/kg per rectum q 8 h.

Notes:
- Solutions not specifically prepared for IV injection should be filtered as administered by slow IV injection (or not administered at all by this route).
- May cause diarrhoea in some horses, especially if intestinal function is already impaired (e.g. after colic surgery).
- Used to reduce ammonia-producing organisms in large intestine in cases of hepatic encephalopathy.

Polymyxin B
POM V

Indication: Although an antibacterial with a Gram –ve spectrum, it is only used in cases of ongoing endotoxaemia in horses.

Presentations: Powder for reconstitution and injection.

Ophthalmic preparations.

Dose: 1000–6000 IU/kg q 8–12 h.

Notes:
- Risk of nephropathy.
- Binds only to circulating endotoxin.

Rifampicin/rifampin
POM V

Indications: Broad-spectrum antibiotic. Particularly indicated for *Rhodococcus equi* (with erythromycin). Treatment of tuberculosis.

Presentation: 150+300 mg capsule, oral.

Dose: 5–10 mg/kg po q 12 h.

Notes:
- Rapid resistance – never use as single drug; use with erythromycin (qv) (synergistic effect). Excellent lipid solubility and cell/tissue-penetrating properties. Good penetration of caseous and purulent material.
- May cause red discoloration in urine. Very safe, even over long courses.
- Prolonged courses usually required.
- Expensive.

(c) Compound Antibacterials

Mixing antibiotics cannot, generally, be recommended. However, several mixtures are so commonly used together that they are sold as an individual product. The use of penicillin and aminoglycoside is well documented due to their complementary bactericidal activity against Gram +ve and –ve organisms, respectively. It should be noted, however, that, although therapeutic levels of procaine penicillin are maintained for 24 hours, levels of aminoglycoside fall to below minimal inhibitory concentration (MIC) within 12 hours. They still remain useful in equine practice.

Penicillin + neomycin
POM V

Indications: Infections due to sensitive Gram +ve and Gram –ve organisms.

Presentations: 100 mg/mL neomycin sulphate + 200 mg/mL procaine benzylpenicillin; 100 mL multidose vials.

Dose: 0.05 mL/kg q 24 h by IM injection.

> **Notes:**
> - Not IV administration.
> - Causes local pain and reaction after 4–5 days.

Penicillin + streptomycin
POM V

Indications: Infections due to sensitive Gram +ve and Gram –ve organisms.

Presentations: 250 mg/mL dihydrostreptomycin sulphate + 200 mg/mL procaine benzylpenicillin; 100 mL multidose vials.

Dose: 0.04 mL/kg q 24 h by IM injection.

> **Notes:**
> - Not IV administration.
> - Causes local pain and reaction after 4–5 days.

(d) Antifungal Agents

Amphotericin B
POM V

Indications: Active against yeasts and fungi. Deep or systemic mycoses. Histoplasmosis, blastomycosis.

Presentation: 50 mg injection single-dose vials, supplied as powder for reconstitution.

Dose: 100 mg test dose. 0.2 mg/kg increasing to 0.5–1.0 mg/kg over 2 days. Given as very dilute IV solution (0.1 mg/mL in 5% dextrose saline drip).

Notes:
- Very light sensitive (protect from light at all times).
- Nephrotoxicity common if prolonged course. May be given alternate days to reduce toxic effects. Monitor renal function. Dilute to avoid cardiac toxicity. May be given with corticosteroids to reduce adverse effects during administration.

Enilconazole
POM *V*

Indication: Treatment of dermatomycosis.

Presentation: 10% concentrate for cutaneous emulsion.

Dose: Dilute 1:50 in water. Apply at 3–4 day intervals.

Note:
- Remove crusts before use.

Fluconazole
POM *V*

Indication: Systemic mycosis.

Presentation: 150 mg tablets.

Dose: 14 mg/kg as loading dose, then reduce to 5 mg/kg po q 24 h.

Note:
- Potentially hepatotoxic. Long treatments usually needed.

Griseofulvin
POM *V*

Indications: Systemic treatment of dermatomycoses.

Presentations: Powder containing 7.5% griseofulvin.

Dose: 10 mg/kg po q 24 h for 7–14 days.

Notes:
- NOT TO BE USED during pregnancy, wear impervious gloves to handle.
- Reduced effect if concurrent phenylbutazone. Effect slow to develop. No action against systemic mycoses due to *Candida*, *Aspergillus*, blastomycoses, etc. Generally need longer dosing periods than manufacturer's recommendation.
- Should not be handled by women of childbearing age.

Itraconazole
POM V

Indication: Systemic mycosis.

Presentation: 100 mg tablets.

Dose: 5–10 mg/kg po q 24 h.

> **Note:**
> ● Oral absorption low and variable.

Ketoconazole
POM V

Indications: Fungistatic. Systemic treatment of dermatomycoses. Also topical treatment of fungal infections (*Aspergillus* spp. require high doses).

Presentation: 200 mg tablets.

Dose: 30 mg/kg po q 12–24 h. Dissolve in 0.2 mmol/L HCl and administer by stomach tube.

> **Note:**
> ● No products licensed for horses in UK. Not for use in pregnant animals. Can reduce testosterone synthesis in breeding males. Possible hepatotoxicity. Not to be used with H_2-blockers, anticholinergics or antacids (increases stomach pH – inhibits absorption of conazoles).

Miconazole
POM V

Indication: Topical treatment of dermatomycoses.

Presentation: Shampoo containing chlorhexidine gluconate 2%, miconazole nitrate 2%; 250 mL bottle.

Dose: Shampoo twice weekly until symptoms subside and negative dermatophyte culture.

> **Note:**
> ● Remove crusts before use.

Natamycin
POM V

Indications: Topical and environmental treatment of dermatomycoses.

In keratomycosis effective against *Fusarium* spp.; less effective against *Aspergillus* and yeasts.

Presentation: Dry powder for resuspension.

Ophthalmic preparation.

Dose: Dilute powder until 0.01% concentration. Sponge onto skin or spray. Wood, leather and metal can be sprayed. Repeat after 4–5 days.

> **Note:**
> - Water quality important and method of suspension significant. Apply by spray – use facemask for personal protection. 10 L suspension (10 g) effective for two horses or one horse and stable (apply with spray, not aerosol generator).

Potassium iodide

Indication: Systemic mycosis.

Presentations: Powder or crystals.

Dose: 20–30 mg/kg po q 24 h.

> **Notes:**
> - Do not use in pregnant mares and foals!
> - Stop if signs of iodism are seen (lacrimation, productive cough and a dry, scurfy coat with some hair loss).

Voriconazole
POM *V*

Indication: Systemic mycosis.

Presentations: 50 and 200 mg tablets.

Solution for injection 200 mg/vial.

Ophthalmic preparation.

Dose: 2–4 mg/kg po q 24 h.

1 mg/kg IV q 24 h.

> **Note:**
> - Wide spectrum of activity.

(e) Antiprotozoal Drugs
Diclazuril
POM V

Indication: Treatment of equine protozoal myeloencephalitis (EPM).

Presentation: 1.56% pellets for oral administration.

Dose: 1–7 mg/kg po, sid for 21 days.

> **Note:**
> - May have to be administered by stomach tube.

Imidocarb
POM V

Indications: Treatment of babesiosis due to *B. equi* and *B. caballi*. Also some effect in treatment of trypanosomiasis.

Presentation: 12% solution for injection, 100 mL multidose vials.

Dose: 2 mg/kg deep IM q 24 h on two consecutive days for *B. caballi*.

B. equi: Four doses of 4 mg/kg IM 72 hours apart (this protocol may not eliminate the parasite consistently).

Note:
- Severe local reactions are common (with subsequent abscess formation) – consider brisket site and vary site for subsequent injections.

Isometamidium
POM V

Indications: Infections due to *T. brucei*, *T. vivax* and *T. congolense*.

Dose: 0.25–2 mg/kg IM injection.

Note:
- Drugs have been used for many years and resistance is commonly encountered.

Metronidazole (see Antibacterials)
POM V

Indications: Narrow spectrum including protozoa (*Giardia* and *Trichomonas* spp.).

Nitazoxanide
POM V

Indications: Treatment of EPM.

Presentation: Paste for oral administration.

Dose: 50 mg/kg po, once a day for 28 days.

Note:
- Side effects include fever, diarrhoea, colic oedema and laminitis.

Ponazuril
POM V

Indications: Treatment of EPM.

Presentation: 15% paste for oral administration.

Dose: 5 mg/kg po, once a day for 28 days.

Note:
- Few side effects except for uterine oedema.

Pyrimethamine
POM *V*

Indications: Toxoplasmosis. EPM (with sulphonamides).

Presentation: 25 mg tablets.

Dose: 0.1–1 mg/kg po q 24 h.

> **Note:**
> ● Prolonged courses possible (over 2–3 months). If used with sulphonamides, may cause leucopaenia, thrombocytopaenia and anaemia. Synergistic with sulphonamides in activity against toxoplasma.

Quinapyramine
POM *V*

Indications: Infections due to *T. equiperdum*. Also for *T. brucei*, *T. vivax* and *T. congolense* when treated in addition with homidium chloride at 1 mg/kg.

Dose: 3–5 mg/kg every 6 hours SC or deep IM, divide dose between sites due to severe local reaction.

> **Note:**
> ● Drugs have been used for many years and resistance is commonly encountered. *T. equiperdum* infections should not be treated due to risk of developing carrier status.

Suramin
POM *V*

Indications: Infections due to *T. evansi* and *T. equiperdum*.

Dose: 7–10 mg/kg slow IV, second treatment 1 week later.

> **Note:**
> ● Drugs have been used for many years and resistance is commonly encountered.

(f) Anthelmintics

> **Note:**
> ● Regular worm egg counts and tapeworm serology should be used to monitor the effects of anthelmintic programmes and the occurrence of resistance. Routine worming programmes should be adjusted to suit the circumstances and the efficiency of clean pasture management. Full therapeutic doses should be used at all times.

Table 3.8 Some of the common, currently available anthelmintics for horses in the UK

Drug	Presentation	Dose rate (mg/kg)	Activity/comments
Piperazine	Salt for admin via tube/in feed	200–250	P. equorum good effect Cyathostomes (adult)
Thiabendazole[a] (tiabendazole)	Paste/powder	44–50 440	Adult strongyles Larvicidal at high doses
Mebendazole[a]	Paste/granules	5–10	Broad-spectrum. Not larvicidal
Fenbendazole[a]	Paste/granules	7.5 50 30 q 48h	Broad-spectrum Strongyloides Larvicidal at high doses/frequencies
Oxibendazole	Oral paste	10–15	Broad-spectrum Strongyles, P. equorum good
Pyrantel	Paste/granules	19 40	Adults Strongyles/ cyathostomes only A. perfoliata tapeworms
Ivermectin	Paste	0.2	Larvicidal Broad-spectrum NB: injectable forms very dangerous (can be given by mouth) Can cause drug eruptions used IV
Moxidectin	Oral paste	0.4	Broad-spectrum as for ivermectin More persistent than ivermectin so resistance more likely to develop

The list is not complete and mention is not to be taken as endorsement of the product.
[a]Benzimidazole resistance is widespread – cross resistance in the group is also possible.

Fenbendazole
POM VPS

Indications: Anthelmintic treatment and control programmes for all types of helminth parasites of horses.

Presentations:

Paste in dosing syringe (graduated kg).

10 g sachets (granules [22%]) for in-feed administration.

Drench for oral administration (10%).

Double-dose formulation for 5-day course to treat larval cyathostomosis/strongylosis.

Dose: Routine worming 5–7.5 mg/kg po.

Parascaris equorum 10 mg/kg.

Larval cyathostominosis 10 mg/kg po, for 5 consecutive days.

Table 3.9 Dose requirements for fenbendazole use in anthelmintic treatment

	Dose
Routine worming	7.5 mg/kg
Cyathostome spp.	30 mg/kg
Migrating *Strongyle* larvae	60 mg/kg once or 7.5 mg/kg daily for 5 days or 50 mg/kg for 3 days
D. arnfieldi	15 mg/kg
Parascaris equorum	10 mg/kg
Strongyloides westeri	50 mg/kg
Verminous arteritis	50 mg/kg q 24 h × 3

Note:
- Larval cyathostominosis resistance very common.

Ivermectin
POM VPS

Indications: Treatment/control of all major helminth parasites including lungworm. Treatment of lice and mange. Treatment of cutaneous and gastric habronemiasis, thelaziasis. Treatment and control of bots. Effective against microfilaria (*Onchocerca*, etc.).

Presentations: Paste for oral administration in graduated syringe (kg) (1.87% w/w).

Contents of syringe treats 600 kg.

Dose: 0.2 mg/kg po lasts 6–8 weeks.

Notes:
- Parenteral administration may cause severe life-threatening reactions. IV use has been reported to be safe but not licensed – this route is not recommended. Injectable form may be given po at 200 µg/kg. 'Pour-on' forms may be effective against lice/mites but can cause moderate/severe skin reactions.
- NOT effective against equine tapeworms (*Anoplocephala* spp.) or encysted Cyathostomin larval stages.
- Environmental considerations – dispose of dung carefully (extremely dangerous to fish/aquatic life).

Levamisole
NFA-VPS

Indications: Treatment/control of adult strongyles. Possible immune stimulatory properties (intractable infections and immune compromise).

Presentations: 7.5% solution for SC injection, oral drench (1.5% w/v).

Dose: 8 mg/kg po.

Immunostimulant 8–11 mg/kg orally q 24 h for 14 days.

Note:
- Anthelmintic effects poor and not licensed for horses (useful in treatment of lungworm in donkeys).

Mebendazole
POM VPS

Indications: Treatment of helminthiasis (strongyles and cyathostomes), mature and larval *Parascaris equorum*, adult *Oxyuris equi*, *Dictyocaulus arnfieldi* at special dose rate.

Presentations: Graduated (kg) syringes – 4 g micronised mebendazole in 20 g paste.

Sachets containing 20 g mebendazole for in-feed use.

Dose: 8.8 mg/kg. Repeat every 6 weeks.

15–20 mg/kg daily for 5 days for *Dictyocaulus arnfieldi*.

Notes:
- Safe for pregnant mares and foals. May cause mild diarrhoea if overdosed. Pregnant donkeys should NOT receive the higher dose regime.
- NOT for use in horses intended for human consumption.
- Resistance patterns not yet clear.

Moxidectin
POM *VPS*

Indications: Broad spectrum of activity and wide safety margin. 13-week duration of action (may favour resistant organisms). Treatment/control of all major helminth parasites including lungworm. Treatment of hypobiotic larvae, lice and mange. Treatment of cutaneous and gastric habronemiasis, thelaziasis. Treatment and control of bots. Effective against microfilaria (*Onchocerca*, etc.).

Presentation: Graduated syringe for oral administration up to 600 kg horse.

Dose: 0.4 mg/kg.

> **Note:**
> ● Contraindicated in foals younger than 4 months of age due to possible neurological reactions including coma and death due to high lipophilicity.

Oxfendazole
POM VPS

Indications: Treatment/prophylaxis of ascarids, strongyles, *Oxyuris equi* and adult *T. axei*.

Presentations: Oral paste in graduated (kg) syringe (18.5% w/w).

Pellets for in-feed administration (6.8% w/v).

Dose: 10 mg/kg po prn.

> **Note:**
> ● Possible cross-resistance with fenbendazole or specific resistance. Safe.

Oxibendazole
POM VPS

Indication: Routine anthelmintic treatment and control.

Presentation: Oral paste in graduated (kg) syringes (8 g as 30% w/w).

Dose: 10 mg/kg po for roundworms. 15 mg/kg po for *Strongyloides westeri*.

> **Note:**
> ● Possible cross-resistance or specific resistance with fenbendazole but so far not established.

Piperazine BP
POM VPS

Indications: Treatment *Parascaris equorum* plus adult strongyles.

Presentations: Powder for oral dosing.

Paste in graduated (kg) syringe; oral.

Dose: 88 mg/kg po (adipate/citrate). Maximum 30 g for foal, 60 g for yearlings, 80 g adults.

Repeat at 10-week intervals for *Parascaris equorum* in young horses.

Notes:
- No specific equine preparations. Risk of photosensitisation.
- No effect on migrating larvae. Large doses best given by stomach tube.
- If used in heavy parascaris infestations can cause rupture or obstruction of small intestine due to rapid death/detachment of worms.
- Most commercial products have additional anthelmintics (e.g. thiabendazole [tiabendazole], trichlophon, phenothiazine or levamisole).

Praziquantel
POM VPS

Indication: Tapeworm treatment, especially *Paranoplocephala mamiliana*.

Presentations: Oral paste in graduated (kg) syringe; 50 mg tablet oral.

Dose: 1 mg/kg.

Note:
- DO NOT use injectable formulation (except by mouth) – risk of laminitis, etc.

Pyrantel embonate (pamoate)
POM *VPS*

Indications: Treatment/control of strongyles, *Oxyuris*, *Parascaris equi*. Also (at higher dose) effective against *Anoplocephala* spp.

Presentations: Oral paste in graduated syringe (kg) 11.41 g in 22 mL base.

Powder/granules for in-feed administration (76.7% w/w).

Dose: 19 mg/kg routine. 38 mg/kg for treatment of tapeworms.

Notes:
- Safe. No known resistance in adult strongyles (or cyathostomes). Good efficacy against equine tapeworms at higher dose rates.
- Not effective against *Paranoplocephala mamiliana*.

Thiabendazole (tiabendazole)
NFA-VPS

Indications: Treatment of adult helminth parasites. At higher doses effective against migrating strongyle larvae and lungworm.

Presentations: Drench (suspension) for oral administration 17.6% w/v.

Paste for oral administration in graduated syringe (kg) 49.3%.

Dose: Routine worming 44 mg/kg po prn.

Foal ascariasis 88 mg/kg po prn.

Notes:
- Not licensed for equine use.
- Dose of 20 mg/kg po q 24 h for 7–14 days has some antifungal properties.

Triclabendazole
POM V

Indications: Immature and adult stages *Fasciola hepatica*. No activity against nematodes.

Presentations: 10% solution (100 mg/mL) oral suspension.

Dose: 15 mg/kg po.

Note:
- Not licensed for equine use in UK. No information on toxicity.

(g) Ectoparasiticides

Benzyl benzoate
NFA-VPS

Indications: Acaricide for control of mange mites and *Culicoides* spp. irritation and allergy (sweet itch).

Presentations: 25% w/v with emulsifying wax in water powder in shaker; 500 mL and 1.8 kg.

Dose: Applied daily to mane and base of tail as repellent/insecticide.

Notes:
- For topical treatment only. Care should be taken with handling.
- Not very effective in many cases, but others are significantly improved.

Coumaphos
NFA-VPS

Indication: Ectoparasiticide for control of lice.

Presentation: 3% powder in shaker with propoxur 2% and sulphanilamide 5%.

Dose: Repeat at 14-day interval (NOT LESS).

Note:
- For topical treatment only. Care should be taken with handling.

Cypermethrin/permethrin
NFA-VPS

Indications: Ectoparasiticide for control of nuisance flies such as *H. irritans*, *H. bovis*, *G. intestinalis*, etc. Cattle ear tags repellent for flies.

Presentation: 5% emulsifiable concentrate; 250 and 1000 mL.

Dose: Diluted 1:50 with water used as TOPICAL WASH. Applied to mane, neck, etc., at sites of predilection for flies. Repeat 14–28 days.

Horse needs 6+ cattle tags (halter/mane/forelock/tail plaited in).

Note:
● For topical treatment only. Care should be taken with handling.

Doramectin
POM VPS

Indication: Treatment of chorioptic mange.

Presentation: 10 mg/mL injectable solution.

Dose: 0.3 mg/kg, subcutaneous, 2 weeks apart.

Note:
● Not licensed for equine use.

Fipronil
POM V

Indications: Control of mange (chorioptic, sarcoptic, psoroptic), trombiculidiasis and lice.

Presentation: Fipronil 0.25%; 100 and 250 mL solution in hand-held sprayer.

Dose: Clip affected hair if necessary, clean scabs away and then apply directly to affected areas. If lesions generalised, treat half animal then treat other half 1–2 weeks later.

Note:
● Not licensed for equine use.

Piperonyl butoxide
NFA-VPS

Indications: Treatment of *Culicoides* sensitivity, sweet itch and lice.

Presentation: Solution containing piperonyl butoxide 0.5%+pyrethrum extract 0.4%; 500+5000 mL.

Dose: Apply to mane, neck, etc., at sites of predilection for flies. Repeat 14–28 days.

Note:
- For topical treatment only. Care should be taken with handling.

Ivermectin
See sections under endoparasiticides (p. 185).

Moxidectin
See sections under endoparasiticides (p. 187).

INDEX OF DRUGS USED IN EQUINE MEDICINE

Section 8
Blood-modifying agents

HAEMOSTASIS

Haemostasis is the balance between coagulation and fibrinolysis. Vascular injury leads to reflex vasoconstriction and damaged endothelial cells release activating/inhibiting substances of coagulation and fibrinolysis. Platelet plug (primary haemostatic plug) forms following interaction of platelets with a discontinuous vascular surface. The coagulation cascade involves successive activation of circulating inactive clotting factors (zymogens) to the active form.

COAGULATION proceeds through the intrinsic and extrinsic pathways to form factor Xa which then enters the common pathway. The end result of the common pathway is formation of FIBRIN through the action of THROMBIN on FIBRINOGEN. A number of anticoagulant proteins localise coagulation to the site of injury to decrease generalised thrombosis. The two most important anticoagulant groups are the SERPINES and the PROTEIN C system. The serpines comprise ANTITHROMBIN III (AT-III) and HEPARIN COFACTOR II.

FIBRINOLYSIS is activated simultaneously with coagulation and functions to limit the extension of fibrin clots and provide a mechanism for fibrin removal. The physiologically important fibrinolytic protein is PLASMIN. Plasminogen is the circulating zymogen which is activated to plasmin by TISSUE PLASMINOGEN ACTIVATOR (t-PA). ANTIFIBRINOLYTIC PROTEINS, namely PLASMINOGEN ACTIVATOR INHIBITOR and α-ANTIPLASMIN (AP), prevent premature and excessive clot lysis.

(a) Anticoagulants (*In Vivo*)
Primarily used to prevent development and progression of thrombi. Heparin acts directly on the coagulation process and has a quick onset of action. The coumarin derivatives act indirectly as vitamin K antagonists; their effect is delayed by 1–2 hours.

Acetylsalicylic acid (see section on NSAIDs, p. 151)

Dalteparin
POM V

Indication: Low molecular weight heparin.

Actions: Used for prophylaxis of coagulation disorders, especially in colic cases, DIC and for prevention of adhesions

Presentation: Preloaded syringes with 2500, 5000, 7500, 10 000, 12 500, 15 000 or 18 000 IU. Multidose vial with 10 000 or 25 000 IU/mL.

Dose: 50–100 IU/kg subcutaneous q 24 h.

Note:
- Does not produce decreases in PCV (unlike unfractioned heparin).

Heparin sodium
POM V

Actions:

1. Prevents formation of stable fibrin clots. Main coagulation effect is through binding with antithrombin III (endogenous anticoagulant protein) thereby increasing the latter's coagulation inhibitory effect by 2000 times. AT III is the main thrombin inhibitor; therefore, increased activity of AT III results in decreased fibrin formation. Heparin also decreases platelet aggregation, increases levels of plasminogen activator and increases the levels of tissue factor inhibitor.

2. Liberates lipoprotein lipase which decreases serum triglyceride levels (treatment of hyperlipaemia).

Indications: Thromboembolism (prevention of further clot formation); DIC; prevention of *in vitro* or *in vivo* coagulation; maintenance of intravenous catheters; prevention of abdominal adhesions following laparotomy; hyperlipaemia.

Presentation: None licensed for horses in the UK. Formulations are designed for catheter flushing, not therapeutic.

Heparin Na: 1000, 5000, 10 000, 25 000 IU/mL as 1–5 mL multidose vials.

Contraindications: Hepatic disease, haemorrhage.

Dose: Anticoagulation: 25–100 IU/kg q 8–12 h IV/SC (in conjunction with FRESH plasma as a source of AT III).

Peritoneal lavage: 50 IU/kg in electrolyte lavage solution.

Catheter management: 5–12.5 IU/mL.

Notes:
- No effect on clotting factor concentrations. (No innate anticoagulant activity – only potentiates other anticoagulants.) Does not lyse clots!
- Do not use IM – may cause haematomas. SC may be used but may cause painful swelling at the injection site. May be given by constant IV infusion.
- Useful as adjunct for DIC/hyperlipaemia but primary treatment should be aimed at underlying cause. PROTAMINE SULPHATE is specific antagonist.

Protamine sulphate
POM V

Indications: Heparin overdose, conditions of excessive coagulation.

Actions: Anticoagulant when given alone. When given with heparin, stable salt is formed (reducing anticoagulant effects of both). Antagonises effect of heparin sulphate within 5 minutes.

Effect lasts approximately 2 hours.

Presentation: 10 mg/mL injection (5 mL multidose vial).

Dose: 1 mg protamine inactivates 100 IU heparin sulphate.

Max dose 100 mg very slow IV.

Note:
- Beware of anaphylaxis. Incompatible with benzyl and procaine penicillin.

Warfarin
POM V

Indication: Treatment of thrombotic conditions.

Actions: Coumarin derivative. Inhibits the hepatic synthesis of vitamin-K-dependent clotting factors. Onset of action 6–12 hours, maximum at 2–3 days.

Presentation: 1, 3, 5 mg tablets, oral.

Contraindications: Purpura, malnutrition, haemorrhage, late pregnancy.

Dose: 0.018–0.75 mg/kg po q 24 h. Start with lower dose and increase by 20% until first stage prothrombin time has increased by 2–4 seconds.

Notes:
- Well absorbed orally, highly bound to plasma albumin.
- Test FIRST STAGE PROTHROMBIN TIME before instigating programme and monitor regularly.
- Treatment for navicular disease: Mainly superseded by other drugs. Maintain steady 50% increase in PT. Variations (wide) may occur related to dietary intake, work and other medications.
- Do not use with phenylbutazone or other non-steroidal drugs likely to induce ulceration of stomach or intestinal tract – risk of haemorrhage.

(b) Coagulants
Aminocaprioc acid
POM V

Indication: Antifibrinolytic agent, used for treatment of excessive bleeding.

Presentation: Solution for injection (250 mg/mL).

Dose: 20–40 mg/kg, diluted in 1–3 L of saline, given by slow IV infusion.

CRI: 52.5 mg/kg in 15 minutes, then reduce to 0.25 mg/kg/minute.

Note:
- Short action so CRI preferred.

Etamsylate
POM V

Indication: Increases capillary endothelial resistance and promotes platelet adhesion, used for treatment of excessive bleeding.

Presentation: Solution for injection (100 mg/mL).

Dose: 10–15 mg/kg IV.

> **Note:**
> ● Used for EIPH prophylaxis.

Vitamin K_3 (menadione)
POM V

Indication: Anaemia caused by haemorrhagic diathesis, warfarin antagonist.

Action: Vitamin K required for synthesis of blood clotting factors by the liver.

> Not recommended for use in horses as nephrotoxic.

Vitamin K_1 (phytomenadione)
POM V

Indications: Antagonist for warfarin overdose/poisoning, haemorrhage and anaemia caused by haemorrhagic diathesis.

Action: Vitamin K required for synthesis of blood-clotting factors by the liver.

Presentation: 10 mg/mL ampoules (1 mL).

Dose: 0.5–1.0 mg/kg daily in divided doses IM/SC.

> **Note:**
> ● May cause anaphylaxis if given IV. Treatment of warfarin (and other coumarin derivative) toxicity may require concurrent blood transfusion.

(c) Haematinics

Agents that increase the haemoglobin level and the number of erythrocytes. They are used in the treatment of some types of anaemia. Haematinic drugs should be used in conjunction with identification and treatment of the cause of anaemia. Most haematinics are compounds of vitamins and minerals (see Vitamin Preparations, below).

Iron
AVM-GSL

Indications: Iron-deficient conditions only (e.g. chronic GI parasitism, neoplasia).

Actions: Required for haemoglobin synthesis.

Presentations: Many products available for oral use.

Dose: As stated on particular formulation.

Note:
- Intestinal absorption of iron can increase with increased demand; therefore, usually requires chronic disease/dietary deficiency before clinical signs develop. Indiscriminate supplementation should be avoided due to risk of toxicity, especially in foals. Diagnose deficiency using serum iron concentration, total iron binding capacity or bone marrow biopsy. Most products available as part of 'multi-supplements'.

(d) Immunosuppressive Drugs

Azathioprine
POM V

Indications: Immune-mediated disorders. Used as an antifibrotic in some hepatic conditions.

Presentation: 50 mg tablets.

Dose: 3 mg/kg q 24 h po.

Note:
- Very low bioavailability so questionable efficacy.

Gold salts: Aurothioglucose and aurothiomalate
POM V

Indications: Used in cases of pemphigus foliaceus refractory to other immunosuppressive drugs.

Presentation: 50 mg/mL solution for injection.

Dose: 1 mg/kg IM every 3 weeks.

(e) Miscellaneous

Pentoxifylline
POM V

Indications: EIPH, endotoxaemia, acute laminitis, inflammatory conditions, navicular disease.

Actions: Phosphodiesterase inhibitor. Increases the deformity of red blood cells and decreases blood viscosity (rheologic agent). Potentially may decrease pulmonary vascular pressures during exercise. In endotoxaemia, reduces production of lipopolysaccharide-induced cytokines and thromboxanes. Bronchodilating properties.

Inhibits neutrophil recruitment to inflammatory sites. Immunomodulatory effects that potentiate the effectiveness of traditional immunosuppressive drugs.

Dose: 8.5 mg/kg q 12 h po.

Note:
- Most extensive use has been as adjunct to prevention of sequelae of endotoxaemia. Efficacy in EIPH and navicular disease debatable. Further research is required to establish therapeutic potentials. (Use as a rheological agent has been suggested in foetal compromise. Anti-inflammatory properties may be useful in the treatment of heaves. Some refractory immune-mediated conditions may respond to addition of pentoxifylline to the treatment regime, e.g. equine pastern dermatitis.)

(f) Vitamin Preparations

Vitamin B group and vitamin C are water-soluble. Vitamins A, D, E and K are fat-soluble. Vitamin deficiency is uncommon if a good-quality diet is fed. Supplementation may be useful in chronic debilitating diseases (e.g. chronic diarrhoea).

Biotin

No applicable category.

Indication: Foot care supplement.

Signs of deficiency: Anorexia; poor growth; dry, staring dermatitis; ulceration and inflammation of the oral mucous membranes; cracking of the soles and tops of the hooves; soft rubbery soles.

Presentation: Many products available, e.g. cubes containing 7.5 mg biotin per cube for in-feed administration.

Dose: 1–3 cubes daily in feed. Not established.

Note:
- Only the isomer D-biotin contains vitamin activity. Deficiency is uncommon in horses as requirements are usually met by large intestinal organisms. Stress, growth, lactation or chronic disease may increase requirements. Polyuric renal disease may increase urinary excretion. Often mixed with other vitamin/mineral supplementation. Supplementation in horses without biotin deficiency may result in improvement in hoof quality.

Methionine BP

No applicable category.

Indications: Treatment of refractory laminitis and poor hoof quality. Hoof wall defects. Re-establishment of depleted keratin sulphate.

Presentations: Many products available, including compound hoof preparation, oral powder biotin 1 mg, methionine 600 mg, zinc gluconate 67 mg/g.

Dose: 15 g of powder daily.

Note:
- Safe but unreliable/poorly documented benefit. Efficacy may be improved if given in combination with biotin.

Vitamin B₁ (thiamine HCl)
POM V

Indications: Bracken poisoning, thiamine deficiency syndromes caused by thiaminase activity.

Presentation: 100 mg/mL aqueous solution; 50 mL multidose vial.

Dietary sources: Cereal grains and their by-products and oilseed meals relatively rich dietary sources of thiamine. The levels of thiamine are related to the protein content. Thiamine in forage decreases with maturity of the plant. Usually readily digested and absorbed (up to 25% of free thiamine produced in the caecum is absorbed). Gastrointestinal disease may impair enteric flora thiamine synthesis and absorption.

Signs of deficiency: Usually caused by thiaminase in bracken fed in the hay. Lethargy, anorexia, weight loss, ataxia, cardiac arrhythmias, muscle tremors and convulsions.

Dose: 0.25–1.25 mg/kg q 12 h IM or slow IV injection, for up to 7 days.

Note:
- IV injections may result in anaphylactic reactions. Avoid IV use if possible – give very slowly.

Vitamin B₁₂ (cyanocobalamin)
POM V

Indications: Vitamin B₁₂ deficiency conditions, anaemia.

Presentations: Many products available, including B₁₂ injection 1000 μg/mL; 1 mg/mL cyanocobalamin; aqueous red solution; 50 mL multidose vials.

Sources: Solely from bacterial synthesis. Plant materials contain virtually none. Requirements met by large intestinal organisms. Requires adequate dietary cobalt for absorption.

Signs of deficiency: Inappetence, anaemia, dermatitis, rough hair coat, wasting and death.

Dose: Foals 0.5–1 mL; horses 1–3 mL. One to two times weekly, SC or IM injection. 0.5–1.5 mg/kg one to two times weekly.

Note:
- Vitamin B₁₂ deficiency is rare. May occur in chronic gastrointestinal disease due to disruption of normal synthesis by large intestinal bacteria. Anaemia in deficient states is due to inadequate synthesis of nucleic acid precursors for haematopoiesis. Often combined with iron supplements. Commonly administered as metabolic/appetite stimulant (very questionable efficacy!).

Vitamin B complex
POM V

Indications: Stress, toxic or deficiency conditions. Supportive therapy for chronic nutritional deficiency syndromes.

Presentations: Many products available (e.g. aqueous solution of vitamin B_{12}, riboflavine BP, pyridoxine BP, nicotinamide BP, minerals and amino acids for injection).

Dose: Administered once every 48 hours by slow intravenous injection or slow intramuscular injection until a maximum of five doses has been administered. Dose depends on formulation.

Note:
● Preparations containing thiamine may cause anaphylactic shock in some animals. Slow IV (should be diluted with saline). Do not mix with other substances. IM injection may result in large local reactions. Some products containing mixed vitamins do not contain thiamine.

CHECK contents of formulation/product and specific instructions from manufacturer before using any of these products – they vary widely in content and indications!

Vitamin E/selenium
POM V/GSL

Indications: Prophylaxis and treatment of selenium and vitamin E deficiency syndromes including nutritional muscular dystrophy and exertional rhabdomyolysis syndrome (ERS).

Presentations: Many products available and various forms for oral use (e.g. white sterile suspension containing 0.5 mg/mL selenium and 150 mg vitamin E/mL for IM use).

Dietary sources:
Vitamin E: Plants, especially young green plants and cereal grains. Wheat germ oil most concentrated natural source (soybean, peanut and cottonseed oil also rich sources).

Selenium: Plant concentration varies widely with soil content and plant species.

Note:
● Monitor blood levels before and during treatment. May cause marked local reaction. Do not exceed recommended daily amount of selenium as toxicity can develop (RDA = 0.2–0.3 mg/kg diet dry matter). Consider dietary route for maintenance of selenium/vitamin E.

Dose: Vitamin E: 5000–7000 IU/day.

(g) Electrolytes/Fluids

Table 3.10 Parenteral fluids comparison (milli-equivalents/L): sodium chloride solutions

Solution	Na (mEq/L)	Cl (mEq/L)	Osmolality (mOsm/L)	Available as: (L)
0.2%	34	34	69	3 mL
0.45%(½N)	77	77	155	0.25/0.5/1.0
0.9%(N)	154	154	310	0.25/0.5/1.0/5.0
3%	513	513	1030	0.25/0.5/1.0
7%	1197	1197	2394	0.5/1.0

Table 3.11 Parenteral fluids comparison (milli-equivalents/L): dextrose solutions

Solution (%)	Dextrose (g/L)	Calories (kcal/L)	Osmolality (mOsm/L)	Available as: (L)
2.5	25	85	12,669	0.25/0.5/1.0
5	50	170	253	0.25/0.5/1.0
10	100	340	505	0.25/0.5/1.0/5.0
30	300	1020	1515	0.25/0.5/1.0
40	400	1360	2020	0.4/0.5/1.0

Table 3.12 Parenteral fluids comparison (milli-equivalents/L): dextrose/saline combinations

Solution	Na (mEq/L)	Cl (mEq/L)	Dex (g/L)	Calories (kcal/L)	Osmolality (mOsm/L)	Available as: (L)
25%D 0.45%	77	77	25	85	280	0.25/0.5/1.0
5%D 0.11%	19	19	50	170	290	0.5/1.0
5%D 0.2%	34	34	50	170	320	0.5/1.0
5%D 0.45%½ N	77	77	50	170	405	0.5/1.0
5%D 0.9%(N)	154	154	100	170	560	0.25/0.5/1.0/5.0
10%D 0.45%½ 2 N	77	77	100	340	660	0.25/0.5/1.0
10%D 0.9%(N)	154	154	100	340	815	0.25/0.5/1.0

Table 3.13 Parenteral fluids comparison (milli-equivalents/L): electrolyte/dextrose combinations

| Solution | Dextrose (g/L) | Calories (kcal/L) | Electrolytes (mEq/L) | | | | | | | Tonicity | Osmolality (mOsm/L) | Other additives/ presentation (volume of packs in L) |
			Na	K	Ca	Cl	Lact	Acet			
Ringer	–	–	147	4	2	155	–	–	–	308	(0.5/1.0)
Hartman/ Ringer/lact	–	–	131	5	2	111	29	–	Iso	278	Isolec (0.5/1.0)
Darrows	–	–	121	35	–	103	53	–	Iso	312	(1.0)
Duphalyte	5	19	18	3	1	5	–	18	Iso	–	+Vitamins/amino acids (0.5/1.0)
Polyfusin-Bicarb	–	–	1000	–	–	–	–	–	Hyper	2000	100 mM/L bicarbonate (0.2/0.5)
KCl	–	–	2000	–	–	2000	–	–	Hyper	4000	(0.025/0.05)
Na Lact IV Hartman	–	–	133	5	2	111	31	–	Iso	282	3.0/5.0 Isolec/Ivex

Table 3.14 Parenteral fluids comparison (milli-equivalents/L): plasma expanding solutions

| Solution | Dextrose (g/L) | Calories (kcal/L) | Electrolytes (mEq/L) | | | | | | Tonicity | Osmolality (mOsm/L) | Other additives/ presentation (volume of packs in L) |
			Na	K	Ca	Cl	Lact	Acet			
Haemacell	–	–	145	5	6	156	–	–	Iso	312	3.5% Polygeline (0.5)
Gelofusin	–	–	77	–	–	62.5	–	–	Iso	200	3% Succinylated gelatin (0.5)

Pharmaceutical companies in the UK producing fluids for parenteral use
These manufacturers will alter their fluids from time to time and some are
prepared to manufacture solutions specifically for veterinary/equine use. This
usually means larger volumes in packs rather than alteration in the specific fluid
requirements.

1. Animalcare Ltd

   10 Great North Way

   York Business Park

   Nether Poppleton

   York YO26 6RB

   (Tel: 01904-487687; Fax: 01904-487611)

2. Zoetis UK Ltd

   6 St Andrew Street

   London EC4A 3AE

   Tel: 0845 300 8034; Fax: 01737 332521

3. Ivex Pharmaceuticals Ltd

   Old Belfast Rd

   Mill Brook

   Larne

   Co Antrim, Northern Ireland BT40 2SH

   (Tel: 028 2827 3631; Fax: 028 2827 3719)

4. Vet-2-Vet Marketing

   PO Box 98

   Bury St Edmonds, Suffolk IP33 2QN

   (Tel: 01284-767721; Fax: 01284-700047)

5. Fresenius Kabi

   Cestrain Court

   Eastgate Way

   Manor Park

   Runcorn, Cheshire, WA7 1NT

6. B. Braun Medical Ltd

   Thorncliffe Park

   Sheffield, S35 2PW

Equipment for fluid administration

Specialised requirements for fluid administration required for equine practice. It is impractical to administer large volumes of fluid from 0.5 or 1.0 L bags. Indwelling catheters are virtually compulsory when administering more than 1–2 L of fluid (almost always the case). 'Off-the-needle' administration is dangerous, ineffective, inefficient and often counterproductive. Requirements:

1. Gyro fluid hanger (Vet-2-Vet).
2. Fluids in suitable volumes (see above).
3. Stat Large Animal I-V Set (Vet-2-Vet).
4. Transfer sets (×2) (Vet-2-Vet).
5. IV catheter of suitable diameter – consider 2/3 port long-stay catheters if prolonged usage expected.
6. Extension set.
7. Swivel(s) (usually available from local yachting shop).
8. Securing tape and suture materials.

Colloidal IV solutions

Indications: Life-threatening circulatory shock. For rapid blood volume replacement therapy and to increase colloid oncotic pressure in conditions in which this is low (protein losing pathologies). Usually use with crystalloids.

Dextrans

POM *V*

Polysaccharides composed of chains of glucose.

Presentation: 10% and 6% solution in saline.

Notes:

- Antithrombotic effect.
- Uncommon complication of dextran administration in human medicine is acute renal failure.

Starches

POM *V*

Modified polymers of amylopectin.

Indications: As above.

Presentation: Different presentations according to average molecular weight, molar substitution, concentration, etc.

Dose: Hetastarch: up to 10 mL/kg/day IV.

Notes:
- Theoretical risk of increasing bleeding time.
- There are currently discussions regarding its removal from the market due to adverse effects in human medicine.

Parenteral feeding fluids
POM V

Complex area: For a full discussion the reader is directed to: K.G. Magdesian in *Vet Clin Equine* 2003; 19: 617–44.

Indications: Injectable solution of electrolytes, vitamins, amino acids, dextrose. Supportive therapy.

Presentation: Multiple products available.

Dose: Aim initially to provide resting digestible energy (DE_r) requirements.
$$DE_r = BW(kg) \times 0.021 + 0.975 = (Mcal/day).$$

Afterwards, if tolerated, try to increase to DE maintenance.

$$DE_m = BW(kg) \times 0.03 + 1.4 = (Mcal/day).$$

Protein requirements: $40 \times DE$ (g/day).

Notes:
- *Slow* IV only. Not remotely sufficient for daily fluid maintenance requirements or for total parenteral/intravenous nutrition.
- **Supportive treatment only.**

e.g. for 500 kg horse:

$$DE_r = 500 \times 0.021 + 0.975 = 11.5 \, Mcal/day.$$

$$DE_m = 500 \times 0.03 + 1.4 = 16.4 \, Mcal/day.$$

Protein requirements: $40 \times 16.4 = 656 \, g/day$.

INDEX OF DRUGS USED IN EQUINE MEDICINE

Section 9
Vaccines/antisera

African horse sickness vaccine
Indication: Prophylaxis for African horse sickness.

Presentations: Freeze-dried pellet of live virus particles of modified strains (8 strains included – covers 43 recognised antigenic types). Reconstituted with water provided. Single-dose vials 5 mL.

Dose: 5 mL IM VACCINE 1, followed 4 weeks later by:

5 mL IM VACCINE 2.

Annual boosters may be as above but may be combined as single dose.

> **Note:**
> * Poor/unreliable efficacy, REST imperative for entire course. Some severe reactions. Many vaccinated horses show mild forms of the disease when subsequently challenged by virulent strains of the virus.

Botulism antiserum
POM *V*

Indication: Treatment of botulism.

Presentation: Polyvalent A/B/C available.

> **Notes:**
> * Anaphylaxis possible (rare). Dubious efficacy.
> * Expensive in UK and difficult to obtain.

Equine herpes virus vaccine
POM *V*

Indications: Infections with EHV-1 and EHV-4 may cause respiratory disease, abortion, neonatal death and paresis. The respiratory form, known as equine viral rhinopneumonitis, is characterised by fever, coughing and nasal and ocular discharge.

Presentations: Inactivated liquid vaccine. Single-dose vial. For active immunisation of horses to reduce clinical signs due to infection with EHV-1 and -4 and to reduce abortion caused by EHV-1 infection.

Dose:

Respiratory disease: first injection from 5 months of age; second injection 4–6 weeks later and then boosters every 6 months.

Abortion: vaccinate mare in 5th, 7th and 9th months of pregnancy.

> **Note:**
> - Not licensed for prevention of neurologic disease.

Equine viral arteritis vaccine
POM V

Indications: Prophylaxis for equine viral arteritis, a contagious disease of worldwide distribution. Most horses develop subclinical infection, but some may exhibit clinical signs of fever, depression and peripheral oedema. Mares may abort and stallions frequently become long-term carriers. Transmission by the respiratory route occurs during acute infection and by the venereal route through semen from chronically infected stallions.

Presentation: Inactivated virus adjuvanted vaccine in 1 mL vials.

Dose: Two doses at 3–5 week intervals and then boosters for challenged animals at 6-month intervals.

> **Notes:**
> - Antibody produced by either vaccine or natural infection is not distinguishable.
> - Major use is to prevent/control shedding in infected stallions.
> - Vaccinate stallions at least 3 weeks before breeding. Vaccinate maiden mares or while open at least 3 weeks before breeding. Pregnant mares should not be vaccinated.
> - Some countries prohibit the importation of animals seropositive to EVA without veterinary certification of vaccination. Therefore, veterinarians are advised to ensure an animal is seronegative before vaccination; the test is available from the Animal Health Trust, UK.

Consult Code of Practice for Control of Equine Viral Arteritis (British Horseracing Board) – issued annually.

Consult with Ministry or British Equine Veterinary Association in UK if you suspect a case!

Influenza vaccine
POM V

Indication: Prophylactic vaccination for equine influenza.

Presentation: Single-dose vials for injection.

Table 3.15 Antigen inclusion in some commercial influenza vaccines

Name	Prague/ Newmarket (IA/E1)	Brentwood (IA/E2)	Miami (IA/E2)	Suffolk (IA/E2)	Borlange (IA/E2)
Prevac Pro	⊕		⊕	⊕	
Duvaxyn IE-Plus	⊕			⊕	
EquipF	⊕	⊕			⊕

Dose: Single-dose 1 mL vials or preloaded syringes IM.

Two injections 4–6 weeks apart; primary booster 6 months later; then yearly boosters:

FEI COMPETITIONS

First primary	Day 0
Second Primary	21–92 days after first
Booster Primary	Within 6 months and 21 days of second vaccine
Annual Booster	≤365 days

But must have had both primary or a booster within 6 months and 21 days of arrival at FEI competition

JOCKEY CLUB REGULATIONS

First Primary	Day 0
Second Primary	21–92 days after first
Booster Primary	150–215 days from second
Annual Booster	≤365 days

- If overdue (even by 1 day) whole course to start again. Anniversary acceptable.
- No horse whose vaccination was given less than 7 days previously may be presented at a meeting.
- Foals: start around 4–6 months.
- Note antigenic drift makes a particular vaccine less effective in time.
- Combined equine influenza virus and tetanus vaccines may be used for the initial course and every alternate annual booster vaccination.

Rabies vaccine
POM V (Ministry permission)

Indications: Prophylaxis for rabies. Neurotropic disease capable of affecting virtually all mammals.

Presentation: Inactivated virus in single-dose vials.

Dose: 1 mL dose administered IM with annual boosters. Usually vaccinated at 6 months of age or may be vaccinated at 2 months and then again at 6 months.

Note:
- In UK must have specific reason for its use. Ministry permission must be obtained and an authority issued before purchase of vaccine possible. Efficacy excellent in horses.

Rotavirus vaccine
POM V

Indications: Vaccination of pregnant mares to provide passive transfer of antibodies to foals to reduce the risk of diarrhoea caused by equine rotavirus.

Presentation: Inactivated liquid vaccine in single-dose syringes.

Dose: 1 mL dose of the vaccine administered at the 8th, 9th and 10th month of each pregnancy.

Strangles vaccine
POM V

Indications: Prophylaxis for strangles (*Streptococcus equi*) infection.

Presentation: Live modified bacteria.

Dose: 1 mL dose of the live modified bacterium administered into the upper lip mucosa.

Primary vaccination from 4 months of age.

Two to three doses at 4-week intervals.

Boosters every 3 months to maintain immunity or in face of outbreak.

Note:
- Some local reactions are often encountered (localised lumps usually).

Tetanus antiserum
POM V

Indications: Prophylaxis and treatment of tetanus. Animals that have not been vaccinated or whose immune status is doubtful should be given antitoxin prophylactically when exposed to risk of infection (e.g. following injury). If desired, toxoid may be given simultaneously at a separate injection site using a different syringe.

Presentation: Refined concentrated hyperimmune serum produced in horses containing 50 000 IU in 50 mL multidose vials.

Dose: Prophylaxis: 5000–10 000 IU (total) SC single dose lasts 4–5 weeks.

Treatment: 100 IU/kg IV repeated daily.

(± intrathecal injection).

Note:
- Anaphylaxis possible (rare). Use care with asepsis. Do not use pre-opened bottles for intrathecal use.

Tetanus toxoid
POM V

Indications: Prophylaxis for tetanus.

Presentation: Single-dose vials or preloaded syringes 1 mL injection.

Dose: 1 mL dose given deep IM. Initial course: two doses 4–6 weeks apart. Booster given at 6–12 months, then biannually.

Foals can be vaccinated from 5 months of age but may be vaccinated from 6 weeks of age according to expected passive immune status.

Pregnant mares can be vaccinated 4–8 weeks before due date to boost colostral antibody production.

Note:
- Very safe/effective.

Part 3 INDEX OF DRUGS USED IN EQUINE MEDICINE

Section 10
Miscellaneous drugs/medications and other materials

Including:

(a) Local anaesthetics

(b) Eye preparations

(c) Skin preparations

(d) Joint preparations

(e) Antidotes and antitoxins

(f) Suture materials

(g) Cytotoxic and anticancer drugs

(a) Local Anaesthetics
Bupivacaine
POM V

Indications: Local, perineural and regional anaesthesia. Most suited to providing therapeutic rather than diagnostic anaesthesia, particularly postoperatively. In lameness workups, it may also be useful to provide prolonged anaesthesia in one or more regions in order to assess lameness at a distant site, e.g. in another limb.

Presentation: 0.5% solution in single-use ampoules.

Dose: As for 2% lidocaine (lignocaine). Toxic dose 1–4 mg/kg.

> **Note:**
> ● Long duration – up to 6 hours. Slower onset of action.

Lidocaine (lignocaine) HCl
POM V

Indications: Local analgesia, perineural regional anaesthesia, epidural anaesthesia, intravenous regional anaesthesia (IVRA) (Bier's block), control of intraoperative cardiac fibrillation, post-operative ileus (see Intestinal stimulants, p. 137).

Presentations: Aqueous 2% solution for injection. Sterile multidose vials.

Dose: Variable according to site and purpose (see Nerve block sites, p. 379). Epidural anaesthesia: use only 4–7 mL (small space). Toxic dose 4–10 mg/kg.

215

Notes:
- Use only specified forms for epidural use (preservative free). Lasts 30–40 minutes (2× with adrenaline [epinephrine] added).
- Poor penetration through fascial planes so accurate placement important. Very stable solution – can be boiled without effect (NB: adrenaline [epinephrine] labile).
- Check if *adrenaline (epinephrine)* added to preparation. Formulations with adrenaline (epinephrine) may hinder wound healing by vasoconstriction if injected at the site of the injury.

Mepivacaine
POM *V*

Indications: Amide local anaesthetic. Prolonged action. Little irritant/toxic effect in joints or epidural space. Non-irritant in tissues. Causes little overall effect on vascular tone; therefore, no adrenaline (epinephrine) needed to prolong its effect.

Presentation: 2% solution in sterile multidose (10, 20, 50 mL) vials. NB: contains no antimicrobial preservatives; therefore, vial should be discarded following withdrawal of the required dose.

Dose: Epidural: 3–5 mL (20–30 minutes onset).

Regional: 3–20 mL (30 minutes onset).

Intra-articular: 3–30 mL (15 minutes onset).

Note:
- Safe. Avoid IV. Duration approximately 2 hours.

Proxymetacaine HCl
POM *V*

Profile: 0.5% solution for surface analgesia of the eye.

Rapid onset (10 seconds), lasts for 15 minutes.

(See Eye preparations, p. 225).

EM LA cream
POM *V*

Indication: For topical anaesthesia.

Presentations: Lidocaine (lignocaine) 2.5%, prilocaine 2.5%; 5, 30 g.

Dose: Onset of action up to 45 minutes, but some effect after 5 minutes.

Note:
- Eutectic Mixture of Local Anaesthetics. An emulsion of prilocaine and lidocaine (lignocaine) bases, which forms a constant melting point mixture (eutectic mixture), of lower melting point than either of the constituents. Absorbed more rapidly across mucosae and should not be administered by this route.

(b) Eye Preparations

Eye preparations with preservatives may be less safe than those without – some horses will react inordinately to the preservatives and give the impression that the drugs are not effective. If possible, choose preservative-free formulations whenever possible. Ointments generally preferable – prolonged contact and ease of administration.

1. Antimicrobials

Acyclovir
POM *V*

Actions: Antiviral.

Indication: Treatment of viral (herpes) keratitis.

Presentation: White sterile eye ointment (3%) in 4.5 g tube (human preparation).

Dose: Apply 1–2 cm ribbon q 4 h.

> **Notes:**
> - Transient mild discomfort. Disappointing results in treatment of putative herpetiform keratitis.
> - Do not use cutaneous formulation for eyes as it is an irritant.

Chloramphenicol
POM *V*

Actions: Broad-spectrum bacteriostatic antibiotic. Effective against many Gram +ve, Gram –ve and anaerobic infections.

Indications: Use only for chloramphenicol-sensitive infections. Good penetration through intact corneal epithelium, useful in cases of stromal abscess.

Presentations: 1% ointment and 0.5% drops.

Dose: Apply q 6 h (minimal) and continue until 48 hours after recovery.

> **Notes:**
> - USE GLOVES – very slight risk of aplastic anaemia!
> - **Contraindications**: Preparations with hydrocortisone are contraindicated if infection/ulcers.
> - Not for horses for human consumption.

Ciprofloxacin
POM *V*

Action: Broad-spectrum fluoroquinolone antibacterial.

Indications: Bacterial eye infections with sensitivity to ciprofloxacin. Good penetration through intact corneal epithelium, useful in cases of stromal abscess and reservoir effect in stroma.

Presentation: 0.3% drops.

Dose: Apply q 6–8 h.

> **Note:**
> ● Fluoroquinolones should not be used as first-line antibiotic for ocular bacterial infections.

Gentamicin
POM *V*

Action: Broad-spectrum aminoglycoside antibiotic. Best activity against aerobic Gram −ve bacteria and mycoplasma. Also active against *Pseudomonas*, *Proteus*, *Staphylococcus* and *Corynebacterium*.

Indication: Bacterial eye infections with sensitivity to gentamicin.

Presentation: 0.3% drops.

Dose: Apply 10 drops q 6 h pnr.

> **Note:**
> ● Broad spectrum. Frequently used as first-line antibiotic for ocular bacterial infections.

Fusidic acid

Action: Steroidal antibiotic chemically related to cephalosporin. Narrower spectrum compared to other antibacterials.

Indication: Bacterial eye infections.

Presentation: Viscous eye drops, 3 g.

Dose: q 12 h.

Idoxuridine
POM *V*

Actions: Antiviral.

Indication: Specific anti-herpes drug particularly effective in the treatment of putative herpetiform keratitis.

Presentation: 0.1% clear drops or ointment.

> **Note:**
> ● Prolonged or repeated treatment likely to be needed but viral keratitis should respond within a few days. If no response after 2–3 days reconsider diagnosis.

Miconazole
POM *V*

Actions: Antifungal.

Indications: Broad spectrum antifungal, frequently used as first choice in keratomycosis cases.

Presentation: 1% IV preparation.

Note:
- Does not penetrate intact corneal epithelium.

Natamycin
POM *V*

Actions: Antifungal.

Indications: Effective against *Aspergillus* spp. and *Fusarium* spp., but not as effective against yeasts.

Presentation: 5% topical solution.

Note:
- Should be stored in the dark.

Neomycin

Action: Broad-spectrum antibiotic (aminoglycoside). Best activity against aerobic Gram –ve bacteria and mycoplasma.

Indications: Frequently used as combination with bacitracin (Gram +ve and spirochetes) and polymyxin B (Gram –ve). Also used to provide antibiotic cover for corticosteroid preparations.

Presentation: Combination of neomycin–bacitracin–polymyxin. See 'Corticosteroids' for combination preparations containing corticosteroids.

Note:
- Preparations containing corticosteroids contraindicated if infection/ulcers. Check formulation carefully before use.

Ofloxacin (see Ciprofloxacin, p. 217)

Tobramycin
POM *V*

Action: Aminoglycoside antibiotic. Similar to gentamicin but more potent activity against *Pseudomonas*.

Indication: 'Melting ulcer' caused by *Pseudomonas*.

Presentation: 0.3% drops. Presentation also available in combination with dexamethasone.

Dose: Apply every 2–4 hours.

Note:
- Preparations containing corticosteroids contraindicated if infection/ulcers. Check formulation carefully before use.

Voriconazole
POM V

Actions: Antifungal.

Indication: Broad spectrum antifungal.

Presentation: 1% topical solution.

Note:
- Very expensive!

Table 3.16 Rational use of topical antibiotic therapy in ulcerative keratitis

	Likely organisms	Antibiotic	Culture/sensitivity	Further tests
Infectious keratitis	Usually initially Gram +ve. Intensive antibiotic therapy causes rapid involvement of Gram –ve organisms. In severe keratitis hourly therapy may be required	Gentamicin (±chloramphenicol) or neomycin–bacitracin–polymyxin B combination	Swab from margin of ulcer before any topical agents are applied (use AP block and sedation)	Corneal scraping following application of local anaesthetic – direct microscopy
Melting ulcer	Pseudomonas Bacillus (NB: Possible fungi)	Tobramycin and EDTA plasma (anti-collagenase)	As above	As above

2. Mydriatics

These are used for diagnostic and therapeutic purposes where maximal pupillary dilatation is required.

The duration and extent of action of all agents are variable. Tropicamide acts within 10–15 minutes and lasts for 1–2 hours (maximum) while atropine may take longer to work and the mydriasis and cycloplegia may last for days or even longer. **Due to its duration of action, atropine is contraindicated as a diagnostic mydriatic.** Remember that a horse with dilated pupils is likely to be photophobic and suffer pain in bright light:

- Cholinergic antagonists block muscarinic receptors on sphincter muscle of the iris and ciliary muscles causing paralysis.
- Adrenergic agonists stimulate contraction of radial muscles of the iris (minimal effect on ciliary muscle).

Adrenaline (epinephrine) BP 1%
POM *V*

Action: Adrenergic agonist. Clear 1% stable solution as drops.

Indication: Miosis refractory to atropine treatment.

Dose: 2–4 drops q 6 h.

> **Notes:**
> - Mydriasis more rapid than atropine and reversed with physostigmine.
> - Keep patient out of direct sunlight (preferably in darkened box).
> - Useful to reduce intra-ocular pressure.
> - Strong mydriatic effect.
> - Initial discomfort following application.

Atropine sulphate BP
POM *V*

Action: Cholinergic antagonist.

Indications: Uveitis and other painful conditions of the eye producing miosis.

Presentations:

Human preparation: 1% drops, 0.5 mL, single use.

Atropine eye ointment (non-proprietary) 1% 3 g.

Other human preparations available as multidose bottles.

Side effects: Ileus may develop with prolonged use.

> **Notes:**
> - Administer frequently until effect is present and then use very sparingly to maintain mydriasis (often every second day is enough). Prolonged mydriasis (5–7 days) may follow single dose.

- Keep patient out of direct sunlight (preferably in darkened box) when mydriatic effects are present.
- Do NOT use atropine as an ophthalmic diagnostic agent – effects may be prolonged and severe mydriasis and cycloplegia can be present for days!

Phenylephrine
POM V

Action: Adrenoceptor agonist.

Indication: Uveitis/pain/glaucoma, etc. Aid to diagnosis of grass sickness.

Dose: Apply 2–4 drops q 4–6 h.

Notes:
- Marked but short-acting mydriatic. Rebound miosis/irritation/corneal oedema. Keep patient out of direct sunlight (preferably in darkened box).
- Useful aid to diagnosis of grass sickness. The disease is characterised by mild/moderate ptosis and this is reversed if phenylephrine is instilled into the conjunctiva.[2]

Notes:
- Phenylephrine eye drops can be used as an aid to diagnosis of grass sickness. The method is a useful one but it is possibly difficult to interpret. Therefore, the method must be followed precisely.

  (i)   Do not sedate the horse with acepromazine or an α_2 agonist for at least 6 hours prior to the test.

  (ii) Assess the patient's eyelash angles in a frontal plane in both eyes (angle with respect to the horizontal, which is the normal position of a resting normal eyelid).

  (iii) Dilute 10% phenylephrine to 0.5% solution with sterile saline (NOT water).

  (iv) Apply 0.5 mL to the conjunctival sac of one eye only.

  (v)   Reassess the eyelash angle in the same way as previously after 30 minutes.

- Interpretation:

  Positive result (i.e. the horse probably has grass sickness) is shown by a reduction in the degree of ptosis (i.e. a widening of the palpebral fissure). The eyelashes on the treated eye will be in a more elevated (normal) position when compared to the untreated eye.

---

[2]Hahn CN, Mayhew IG (2000). Phenylephrine eye drops as a diagnostic test in equine grass sickness. *Veterinary Record* 147 (21): 603–606.

Tropicamide
POM V

Action: Synthetic anticholinergic.

Indication: Mydriatic of choice for diagnostic procedures.

> **Note:**
> - Onset in 10–15 minutes and lasts <2 hours (usually).

Presentation: 0.5%, 1% solution as drops.

Dose: 2–5 drops q 1 h pnr.

3. Glaucoma medications

These decrease intra-ocular pressure (IOP) by reducing aqueous humour production. Some can be absorbed via the nasolacrimal duct into the circulation and induce systemic effects. The effects of these drugs are poorly defined in horses and are, in any case, seldom required except in a referral situation.

Dorzolamide
POM V

Indications: Reduction of IOP.

Actions: Carbonic anhydrase inhibitor, reduces aqueous humour production.

Presentation: 2% drops in aqueous solution.

Dose: Apply 1–5 drops pnr.

> **Note:**
> - Commercial formulation available in combination with Timolol (2% Dorzolamide+0.5% Timolol).

Timolol maleate
POM V

Indication: Reduction of IOP.

Contraindications: Use care in patients with pre-existing cardiovascular, respiratory or metabolic disease. Hypotensive effects are additive with parasympathomimetics and carbonic anhydrase inhibitors.

Presentation: 0.5% drops in aqueous solution.

Dose: Apply 1–5 drops pnr.

> **Note:**
> - Commercial formulation available in combination with Timolol (2% Dorzolamide+0.5% Timolol).

4. Topical anaesthetics

Local anaesthesia of the cornea and conjunctiva can be easily achieved with topical drops. The effects begin within minutes and last 5–10 minutes (depending on the extent of tear dilution/flushing), seldom longer, so prolonged procedures may need repeated doses.

Amethocaine (tetracaine) is faster acting and more powerful than most others. The anaesthetic effects are useful for investigation, procedures, foreign body retrieval and as an adjunct to sedation/general anaesthesia for more detailed procedures.

Lidocaine (lignocaine) hydrochloride (2%) is acidic and should not be used in the eye if any alternative can be found. Formulations with adrenaline (epinephrine) are contraindicated at all times.

Amethocaine (tetracaine)
POM V

Presentation: 0.5% drops.

Dose: Apply 1–5 drops pnr.

> **Note:**
> - Initial discomfort. Effect lasts 5–10 minutes. Protect eye from dust and trauma.

Proxymetacaine HCL/proparacaine
POM V

Dose: 0.5% solution for surface analgesia of the eye. Apply as necessary.

> **Notes:**
> - Rapid onset (10 seconds) lasts for 15 minutes. Commonest surface analgesic for the eye.
> - Solutions inclined to weaken if not stored correctly – keep cool and preferably refrigerated until a minute or two before use.

5. Steroids

Corticosteroid applications to the eye surface carry significant risks when ulceration is present. **They are, therefore, contraindicated in all cases of corneal ulceration (no matter how small/insignificant they might appear to be).** As soon as ulceration is demonstrably absent, corticosteroids may be applied in an attempt to reduce the extent of fibroplasia and leukoma formation. Lesions in the visual axis should probably be treated as early as possible to limit the effects on vision while those away from the axis can be left for longer before steroid administration.

Ocular bioavailability of topical glucocorticoid formulations varies significantly. Lipid-soluble alcohol and ester preparations penetrate the anterior chamber rapidly. Water-soluble preparations have poor penetration of the intact cornea and are more useful for corneal/conjunctival inflammation than uveitis. Ocular inflammation may increase the penetrating ability of all preparations. Potency of corticosteroids can be scored as: hydrocortisone 1, prednisolone 5, β-methasone 25, dexamethasone 25 and flumethasone (flumetasone) 30 (30 is greatest potency). The actual clinical effect will depend upon concentration, formulation and frequency of application.

Frequency of application varies with severity and nature of problem. Hourly medication may be required in the initial stages of acute anterior uveitis whereas chronic superficial keratitis may be treated on alternate days for prolonged periods.

Notes:
- Repeated detailed examination is essential for any eye case receiving prolonged corticosteroid medication.
- There is a tendency for horses on prolonged corticosteroids and antibiotics to develop serious corneal fungal infections.

Dexamethasone
Action: Anti-inflammatory.

Indications: Treatment and control of corneal/conjunctival inflammation. Anterior uveitis. Immune-mediated keratopathy.

Dose: Sterile 0.1% solution as drops or ointment (+neomycin+polymyxin B and hypromellose).

Apply 2–4 drops q 4 h pnr.

Contraindications: Infection/ulcers.

Note:
- Good penetration when formulated as a suspension with efficacy similar to 1% prednisolone acetate.

Prednisolone
POM V

Action: Anti-inflammatory.

Indications: Treatment and control of corneal/conjunctival inflammation. Uveitis. Immune-mediated keratopathy.

Contraindications: Infection/ulcers.

Dose: 1% prednisolone acetate solution. Apply as necessary.

Note:
- Potent anti-inflammatory. Probably the best topical steroid for ophthalmic use. Prednisolone acetate is lipid soluble and gives good penetration. 1% prednisolone acetate solution drug of choice in uveitis. Use with antibiotic preparation. Prednisolone sodium phosphate less penetration than acetate.

6. Non-steroidal anti-inflammatory drugs

The pharmacokinetics and bioavailability of ocular NSAIDs are unknown in the horse. Generally, they are presumed to reach higher local therapeutic levels than oral or parenteral drugs.

Subconjunctival injection of parenteral formulations is not recommended as they are potentially very irritating. Efficacy of topical NSAIDs is significantly less than glucocorticoids. Drug of choice if ocular infection is a concern. Use care if ulcerative keratitis is present as they can delay corneal healing.

Comparisons of the efficacy of the different topical NSAIDs have not been made in the horse. Optimal therapeutic protocols are not established. Dosing will depend on severity of the condition and clinical response. Acute uveitis may require hourly dosing initially. Often combined with systemic NSAIDs therapy for maximum effect.

Diclofenac
POM V

Indications: Anterior uveitis, equine recurrent uveitis, traumatic and non-ulcerative keratitis and keratouveitis.

Presentation: 0.1% eye drops.

Dose: Apply q 12 h pnr.

Notes:
- Useful non-steroidal drug that inhibits miosis and provides topical anti-inflammatory effects.
- Used when corticosteroids are contraindicated.
- Relatively expensive.

Flurbiprofen
POM V

Indications: Anterior uveitis, equine recurrent uveitis, traumatic and non-ulcerative keratides and keratouveitis.

Presentation: 0.03% drops.

Dose: Apply q 12 h pnr.

Notes:
- Useful non-steroidal drug, which inhibits miosis and provides topical anti-inflammatory effects.
- Used when corticosteroids are contraindicated. Relatively expensive.

7. Artificial tears/lubricating solutions

Tears are a complex physiological solution – not just saline! Ocular lubricants are designed to correct unstable or deficient precorneal tear film in which the aqueous, mucoid or lipid components may be deficient. *Carbomers (polyacrylic acid), polyvinyl alcohol, polyethylene glycol* and *dextran* can assist the tear film to spread more evenly over the eye when mucus production is either deficient or unevenly distributed over the corneal epithelium. *Saline* drops will inhibit lipid secretion by the meibomian glands.

Care should be taken to avoid contamination of bottles. Discard partially used open bottles.

Hypromellose USP

Indications: Lubrication for eye where xerophthalmia or keratoconjunctivitis sicca present.

Presentations: Eye drops 0.3%.

Dose: As required. Apply frequently (q 2–3 h minimum) pnr.

> **Note:**
> - Often used to dilute complex medication collyrium for topical treatment.

Liquid paraffin
POM V

Indications: Used as required to provide lubrication when keratoconjunctivitis sicca (dry-eye) conditions are present (i.e. tear deficiency). Often used to protect eyes during anaesthesia.

Presentation: Preservative-free ointment in 5 g tube.

Dose: Apply as necessary.

Polyacrylic acid (carbomer)
POM V

Indications: Very effective eye lubrication when dry-eye or unstable tear film conditions are present.

Presentation: Sterile, colourless liquid gel containing 2.0 mg/g carbomer 940. 10 g tube.

Dose: Apply 2–4 drops q 8 h.

> **Note:**
> - Probably the best eye lubricant/artificial tear solution. Mild initial transient irritation may occur.

Polyvinyl alcohol

Indications: Used as required to provide lubrication when keratoconjunctivitis sicca (dry-eye) conditions are present (i.e. tear deficiency).

Dose: Apply 8–10 times a day.

8. Anti-collagenases

Corneal ulcers can be complicated by corneal stromal melting or keratomalacia which occurs as a result of imbalances between naturally occurring proteinases and their inhibitors. These proteinases are produced by corneal epithelial cells, fibroblasts, inflammatory cells and microorganisms and can result in the destruction of the corneal stroma in a very short period of time. Aggressive therapy is essential to prevent this corneal melting.

Acetylcysteine
POM V

Indications: Potent/specific anti-collagenase. Specific mucolytic and lubricant properties. Used for control and treatment of melting ulcers. Tear deficiency.

Dose: 5% acetylcysteine w/v in hypromellose base 2–6 drops q 2 h for melting ulcers, q 6 h for dry-eye syndromes.

EDTA
Not classified

Indications: Anti-collagenase. Control and treatment of melting ulcers.

Dose: Add 5 mL sterile saline to 10 mL EDTA Vacutainer (BD Ltd) (ideally 2% solution of EDTA). Apply as drops q 2 h.

> **Note:**
> ● Alternatives – Solution of acetylcysteine, serum, tetracyclines.

9. Miscellaneous drugs

Cyclosporin (ciclosporin) A
POM V

Indications: Licensed for use in treatment of keratoconjunctivitis sicca in dogs. Known to have similar effect on tear production in horses. Used in the treatment of immune-mediated keratopathies.

Presentation: 2% ointment.

Dose: 4–6 drops every 6 hours.

> **Note:**
> ● It does not penetrate intact corneal epithelium; no effect in cases of uveitis when applied topically.

Hyperosmotic saline ointment
POM *V*

Indications: Used symptomatically to reduce corneal oedema to allow effective examination of the anterior chamber. Reduces secretions of lipid by meibomian glands.

Dose: 5% saline ointment applied q 8–12 h.

10. Ophthalmic stains

Fluorescein
POM V

Indications: Diagnostic solution for detection of corneal ulceration and patency of nasolacrimal duct (may take 5–15 minutes to pass down duct).

Dose: Single-use sterile drops (1%, 2%) or impregnated paper strips (1 mg).

Notes:

- Conjunctival abrasions stain faint green, corneal ulcers stain bright green. Avoid bacterial contamination. May be irritant (consider use of topical anaesthetic).
- Seidel's test: used to detect aqueous humour leakage.
- Tear film break up time: time required for a dry spot to appear on the surface of the fluorescein (normally 10–12 seconds).

Rose Bengal BP
POM V

Indications: Diagnostic solution for detection of necrotic tissue (devitalised epithelium) and abnormal precorneal tear film. Also used for detection of neoplastic areas (squamous cell carcinoma) on the ocular surface.

Dose: Single-use sterile drops (1%) in single-dose dropper sachets or impregnated paper strips.

Note:

- Somewhat irritating.

(c) Skin Preparations
1. Disinfectants and antiseptics

Definitions:

- *Antiseptic*: A preparation that inhibits the growth of microorganisms and that is suitable for application to wounds or broken skin without significant harmful effects.
- *Disinfectant*: A preparation that inhibits the growth of microorganisms and that is not suitable for the application to wounds or broken skin because it is too strong or is otherwise harmful to the health of the tissue.
- *Germicide*: Preparation that kills microorganisms outright. This is a largely discredited name.

Note:

- Modern wound management/tissue viability studies suggest that almost all chemicals applied to wounds have some harmful effects. Acceptable antiseptics have minimal harmful effects in the concentrations that are used clinically. Often higher concentrations will have a dramatic and significantly increased harmful effect even up to the point of causing tissue necrosis.

Chlorhexidine

GSL

Indications:

- Topical antiseptic.
- Disinfection of wounds, burns, surgical scrub.
- Adjunct to treatment of ringworm (with enilconazole).
- Variable activity against viruses and fungi.

Presentations: Pink lathering solution (5%) or pink alcoholic solution (5%).

Use: On broken skin use a 1:100 dilution of the solution (do not use the alcoholic solution).

Effective navel dip solution (0.5%) chlorhexidine solution can be made up by diluting with sterile water. This solution has a residual effect for up to 3 hours and should therefore be repeated at 3–4-hour intervals over the first 24 hours.

Notes:

- **DO NOT mix with other antiseptics/disinfectants.**
- Rapid onset of action and some residual effect (for up to 2 hours) by binding to cell surfaces.
- Can be advantageous in preparation of elective surgical sites under bandages (e.g. foot and skin preparation).

Povidone iodine

GSL

Indications:

- Broad-spectrum antibacterial effect with some antifungal, antiprotozoal and antiviral effects.
- For application on wounds, wound ointment, endometritis, surgical preparation, obstetric manipulation and routine skin care.
- The antiseptic solutions are commonly used for navel dipping in neonatal foals (see below under Notes).
- The scrub should be used on heavily contaminated sites before the solution.
- The antibacterial effect is reduced by contact with pus and exudates and there is no significant residual effect. Therefore, regular reapplication may be necessary depending upon the degree of wound exudation.

Presentations: Antiseptic solution – non-lathering (1% available iodine); surgical scrub – lathering solution (0.75% available iodine); antiseptic ointment for wound application.

Use: Surgical scrubs (soap-based solutions) are widely used.

For wound management the dilution needs to be high – the solution used for irrigating wounds should not appear any stronger than a very weak tea.

Notes:

Navel dips require strong solutions to be effective and these can cause desiccation and necrosis of the navel remnant. In general, this use is to be avoided. Not only does it not protect the umbilical remnants from infection (there is no residual effect) but it can cause damage.

- **DO NOT mix with other antiseptics, soap or detergents; doing so reduces the available iodine.**
- Rapidly deactivated by organic contact. Colour fades when action lost.
- Therapeutic effect on open wounds has been supported by some reviews but questioned by others because of delayed wound healing.
- Iodine toxicity has been reported – the use of this agent should be avoided on very large wounds.

CAUTION:

(i) The action of iodine solutions relies upon a dilution, strong solutions are less effective than weak ones!

(ii) Under no circumstances should the 7% iodine solutions be used on the navel of neonatal foals. It will cause serious necrosis.

(iii) Under no circumstances should iodine solutions be used to flush/irrigate the guttural pouches. Serious and permanent nerve damage can occur.

NB: Alcohol dries skin cells and delays wound healing. Alcohol-based preparations should be restricted to prophylactic skin disinfection before needle insertions or surgical procedures.

2. Astringents

Malic acid

Indications: Debriding and cleansing agent for skin wounds, particularly when necrotic tissue is present (encourages sloughing). The agent is mildly antibacterial. It discourages granulation tissue formation and so should only be used in the debridement phase of wound healing.

Good action against *Pseudomonas* organisms.

Presentations: Solution 2.25% 100/350 mL plastic squeeze bottles. Cream 30 and 100 g tubes.

Dose: Use as necessary.

Notes:

- Avoid eye contact.
- Do not mix with other agents.
- Should not be used for cleansing fresh wounds (too acidic).
- The compounds should be used carefully after balancing the significant disadvantages with the perceived advantages. In some cases, wound infection must be controlled quickly regardless of the potential harmful effects on tissues.

3. Antibacterials

As a general rule, antibiotics should not be applied topically but given systemically. There are two main hazards associated with their use – resistance and sensitivity/untoward reactions. Controlled use of topical antibiotics will eliminate some of the problems caused by plasmid transfer and induction of antibiotic resistance by inappropriate use; this will reduce sensitivity reactions, which cause considerable harm and delay healing.

Silver sulphadiazine (sulfadiazine)
POM V

Indications:

- Silver metal or its salts have significant bacteriostatic and bactericidal, as well as some antifungal, properties.
- Broad-spectrum antibacterial function when applied topically.
- Used to treat a variety of wounds where infection may prevent wound healing.
- Significant beneficial effect on *Dermatophilus congolensis*.
- Very helpful in burn wound management.

Presentation: A hydrophilic cream containing 1% silver suphadiazine (sulfadiazine).

> **Note:**
> - To be used under a non-adherent dressing or directly on open sites.

Honey
Indications: Antibacterial action is due mainly to hydrogen peroxide which is liberated by enzyme reaction. Some types of honey may also contain other natural antibacterial substances. Bacterial growth will not be supported because of the high osmotic pressure of the honey. Its efficacy is diluted with increasing exudation due to the reduction in the osmotic pressure but the other antimicrobial components in honey will ensure that inhibition is maintained. Good (documented effects) against *Pseudomonas* spp. It is non-irritant and has a low pH.

Presentations: (i) Gel form, antibacterial honey 50 g; (ii) Dressings with impregnated honey are the most convenient method of applying honey to wounds.

> **Notes:**
> - Not all honeys are effective – the right formulation is necessary. If the gel form is used, then the treated area should be covered with a dressing. If the wound is only mildly exudative, then a waterproof dressing may help to maintain the honey at the wound site rather than leaking out.
> - Honey is not appropriate for acute wounds and can actually be harmful to healing if used inappropriately. It is not a universal panacea for wound management.

4. Poultices

Complete poultice dressing
GSL

Indications: Poulticing of infected/inflamed foci in feet and skin. Encourages pus drainage through tissue softening/maceration and osmotic gradient.

Presentation: Single pieces of impregnated bandage with plastic backing sheet.

Use: Change every 24 hours.

> **Notes:**
> - Useful for softening hoof to permit easier paring and debriding. May encourage draining of infected or inflamed sinus tracts.
> - The dressing is not a primary wound dressing and is too acidic for healthy tissues. Application to skin injuries should be used with clinical judgement only.
> - Cover with a bandage to keep the poultice in place.

Kaolin (heavy)
GSL

Indications: Poulticing skin and foot infections.

Presentation: Paste for topical application.

Use: Change as required.

> **Note:**
> - Messy and smelly! Little to commend it!

5. Wound dressings

The ideal wound dressing should:

- maintain a moist environment at the wound interface
- remove excess exudates without allowing 'strike through' to the surface of the dressing
- provide thermal insulation and mechanical protection
- act as a barrier to microorganisms (both directions)
- allow gaseous exchange
- be non-adherent and easily removed without trauma to the wound or the surrounding skin
- leave no foreign particles in the wound
- be non-toxic, non-allergenic, non-sensitising
- be compatible with and support delivery of medications
- be conformable and mouldable to the anatomical outline of the region.

Note:
- No single dressing is appropriate for all wound types and all stages of wound healing.

Hydrogel

Indications: A hydrogel with a high available water content that creates and maintains a moist wound environment at the wound site. Hydrogels debride the wound by hydration and promotion of autolysis.

- They are used on fresh wounds as a protective layer that helps to control infection and prevent further contamination, desiccation and tissue shrinkage.
- It has a useful debriding effect on dry and sloughy wounds.
- It is not appropriate for heavily exudating wounds but can be used for lightly exudative wounds, necrotic or sloughing wounds as well as for protecting granulating wounds.
- It is suitable for many stages of wound healing and even in dry wounds acts as a net donator of moisture.
- Hydrogels can be used where aerobic and anaerobic infection is present and where the patient is receiving systemic antibiotics.

Presentations: (i) Gel form; (ii) non-woven, non-felting dressing impregnated with hydrogel.

Notes:
- Apply to the wound surface, needs to be covered with a sterile dressing.
  - Adhesion to wound surfaces is poor with some particular commercial forms so it is best to apply it to the primary dressing before this is applied to the wound surface. Some forms have a better adhesion but are less effective moisture donators.

Non/low-adherent primary wound dressings (variable absorbency)

Melolin
Indications: For use on non-exudative or very mildly exudative wounds.

This dressing will not absorb excessive exudation, which will cause maceration and so is applicable to non-exudative wounds.

Presentations: (i) Melolin; (ii) melolin on an adhesive dressing retention sheet.

Note:
- Apply to the wound surface as a primary dressing and retain in position with a secondary dressing. Cover with a bandage.

Vapour-permeable dressings
Indications: Hydrophilic polyurethane film that is vapour permeable. Can be used for mild or moderately exudating wounds. There are various forms available.

Presentations:
(i) Vapour-permeable adhesive film dressing with an absorbent pad.
(ii) Film combined with a low-adherent pad. A waterproof, bacteria-proof adhesive dressing.
(iii) The spray forms a transparent and quick drying film which is permeable to moisture vapour and air. The film can be peeled off when completely dry or left to slough off naturally. Can be used on minor wounds or over sutured wounds.

Note:
● Apply to the wound surface and cover with a bandage.

Polyurethane foam

Indications: A hydrophilic absorbent polyurethane dressing. To be used on light to moderately exudative wounds.

Presentations: Comes in various forms. Cavity form is highly absorbent and conformable and can be used for deep wounds.

Note:
● Apply to the wound surface and cover with a bandage.

Calcium/sodium alginate

Indications: Calcium and sodium salts of alginic acid are obtained from seaweed. It is biodegradable and highly absorbent due to a strong hydrophilic gel formation that occurs on contact with wound secretions. Highly absorbent – useful in medium to heavily exudating wounds. Some dressings have haemostatic properties (calcium sodium alginate). Alginates have a significant effect in promoting granulation tissue and so are particularly useful where granulation tissue cover is slow to develop (e.g. exposed periosteum/bone) or inhibited such as in indolent wounds.

Some are combined with silver salts or nanocrystaline silver to impart an antimicrobial effect.

Presentations: (i) Calcium alginate; (ii) calcium sodium alginate.

Note:
● Apply to the wound surface and cover with a bandage. May need saline irrigation for dressing removal. Not suitable for dry wounds or wounds that are covered with hard necrotic tissue because of the marked hydrophilic properties.

Deodorising carbon dressings

Indications: Used in the management of discharging, purulent and contaminated wounds complicated by bacterial infection and offensive odour. The charcoal fibres become microporous and develop thin, slit-like pores. This substantially increases the surface area, making charcoal-based dressings highly absorbent.

Some dressings also absorb bacteria (electrostatic or physiochemical attractions). Some are combined with silver salts or nanocrystaline silver to impart an antimicrobial effect.

Note:
- Apply to the wound surface and cover with a bandage. Do not cut to size.

Silver-coated dressing
Indications: Silver metal or its salts have significant antibacterial properties. Absorbent dressing containing nanocrystalline silver (antibacterial) is widely available. Used for mildly exudative wounds. Silver-impregnated dressings are effective means of controlling even some difficult wound infections including *S. aureus*, MRSA and *Pseudomonas aeruginosa*.

Note:
- Apply to the wound surface and cover with a bandage. Dressings should not be changed too frequently. The change interval will be dictated by the extent of exudates and other factors. These dressings often retain their effects for up to 7 days. They should not, however, be reapplied to a wound after removal.

Wet-to-dry dressings
Indications: Used for sloughing, necrotic wound. Used where mechanical debridement is necessary. The indications for this approach are few.

Presentation: Saline-soaked gauze swabs (can be soaked in a dilute solution of crystalline penicillin).

Note:
- Place onto the wound and cover with a bandage. Do NOT use where mechanical debridement is not directly indicated. These dressings cause significant damage and the disadvantages outweigh the advantages in most circumstances. Usually, there are much better ways of performing the debridement in modern wound management – these dressings are probably best regarded as contraindicated except in particular circumstances. Combination of this dressing method with hypochlorite solutions (e.g. EUSOL) are specifically contraindicated in equine wound management.

Absorbent dressings
These should only be used over a dressing and should NOT be placed directly onto a wound.

Absorbent cotton
Indications: Absorbent dressing.
Presentation: Rolls or balls.

> **Note:**
> - Do not place directly over a wound. They can be used as dressings to provide padding or protection.

Gamgee
Indications: Pad of cotton wool enclosed in cotton gauze. Soft and absorbent, allows strike through.

Presentation: Rolls.

> **Note:**
> - Do not place directly onto a wound. Gamgee should not be used as padding in dressings as it is difficult to apply without kinks and folds, increasing the risk of bandage sores.

Nappy
Indications: Used for highly exudative wounds.

Presentation: Commercially available.

> **Note:**
> - Do not place directly onto a wound. Dressings on highly exudative wounds should be changed frequently.

Table 3.17 Rational dressing selection for uncomplicated skin wounds

Wound dressing	Dry non-discharging (surgical) wound	Dry non-exudative (healthy) wound	Epithelialising (healthy) wound	Granulating (healthy) wound	Mildly exudative wound	Moderately exudative wound	Severely exudative wound	Haemorrhagic wound	Cavity wounds	Infected/purulent exudative wound	Necrotic wound
Hydrogel	✓	✓	✓	✓	✓				✓	✓	✓
Melolin	✓	✓	✓	✓	✓						
Vapour permeable	✓	✓	✓		✓	✓					
Allevyn			✓	✓	✓	✓	✓ (Cavity)		✓ (Cavity)	✓	
Calcium alginate			✓	✓	✓	✓	✓	✓	✓	✓	✓
Carbon-based dressing						✓	✓	✓	✓	✓	✓
Silver-based dressing					✓					✓	
Honey dressing						✓	✓		✓	✓	✓
Wet-to-dry dressing											✓
Comments									Provide drainage where possible	Surgical debridement may be necessary	Surgical debridement may be necessary

6. Casting materials

Orthopaedic felt

Indication: A soft, adhesive sponge to be placed underneath the cast to protect against pressure sores.

Presentation: Sheets of felt that can be easily cut to size.

> **Note:**
> - A strip to be placed at the top of a cast. It should also be placed around the accessory carpal bone, tuber calcis and on the cranial aspect of the hock in full-limb casts.

Custom support foam

Indication: Conforming padding for application under casts or bandages.

Presentation: Impregnated bandages in dehydrated foil wrap (various sizes).

> **Note:**
> - Apply over double layer of stockinet after immersing roll in tepid water for a few seconds (one immersion/squeeze). Bandage around limb using 50% overlap technique. Apply casting material immediately. Cures rapidly, close anatomical fit, good porosity, radiolucent, energy absorbent, rapid drying. Makes cast removal less complicated/dangerous.

Plaster of Paris (calcium sulphate)

Indications: Immobilisation of fractures, granulating wounds, etc.

Presentation: Impregnated bandages in dehydrated foil wrap (various sizes).

> **Notes:**
> - Easy to apply and use – conforms well to limb and cheap. However, it is messy and heavy with a low strength-to-weight ratio. Does not achieve maximum strength until 24 hours after application. Liable to break. Softens on contact with moisture, protective waterproofing is available as emulsion applied after drying.
> - Not recommended.

Thermoplastic casting material

Indications: A linear polyester polymer used for immobilisation of fractures, granulating wounds, etc.

Presentation: Plastic-wrapped plastic mesh bandage.

Note:
- Made mouldable by heating in boiling water for 5–10 minutes. Becomes mildly adhesive and conforming. Sets as placed as it cools. Poor conformation on limb. Best reserved for making 'slabs' and for additional application to foot over synthetic polyacrylic casts.

Synthetic polyacrylic casting material
1. Fibreglass tape impregnated with polyurethane resin

Indications: Immobilisation of fractures, granulating wounds, etc. (see Casting, p. 329).

Presentation: Individual bandages soaked in water immediately prior to use. Different sizes available.

Notes:
- Use proprietary orthopaedic sponge around the top of the cast. The felt should also be used with appropriate cut-out portions over pressure points in full-limb casts (see p. 323).
- A useful tip is to include a moderate layer of toilet tissue over the stockinet/bandage layer so as to facilitate cast removal.

2. Polypropylene mesh impregnated with polyurethane resin

Indications: Immobilisation of fractures, dislocations and granulating wounds, etc. (see Casting, p. 329).

Presentations: Individual bandages soaked in water immediately prior to use. Different sizes available.

Notes:
- Use proprietary orthopaedic felt around the top of the cast. The felt should also be used with appropriate cut-out portions over pressure points in full-limb casts (see p. 329).
- Wear gloves as compound is very sticky and persistent!
- New formulation suitable for making casting slabs (splints) – effective for slab construction (particularly useful for foals with flexural deformities, etc.). Material sprayed with water to dampen and then layered on to conform around the limb sets very hard and allows slab construction.
- A useful tip is to include a moderate layer of toilet tissue over the stockinet/bandage layer so as to facilitate cast removal.

(d) Joint Preparations

Polysulphated glycosaminoglycan (PSGAG)
POM V

Indications: Anti-inflammatory, inhibits degradative proteolytic enzymes, stimulates hyaluronic acid production, stimulates proteoglycan production. Treatment of lameness due to degenerative (aseptic/closed) joint disease. Generally used for mild, chronic joint disease.

Presentations: Intra-articular injection – 250 mg/mL in 1 mL single-dose ampoule. Intramuscular injection – 100 mg/mL in 5 mL single-dose ampoule.

Dose: 250 mg intra-articular injection once weekly for 5 weeks.

500 mg intramuscular injection every 4 days for seven doses.

> **Note:**
> ● Ensure asepsis. DO NOT inject into infected joints or non-infected joints with significant soft tissue inflammation. DO NOT use if renal or hepatic disease. Transient swelling. Discontinue if reaction.

Sodium hyaluronate
POM V

Indications: Anti-inflammatory, protective against cartilage degradation and decreases inflammatory cell migration. Treatment of lameness due to degenerative (aseptic/closed) joint disease. Generally used for acute synovitis.

Presentations:
● Intra-articular – 10 mg/mL in 2 mL single-dose vials.
● Intra-articular – 10 mg/mL in 2 mL preloaded syringes.
● Intra-articular – 50 mg/3 mL preloaded syringe: high molecular sodium hyonate.

Dose: Intra-articular (20 mg small joints/50 mg large joints). Repeat doses at 7–10-day intervals for three to four treatments.

Intravenous 40 mg – single injection.

> **Notes:**
> ● Intra-articular route – ensure aseptic injection. Transient swelling may be produced. No more than two joints to be treated at any one time. Horse should receive 3 days' stable rest and then controlled exercise for 7–10 days after injection. Intravenous route – some reviews support the systemic route of administration, others dispute it.
> ● Useful (but expensive) as anterior chamber dilating agent in eye surgery.

Methylprednisolone acetate
POM V

Indications: Anti-inflammatory, inhibits the production of cartilage matrix. High doses have been associated with articular cartilage disruption. Treatment of lameness due to degenerative (aseptic/closed) joint disease.

Presentation: Intra-articular – 40 mg/mL in 5 mL single-dose ampoule.

Dose: Intra-articular – 80–120 mg joint. Use care when injecting multiple joints, as dose is cumulative. This can be repeated every 3–4 months. Do not exceed a total dose of 120 mg at any one time.

Notes:
- Ensure aseptic injection.
- Risk of laminitis (theoretical).

Triamcinolone acetonide
POM V

Indications: Anti-inflammatory, inhibits the production of cartilage matrix. High doses have been associated with articular cartilage disruption, lower doses have been shown to have beneficial effects on the articular cartilage. Treatment of lameness due to degenerative (aseptic/closed) joint disease.

Presentation: Intra-articular – 40 mg in 1 mL single-dose ampoule.

Dose: Intra-articular – 5–10 mg/joint up to a maximum dose of 18–20 mg.

Notes:
- Ensure aseptic injection.
- Slight risk of laminitis.

Tiludronate
POM V

Indications: Treatment of lameness associated with bone and cartilage reshaping and modelling associated with navicular disease. A possible future treatment for osteoarthritis of the tarsometatarsal and distal intertarsal joints.

Presentation: 50 mg dry substance per vial with 10 mL diluent supplied separately.

Dose: 0.1 mg/kg as an intravenous infusion over 30–60 minutes.

Potential side effects:

1. Hypocalcaemia (over rapid injection) with resulting cardiac dysrhythmia that responds to calcium infusions. Slow injection minimises this possibility.
2. Colic (usually respond to a single injection of an antispasmodic or mild analgesic).

Notes:
- The drug modifies osteoblastic activity preventing resorption of bone and so prevents the decay of the navicular bone. Corrective farriery also necessary to limit the loads on the flexor structures of the foot.
- Do not mix with lactated Ringers solution.
- It should not be used in horses under 2 years of age.

(e) Antidotes and Antitoxins
Adrenaline (epinephrine)
POM V

Indications: Treatment of shock and severe anaphylaxis due to insect bites or zootoxicosis.

Presentation: Clear, aqueous solution for injection. 1 mg/mL (1 in 1000) as adrenaline acid tartrate BP.

Doses: For anaphylaxis: 0.2–0.4 mL/50 kg by IM or SC injection (2–4 mL/500 kg horse).

Table 3.18 Dose rates for IM/SC administration of Adrenalin solution

Body weight (kg)	Dose (µg)	Volume (mL) 1:1000 solution
<300	1000	1.0
300–500	2000	2.0
>500	3000	3.0

Note:
- Intramuscular injection is the route of choice in the management of anaphylactic shock. It has a rapid onset of action and absorption from IM sites is far faster than subcutaneous sites. The IV route should be reserved for absolute emergencies when the circulation is known or suspected to be inadequate.

Activated charcoal
POM V

Indications: Absorption of poisons and toxins in the gastrointestinal tract.

Presentation: Powder or oral suspensions.

Dose: 150–300 g orally pnr.

> **Note:**
> ● Should not be used for treatment of corrosive poisonings.

Dimercaprol (BAL)
POM V

Indications: Heavy metal intoxication (As, Pb, Hg, Sb).

Presentation: Injection in oil.

Dose: 3–5 mg/kg q 6 h IM for 2 days then reducing daily doses over recovery period.

> **Note:**
> ● May be used at low dosages simultaneously with CaEDTA.

Domperidone
POM V

Indications: Fescue toxicosis. Can also be used to promote lactation.

Presentation: 10, 30 and 60 mg tablets.

Dose: 1.1 mg/kg po q 24 h.

> **Note:**
> ● Can also be used to advance ovulation in transitional mares.

Methylene blue
POM V

Indications: Nitrate/Nitrite poisoning.

Presentation: 10 mg/mL injection.

Dose: 8.8 mg/kg IV.

Sodium calcium edetate (calcium edetate)
POM V

Indications: Lead intoxication.

Presentation: 200 mg/mL solution for injection in 5 mL glass ampoule.

Dose: 37.5 mg/kg slow IV q 12 h for 2–3 days, then stop for 2–3 days. Can be repeated if necessary.

> **Note:**
> ● Lower doses may be indicated when other antidotes are given simultaneously. Highly irritant if injected extravascularly.

Sodium nitrite
No applicable category.

Indication: Cyanide poisoning.

Presentation: 30 mg/mL injection.

Dose: 10–20 mg/kg IV.

> **Note:**
> ● Most effective when used with sodium thiosulphate.

Sodium thiosulphate
No applicable category.

Indication: Cyanide poisoning.

Presentation: 250 mg/mL injection.

Dose: 250–500 mg/kg slow IV, may be repeated.

> **Note:**
> ● Seldom in time!

Snake bite antivenom
POM V

Indications: Proven or suspected zootoxicosis.

● *Antivenom*: Can be expensive! Contact for advice:

   LIVERPOOL: 0151-706 2000

   LONDON: 020 7188 5394 or 020 7188 7188

● Adrenaline (epinephrine) IM (see p. 97).

● Cortisone (dexamethasone IV).

(f) Suture Materials

1. *Absorbable*
2. *Non-absorbable*

Size and shape of needle
The ability of a needle to penetrate tissue is dependent on the shape of the point and body.

● *Taper-point* (round-bodied) needles have a sharp point and cylindrical body and are used on non-fibrous tissues such as abdominal viscera.

● *Cutting* needles are used to penetrate dense tissues such as fascia and skin. They may be of the *conventional (side) cutting* or *reverse cutting* type, where the cutting edge is located on the convex side of the needle. The *taper-cut* needle combines the reverse cutting point with a round shaft that is useful in delicate fibrous tissue.

Needles are available in various shapes: *straight, half-curved* or with a *variable curvature*. Wound depth, size and accessibility to suturing are the factors considered when choosing needle shape.

Most modern suture materials have a swaged on needle (atraumatic). This means that the suture is fastened inside the shaft of the needle – the needle has no 'eye'. This usually requires that the full range of suture materials with needles of appropriate types are held ready.

- Dispenser suture materials from a larger pack require eyed needles.
- Sterility is not always maintained unless the dispenser is carefully treated.

See Tables 3.19–3.22 and Figures 3.2 and 3.3

Table 3.19 Absorbable suture materials

Nature	Material	Trade name	Character	Gauges (metric)	$t_{1/2}$ (days)	Absorption (days)	Foreign body response	Handling	Colour
Absorbable	Plain gut	Catgut	Natural	1–3.5	7	90	Severe	Fair to good	Beige
	Coated gut	Chromic catgut	Natural	1–6	14	90	Moderate to severe	Fair to good	Beige
	Glyconate	Monosyn Quick	Synthetic Monofilament	0.7–4	6–7	56	Slight	Good	Beige
		Monosyn	Synthetic Monofilament	0.7–4	14	60–90	Slight	Good	Beige
	Polyglactin 910	Coated vicryl	Synthetic braided-coated	0.4–8	14	60–90	Slight	Good	Purple
	Polyglactin 910	Vicryl Rapide	Synthetic braided-coated	1–4	5	42	Slight	Good	Purple/white
	Polyglycolic acid	Dexon Safil	Synthetic braided	0.7–5	10 18	120 60–90	Slight	Good	Green Violet
	Polydioxanone	PDS Monoplus	Synthetic monofilament	0.4–5	35	182	Slight	Good	Blue Violet
	Polyglyconate	Maxon	Synthetic braided-coated	0.4–8	21	180	Slight	Good	Green
	Polyglycolide	Novosyn	Synthetic braided-coated	0.2–5	21	56–70	Slight	Good	Violet

Table 3.20 Non-absorbable suture materials

Nature	Material	Trade name	Character	Gauges (metric)	$t_{1/2}$ (days)	Absorption (days)	Foreign body response	Handling	Ccolour
Non-absorbable	Polyamide (nyl)	Supramid Ethicon	Synthetic sheathed	0.5–8	n/a	n/a	Moderate, if coating breaks	Good	White
	Polyester	Ethibond PremiCron	Synthetic raided-coated	0.5–7 0.7–7	n/a	n/a	Moderate	Good	Green White
	Polyamide (nyl)	Ethilon Dafilon	Synthetic monofilament	0.1–5 0.1–4	n/a	n/a	Minimal	Fair	Blue Black
	Polypropylene	Prolene Premilene	Synthetic monofilament	1–4 0.2–4	n/a	n/a	Minimal	Poor to fair	Blue
	Silk	Mersilk Silkam	Natural braided	0.2–5 0.4–8	365	>720	Moderate to severe	Excellent	Black White
	Linen	Surgical linen	Natural braided	2–5	n/a	n/a	Severe	Excellent	White
	Stainless steel	Stainless steel wire Steelex	Synthetic	1.5–6 1–3	n/a	n/a	Almost inert	Poor	Metallic

Table 3.21 Suture material size conversion table

Metric size	USP size (synthetic materials)	Actual size
0.2	10/0	0.02
0.4	8/0	0.04
0.7	6/0	0.07
1.5	4/0	0.15
2.0	3/0	0.2
3.0	2/0	0.3
3.5	0	0.35
4.0	1	0.4
5.0	2	0.5
6.0	3	0.6
7.0	5	0.7
8.0	6	0.8

Table 3.22 Suture sizes and types for various tissues

Tissue	Suture size (metric)	Suture type
Skin	3–5	Non-absorbable monofilament
Subcutis	3–3.5	Absorbable monofilament or multifilament
Fascia	3.5–5	Absorbable monofilament or multifilament
Muscle	3.0–3.5	Absorbable monofilament or multifilament
Hollow viscus	3–3.5	Absorbable monofilament or multifilament
Tendon	5	Non-absorbable monofilament
Vessel (ligatures)	3–3.5	Absorbable multifilament
Vessel (sutures)	0.7–1.5	Non-absorbable monofilament
Nerve	0.4–0.7	Non-absorbable monofilament

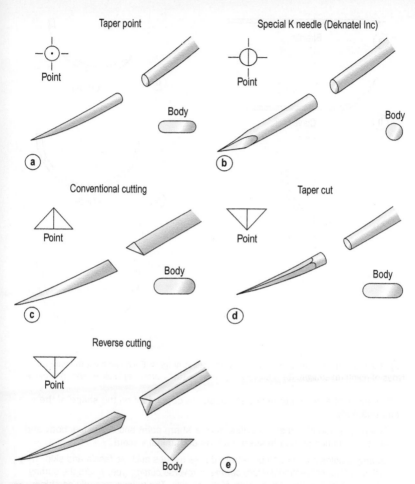

Fig. 3.2 Various needle types commonly used for veterinary surgery. Showing taper point, special K needle (Deknatel Inc.), conventional cutting, taper cutting and reverse cutting needles (top to bottom).

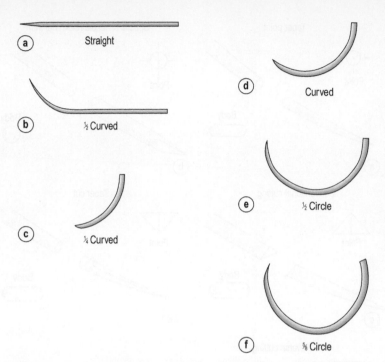

Fig. 3.3 The common needle shapes used in equine surgery. Each can have the various types of point: (a) straight, (b) ½ curved, (c) ¼ circle, (d) ⅜ circle, (e) ½ circle and (f) ⅝ circle.

The ability of a needle to penetrate tissue is dependent on the shape of the point and body.

- *Taper-point* (round-bodied) needles have a sharp point and cylindrical body and are used on non-fibrous tissues such as abdominal viscera.
- *Cutting* needles are used to penetrate dense tissues such as fascia and skin. They may be of the *conventional (side) cutting* or *reverse cutting* type, where the cutting edge is located on the convex side of the needle. The *taper-cut* needle combines the reverse cutting point with a round shaft that is useful in delicate fibrous tissue.

Needles are available in various shapes: *straight, half-curved* or with a *variable curvature*. Wound depth, size and accessibility to suturing are the factors considered when choosing needle shape.

Most modern suture materials have a swaged on needle (atraumatic). This means that the suture is fastened inside the shaft of the needle – the needle has no 'eye'. This usually requires that the full range of suture materials with needles of appropriate types are held ready.

- Dispenser suture materials from a larger pack require eyed needles.
- Sterility is not always maintained unless the dispenser is carefully treated.

(g) Cytotoxic and Anticancer Drugs

The use of cytotoxic drugs in equine practice is not widespread. The reasons for this include:

1. the overall cost of the drugs given the size of the patient
2. the logistics of administration (often require specialist and hospitalisation facilities)
3. the widespread secondary/concurrent effects on other organs/structures
4. the poor results that are achievable overall, regardless of the cost and logistic implications
5. the late presentation of cases (such that the disease is beyond treatment from the point of diagnosis).

Effective cancer therapy is, for all practical purposes, confined to skin and other superficial/accessible tumours. Although generalised neoplastic diseases, such as lymphoma/lymphosarcoma and myeloma, have been treated with systemic chemotherapy, the results have largely been very poor. Temporary remission can be achieved in some cases but cures are very rare. Topical therapy of cutaneous neoplasia is much more practical but melanoma and lymphoma/lymphosarcoma are generally not amenable to therapy. Individual troublesome superficial lesions may be removable surgically.

Reports of effective systemic chemotherapy have been made using a combined 'C-A-P' protocol comprising loading doses of *cytosine arabinoside* (at average dose of 1–2 g total dose subcutaneous or intramuscular once every 1–2 weeks), *cyclophosphamide* (total dose of 1 g IV every 2 weeks, alternating with cytosine arabinoside) and *prednisolone* (1 mg/kg per os every other day). Vincristine (2.5 mg IV) can be added if the cytosine arabinoside is not resulting in remission. Maintenance doses up to 20–30% higher can usually be used without undue side effects. Once remission is achieved, a maintenance protocol is used in which the intertreatment interval is increased by 1 week (except that the prednisolone is maintained every other day throughout). The expected remission periods vary from 6 to 12 months.

Realistically, however, the most practical course is simply to use corticosteroids (either prednisolone or dexamethasone). These drugs have the advantages of being relatively cheap, safe and also suppress the common secondary effects of immune-mediated thrombocytopaenia and anaemia.

Notes:
- Side effects include gastrointestinal derangements (diarrhoea, inappetence and gastric ulceration) and some bone marrow suppression (as detected by routine haematology).
- It is strongly advised to contact a specialist centre before embarking upon any chemotherapy. Even topical drugs may have serious side effects and are often potentially dangerous for the persons handling them, also.

Many of the drugs outlined in the table below have not been described in any numbers in equine oncology. Currently, it is probably best to consult with specialist oncologists for the latest information on their use and recent developments.

Table 3.23 Cytotoxic and anticancer drugs

Drug category	Drug				Tumour types
	Name	Dose (/m²)	Freq	Route	
Alkylating agents	Carboplatin	20 mg		Intralesional	Sarcoid
	Chlorambucil				Squamous cell carcinoma
	Cisplatin	1 mg/mL of tumour			
	Cyclophosphamide	200 mg		IV	Lymphosarcoma
	Lomustine				
	Melaphan				
Antibiotics with antineoplastic effects	Dactinomycin	0.5–0.75 mg	3 weeks	IV	
	Bleomycin				
	Doxorubicin	20–30 mg	2–3 weeks	IV	
	Mitozantrone (mitoxantrone)				
	Mitomycin C			Intralesional Topical (eye)	Sarcoid, melanoma, SCC Squamous cell carcinoma
Plant-derived alkaloids	Vinblastine	0.5 mg	Weekly	po	Lymphosarcoma/ lymphoma
	Vincristine				Plasma cell myeloma

Corticosteroids	Dexamethasone	0.1–0.3 mg/kg	48 hours	Lymphosarcoma
	Prednisolone	1–3 mg/kg	48 hours	Mastocytoma
Antimetabolites	Cytosine arabinoside			
	L-asparaginase	10000–40000 IU		
	5-Fluorouracil		Topical cream (Ophthalmic drops)	Sarcoid Squamous cell carcinoma
	Thiouracil			Basal cell carcinoma
Others	Methotrexate Taxol			
	Asparaginase			
	Heavy metals (Hg/As/Sb)	NA	Various Topical	Sarcoid
	Homoeopathic/ natural		Topical	Sarcoid

SUSPECTED ADVERSE REACTIONS TO DRUGS USED IN THE HORSE

A report should be made in every case if an adverse reaction is suspected during or after the use of any drug. An official report form is available from the VMD (address below):

● The batch numbers and expiry dates MUST be recorded.

● You should record the circumstances of the problem in detail.

● It is sometimes useful to inform the manufacturer also.

The report can be done online:

https://www.vmd.defra.gov.uk/adversereactionreporting/
Pharmacovigilance team: 01932 338427.

Table 3.24 Drugs contraindicated in the horse

Drug	Effects/comments
Amitraz	Colic (due to intestinal stasis) Severe CNS effects Shock
Amoxycillin (amoxicillin)	Severe local reactions Specific IV form may be safe
Cortisone	(see Notes, p. 152) Laminitis (probably an overstated risk) Immunosuppression Exacerbation of corneal ulcers Catabolic effects in horses with weight loss problems
Triamcinolone	Laminitis Immunosuppression Exacerbation of corneal ulcers
Lincomycin	Diarrhoea Colitis Laminitis Shock
Tilcomycin	Severe diarrhoea
Monensin	Severe myocardial degeneration/necrosis
Trimethoprim-sulphur with detomidine	Serious cardiac arrhythmia – risk low but present
Tylosin	Severe diarrhoea if administered by any route (often fatal) Severe local reactions if administered IM
Vancomycin	Theoretically useful in horses but there are NO conditions where this drug should be used in equine practice It is specifically reserved for human use
Enrofloxacin	Severe cartilage defects in young growing horses

Part 4 CLINICAL AIDS

SECTION 16
CURRENT REQUIREMENTS CONCERNING DRUG USAGE AND PASSPORT REGULATIONS IN THE UK
CHECKING THE PASSPORT

The following sections are included here as an *aide memoir* and should be added to by the reader as experience and knowledge is acquired. They are intended to be helpful rather than definitive.

Part 4 CLINICAL AIDS

Section 1
Bodyweight and surface area estimation

BODYWEIGHT ESTIMATION

Estimation of bodyweight is very important for accurate calculation of drugs, particularly when the LD_{50} is low!

Formula for estimation of body weight:

$$\text{Weight (kg)} = \frac{\text{Length (cm)} \times \text{Girth (cm)}^2}{12000}$$

$$\text{Weight (lb)} = \frac{\text{Length (in)} \times \text{Girth (in)}^2}{300}$$

where length = point of shoulder to point of buttock and girth = thoracic girth behind point of elbow.

Note: Where a calculator is available a more accurate weight can be obtained from the following formula:

$$\text{Weight (kg)} = \frac{\text{Length (cm)}^{0.97} \times \text{Girth (cm)}^{1.78}}{12000}$$

where length = point of elbow to point of buttock and girth = umbilical girth (Jones RS et al. *Veterinary Record*, 1990).

SURFACE AREA ESTIMATION

The surface area of an animal is an important (but underused) parameter that is most often used in respect to the use of drugs. Ideally, patients should be dosed according to the surface area expressed in square metres. The value of surface area is that it is a more reliable value than bodyweight and does not vary with changes in body weight. This measurement is only really valuable in some circumstances and little is known about the dose rate of drugs for horses. Nevertheless, this method allows reasonable comparison with other animals.

The surface area of the horse can be calculated with a reasonable degree of accuracy using the formula:

$$\text{Surface area} \left(\text{square metres/m}^2\right) = 2 \times H^2$$

where H = height at the withers in metres (measured accurately if possible).

For Example

A horse measuring 1.6 m (160 cm/16 hh) has a surface area of 5.12 m². If this horse weighed 500 kg, the conventional dose of detomidine of 20 μg/kg would be 20×500 μg (i.e. 10 mg).

From a dose of 2 mg/m² the dose would be calculated as: 5.12×2 mg (i.e. 10.24 mg). In some cases, the weight is the critical measurement but in others, especially toxic and cytotoxic and antimitotic drugs used for chemotherapy for cancer, the surface area is a much better measure (Fig. 4.1).

Alternative calculation for horses from Doyle PS (1998) *Current techniques in equine surgery and lameness*, 2nd edn. NA White, JN Moore, eds. WB Saunders, Philadelphia, pp. 93–97:

$$\text{Body surface area} \left(m^2\right) = \frac{\text{Bodyweight} \left(g^{2/3}\right) \times 10.5}{10^4}$$

where g = girth in cm.

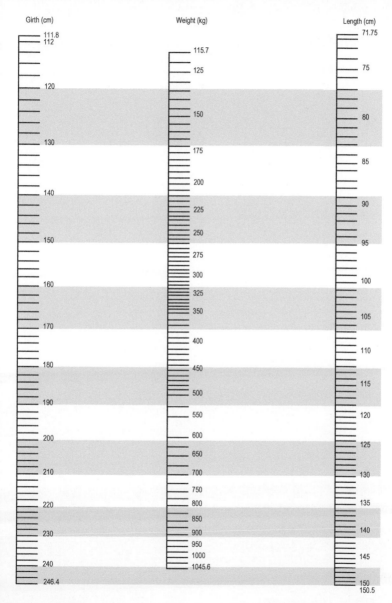

Fig. 4.1 Bodyweight calculator.

Section 2
Imperial–metric conversion

CONVERSION FACTORS FOR VETERINARIANS

Temperature

Table 4.1 Temperature conversion	
Temperature	
Celsius (°C) °C=5/9 (°F)−32	Fahrenheit (°F) °F=9/5 (°C)+32
−273.15	−459.67
−40	−40
−17.78	0
0	32
10	50
20	68
30	86
35	95
36.0	96.8
36.5	97.7
37.0	98.6
37.5	99.5
38.0	100.4
38.5	101.3
39.0	102.2
39.5	103.1
40.0	104.0
40.5	104.9

Continued

Table 4.1 Temperature conversion—cont'd	
Temperature	
Celsius (°C) $°C = 5/9\,(°F) - 32$	Fahrenheit (°F) $°F = 9/5\,(°C) + 32$
41.0	105.8
41.5	106.7
42.0	107.6
42.5	108.5
43.0	109.4
43.5	110.3
44.0	111.2
44.5	112.1
45.0	113.0
45.5	113.9
46.0	114.8
50	122
60	140
70	158
80	176
90	194
100	212
150	302
200	392
300	572
400	752
500	932
600	1112
700	1292
800	1472
900	1652
1000	1832

Mass (Weight)

1 kg = 2.204 lb (pounds)

1 ounce (oz, avoirdupois) = 28.3 g (grams)
1 ounce (oz, troy) = 31.1 g (grams)

1 lb = 16 oz (ounces)
454 g (grams)

1 stone = 14 lb (pounds)
6.35 kg

1 hundredweight (cwt) = 112 lb (pounds)
8 stones
50.8 kg

1 ton (imperial or UK) = 2240 lb (pounds)
160 stones
20 hundredweight (cwt)
1016 kg

1 ton (short ton or US) = 2000 lb (pounds)
907 kg

1 tonne (metric) = 2204 lb (pounds)

Length

1 inch (1″) = 25.4 mm

1 foot (1′) = 12 inches (″)
304.8 mm

1 yard (yd) = 3 feet (′)
36 inches (″)
914.4 mm

1 mile = 5280 feet (′)
1760 yards (yd)
1609 m

Area

1 square inch (sq in.) (sq″) = 645 sq mm
6.45 sq cm

1 square foot (sq ft.) = 929 sq cm
0.0929 sq m

1 hectare (ha) = 2.47 acres

1 acre = 0.4047 hectares (ha)

Volume

1 imperial fluid ounce (fl oz) = 28.41 mL

1 imperial pint = 20 fluid ounces (fl oz)
0.568 L

1 imperial quart = 1.137 L

1 imperial (UK) gallon = 160 fluid ounces (fl oz) = 4.546 L
8 pints
4 quarts

1 US fluid ounce (US fl oz) = 29.6 mL
1 US pint = 16 US fluid ounces (US fl oz) = 0.473 L
1 US quart = 0.946 L

1 US gallon = 128 US fluid ounces (US fl oz) = 3.785 L
8 US pints
4 US quarts

Pressure

Atmospheric pressure = 101 325 Pascals (Pa)
1013 hectopascals (hPa)
1013 millibars (mb)
760 mmHg
14.7 psi (lb/sq″)

1 pound per square inch (psi) (lb/sq″) = 6895 Pascals (Pa) = 0.0704 kg/sq cm

6.895 kilopascals (kPa)

0.0689 bar

Table 4.2 Pressure conversion

Pressure			
Pounds/square inch (psi) (lb/sq″)	kilopascals (kPa)	Bar (bar)	kg/sq cm
0	0	0	0
10	69	0.69	0.70
20	138	1.38	1.41
30	207	2.07	2.11
40	276	2.76	2.81
50	345	3.45	3.52
60	414	4.14	4.22
70	483	4.83	4.93
80	552	5.52	5.63
90	621	6.21	6.33
100	690	6.90	7.04

Table 4.3 Molecular weights

Compound	Molecular weight	Equivalent weight
Sodium chloride	58	58
Sodium bicarbonate	84	84
Sodium acetate (anhydrous)	82	82
Sodium acetate (trihydrate)	136	136
Sodium lactate	112	112
Potassium chloride	75	75
Calcium gluconate	430	215
Calcium lactate (anhydrous)	218	114
Calcium chloride	111	56.5
Magnesium sulphate ($5H_2O$)	246	123

Molecular weights are important in preparation of parenteral fluid solutions.
1 milliequivalent is 0.001 of the equivalent weight in 1 L of water.

Part 4 CLINICAL AIDS

Section 3
SI–old unit conversion factors

- There is no real justification for the use of Imperial units. The only reason these conversions are included here is in the use of older/outdated publications when conversion to SI units may be required to compare values.
- SI units are compulsory in scientific publications. They really are better/easier!
- The SI unit of temperature is degrees Celsius.

Table 4.4 Conversion factors (conventional and SI units)

Component	Conventional unit	Conversion factor	SI unit
Acetoacetic acid	mg/dL	0.098	mmol/L
Acetone	mg/dL	0.172	mmol/L
Acid phosphatase	units/L	1.0	U/L
Alanine aminotransferase (ALT)	units/L	1.0	U/L
Albumin	g/dL	10	g/L
Alcohol dehydrogenase	units/L	1.0	U/L
Aldolase	units/L	1.0	U/L
Aldosterone	ng/dL	0.0277	nmol/L
Alkaline phosphatase	units/L	1.0	U/L
Aminobutyric acid	mg/dL	97	μmol/L
Ammonia (as NH_3)	μg/dL	0.587	μmol/L
Amylase	units/L	1.0	U/L
Androstenedione	ng/dL	0.0349	nmol/L
Angiotensin I	pg/mL	0.772	pmol/L
Angiotensin II	pg/mL	0.957	pmol/L
Anion gap	mEq/L	1.0	mmol/L

Continued

Table 4.4 Conversion factors (conventional and SI units)—cont'd

Component	Conventional unit	Conversion factor	SI unit
Antidiuretic hormone	pg/mL	0.923	pmol/L
Antithrombin III	mg/dL	10	mg/L
Arginine	mg/dL	57.4	µmol/L
Asparagine	mg/dL	75.7	µmol/L
Aspartate aminotransferase (AST)	units/L	1.0	U/L
Bicarbonate	mEq/L	1.0	mmol/L
Bilirubin	mg/dL	17.1	µmol/L
Blood gases (arterial) $Paco_2$	mmHg	1.0	mmHg
pH	pH units	1.0	pH units
Pao_2	mmHg	1.0	mmHg
Cl esterase inhibitor	mg/dL	10	mg/L
C3 complement	mg/dL	0.01	g/L
C4 complement	mg/dL	0.01	g/L
Calcitonin	pg/mL	1.0	ng/L
Calcium	mg/dL	0.25	mmol/L
Carbon dioxide	mEq/L	1.0	mmol/L
Carboxyhaemoglobin	% of haemoglobin saturation	0.01	Proportion of haemoglobin saturation
Carotene	µg/dL	0.0186	µmol/L
Ceruloplasmin	mg/dL	10	mg/L
Chloride	mEq/L	1.0	mmol/L
Cholesterol	mg/dL	0.0259	mmol/L
Citrate	mg/dL	52.05	µmol/L
Copper	µg/dL	0.157	µmol/L
Corticotropin (ACTH)	pg/mL	0.22	pmol/L
Cortisol	µg/dL	27.59	nmol/L
Creatine kinase (CK)	units/L	1.0	U/L

Table 4.4 Conversion factors (conventional and SI units)—cont'd

Component	Conventional unit	Conversion factor	SI unit
Creatinine	mg/dL	88.4	µmol/L
Creatinine clearance	mL/min	0.0167	mL/s
Cyanide	mg/L	23.24	µmol/L
Dehydroepiandrosterone (DHEA)	ng/mL	3.47	nmol/L
Epinephrine (adrenaline)	pg/mL	5.46	pmol/L
Erythrocyte sedimentation rate	mm/h	1.0	mm/h
Ethanol (ethyl alcohol)	mg/dL	0.217	mmol/L
Ferritin	ng/mL	2.247	pmol/L
alpha-Fetoprotein	ng/mL	1.0	mg/L
Fibrinogen	mg/dL	0.0294	µmol/L
Fluoride	mg/mL	52.6	µmol/L
Folate	ng/mL	2.266	nmol/L
Follicle-stimulating hormone	mIU/mL	1.0	IU/L
Galactose	mg/dL	55.506	µmol/L
Glucagon	pg/mL	1.0	ng/L
Glucose	mg/dL	0.0555	mmol/L
Glutamine	mg/dL	68.42	µmol/L
Gamma-glutamyltransferase (GGT)	units/L	1.0	U/L
Glycated haemoglobin (glycosylated haemoglobin A_1, A_{1c})	% of total haemoglobin	0.01	Proportion of total haemoglobin
Haematocrit	%	0.01	Proportion of 1.0
Haemoglobin (whole blood) Mass concentration	g/dL	10.0 0.6206	g/L mmol/L
Haptoglobin	mg/dL	0.10	µmol/L
High-density lipoprotein cholesterol (HDL-C)	mg/dL	0.0259	mmol/L

Continued

Table 4.4 Conversion factors (conventional and SI units)—cont'd

Component	Conventional unit	Conversion factor	SI unit
Hydroxybutyric acid	mg/dL	96.05	μmol/L
Hydroxyproline	mg/dL	76.3	μmol/L
Immunoglobulin A (IgA)	mg/dL	0.01	g/L
Immunoglobulin D (IgD)	mg/dL	10	mg/L
Immunoglobulin E (IgE)	mg/dL	10	mg/L
Immunoglobulin G (IgG)	mg/dL	0.01	g/L
Immunoglobulin M (IgM)	mg/dL	0.01	g/L
Insulin	μIU/mL	6.945	pmol/L
Iron, total	μg/dL	0.179	μmol/L
Iron binding capacity, total	μg/dL	0.179	μmol/L
Lactate (lactic acid)	mg/dL	0.111	mmol/L
Lactate dehydrogenase	units/L	1	U/L
Lactate dehydrogenase isoenzymes (LD_1–LD_5)	%	0.01	Proportion of 1.0
Lead	Mg/dL	0.0483	μmol/L
Leucine	mg/dL	76.237	μmol/L
Lipase	units/L	1.0	U/L
Lipids (total)	mg/dL	0.01	g/L
Lipoprotein (a)	mg/dL	0.0357	μmol/L
Low-density lipoprotein cholesterol (LDL-C)	mg/dL	0.0259	mmol/L
Luteinising hormone (LH, leutropin)	IU/L	1.0	IU/L
Magnesium	mg/dL	0.411	mmol/L
Manganese	ng/mL	18.2	nmol/L
Methaemoglobin	% of total haemoglobin	0.01	Proportion of total haemoglobin
Methionine	mg/dL	67.02	μmol/L

Table 4.4 Conversion factors (conventional and SI units) –cont'd

Component	Conventional unit	Conversion factor	SI unit
Myoglobin	µg/L	0.0571	nmol/L
Norepinephrine	pg/mL	0.00591	nmol/L
Oestradiol	pg/mL	3.671	pmol/L
Oestrone	ng/dL	37	pmol/L
Osmolality	mOsm/kg	1.0	mmol/kg
Oxalate	mg/L	11.1	µmol/L
Parathyroid hormone	pg/mL	1.0	ng/L
Phosphorus	mg/dL	0.323	mmol/L
Plasminogen	mg/dL %	0.113 001	µmol/L Proportion of 1.0
Plasminogen activator inhibitor	mIU/mL	1.0	IU/L
Platelets (thrombocytes)	×10³/µL	1.0	× 10⁹/L
Potassium	mEq/L	1.0	mmol/L
Progesterone	ng/mL	3.18	nmol/L
Prolactin	mg/L	43.478	pmol
Protein, total	g/dL	10.0	g/L
Prothrombin	g/L	13.889	µmol/L
Prothrombin time (protime, PT)	seconds	1.0	seconds (s)
Pyruvate	mg/dL	113.6	µmol/L
Red blood cell count	×10⁶/µL	1.0	× 10¹²/L
Renin	pg/mL	0.0237	pmol/L
Serotonin (5-hydroxytryptamine)	ng/mL	0.00568	µmol/L
Sodium	mEq/L	1.0	mmol/L
Testosterone	ng/dL	0.0347	nmol/L
Thyroglobulin	ng/mL	1.0	µg/L
Thyrotropin (thyroid-stimulating hormone, TSH)	mIU/L	1.0	mIU/L

Continued

Table 4.4 Conversion factors (conventional and SI units)—cont'd

Component	Conventional unit	Conversion factor	SI unit
Thyroxine, free (T_4)	ng/dL	12.87	pmol/L
Thyroxine, total (T_4)	µg/dL	12.87	nmol/L
Transferrin	mg/dL	0.01	g/L
Triglycerides	mg/dL	0.0113	mmol/L
Triiodothyronine			
Free (T_3)	pg/dL	0.0154	pmol/L
Resin uptake	%	0.01	Proportion of 1.0
Total (T_3)	ng/dL	0.0154	nmol/L
Tryptophan	mg/dL	48.97	µmol/L
Tyrosine	mg/dL	55.19	µmol/L
Urea nitrogen	mg/dL	0.357	mmol/L
Vitamin A (retinol)	µg/dL	0.0349	µmol/L
Vitamin B_6 (pyridoxine)	ng/mL	4.046	nmol/L
Vitamin B_{12} (cyanocobalamin)	pg/mL	0.738	pmol/L
Vitamin C (ascorbic acid)	mg/dL	56.78	µmol/L
Vitamin D 1,25-Dihydroxyvitamin D	pg/mL	2.6	pmol/L
25-Hydroxyvitamin D	ng/mL	2.496	nmol/L
Vitamin E	mg/dL	23.22	µmol/L
Vitamin K	ng/mL	2.22	nmol/L
White blood cell count	×10^3/µL	1.0	×10^9/L
White blood cell differential count (number fraction)	%	0.01	Proportion of 1.0
Zinc	µg/dL	0.153	µmol/L

[a]To convert BUN to urea multiply by 2.14.

Part 4 CLINICAL AIDS

Section 4
Restraint of horses

- Horses respond instinctively to stress and fear through fight/flight.
- Instinct ultimately overcomes the best training – don't be convinced otherwise.
- With their large size, rapid responses and agility, ALL horses are inherently dangerous.
- Always establish the degree of restraint essential to guarantee the safety of yourself, lay handlers and the animal before attempting potentially dangerous or painful procedures.
- Don't forget that injuries incurred to people or animals through avoidable inadequacies of restraint are YOUR liability.
- You must be able to JUSTIFY your selection of physical or chemical restraints on physiological and practical grounds.

1. Approach
- Where possible avoid approaching the animal from immediately behind or in front.
- Don't sneak up on it! Talk as you approach to let it know you are there.
- An approach from the left side contacting the animal at the level of the shoulder is ideal.

2. Securing
Headcollar
- When required for restraint the headcollar should be fitted snugly (noseband approximately two fingers below the cranial edge of the masseters with two fingers 'give' between the noseband and nasal bone).
- Leather is preferred to nylon webbing – it will break, as opposed to cut, if the animal panics.
- The lead rope can be threaded through the noseband to provide increased control (Fig. 4.2). Avoid passing ropes through the mouth for this purpose.

Rope halter
- Not ideal as these tighten and may injure the head of a resistant horse.
- Don't use if fashioned from synthetic rope.

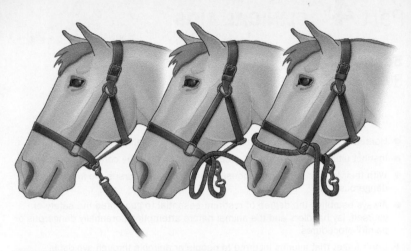

Fig. 4.2 Headcollar lead rope threaded over nose.

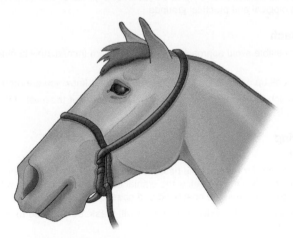

Fig. 4.3 Rope halter lead passes through eye and beneath jaw.

- The lead rope passes through the rope 'eye' and under the nose when correctly fitted (Fig. 4.3).
- Rapidly fashioned from lead ropes when no other form of restraint is available (Fig. 4.4).

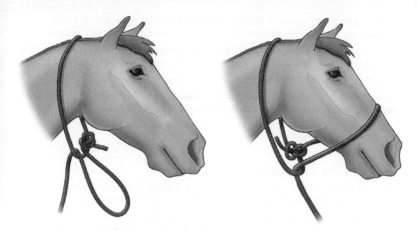

Fig. 4.4 Makeshift halter readily assembled.

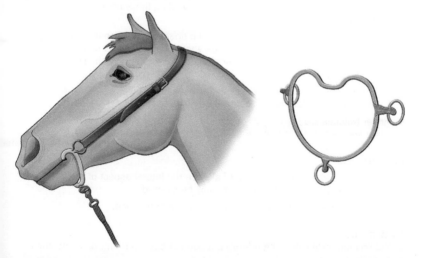

Fig. 4.5 Simple bridle with Chiffney bit.

Bridles

- Any headgear which positions a bit securely in the mouth.
- Pressure applied to the bit is focused on the mouth and the poll to give increased control.
- Simple bridles consist of a single strap and are commonly used with a Chiffney bit (Fig. 4.5) to restrain 'difficult' animals or animals in 'difficult' situations

(e.g. loading into lorries or stocks). BEWARE! This bit is severe and can potentially fracture the mandible if excessive pressure is applied sharply.

● Where riding bridles are used, reins should be removed and a lead rope passed through the near ring, beneath the jaw and attached to the far ring.

● ALWAYS hold bridled horses; NEVER tie them by the bit to walls or gates!

At best, these methods ensure control over the front end of the animal only – a handler at the head cannot control the animal's hindquarters.

3. Added Security
Twitches

● Time-honoured and effective.

● Correct application to the sensitive upper lip greatly increases control, especially where examination or treatments are liable to incur discomfort.

● Loop and pincer twitches are commonly encountered and readily applied singlehanded. The handlers' wrist is passed through the loop twitch before securely grasping the animal's lip in the fingers of the same hand. The loop is manipulated over the hand and secured by twisting firmly until a secure grip is established (Fig. 4.6).

● Repeated flexing of the wrist 'works' the lip snare to enhance its distracting effect and offer further control. Twitches should be held firmly mid-shaft and angled downwards towards the horses' chest. NEVER secure the twitch shaft to the headcollar.

● Makeshift loop twitches are readily and successfully assembled (Fig. 4.7). Avoid the use of nylon rope or baler twine at all costs.

● Pincer twitches are more readily applied but are generally less secure and adapt less readily to animals of different body size (Fig. 4.8).

Neck twitches

● By gripping and twisting a section of skin on the lateral aspect of the horse's neck a small degree of added control may be exerted.

● Particularly useful to aid intramuscular injection at this site.

Ear twitches

● Not recommended. Twisting a firmly gripped ear base certainly distracts some animals but permanent damage can ensue.

Raising a foreleg

● Allows the handler to help limit movement of the horses' hindquarters, but won't necessarily prevent kicking.

● When the leg is raised for an extended period a rope may be attached to a pastern hobble (Fig. 4.9) and released if the horse attempts to go down.

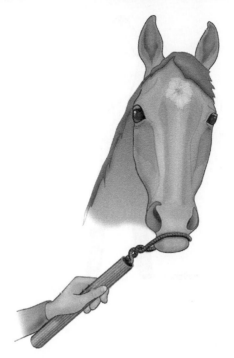

Fig. 4.6 Loop twitch positioned correctly on lip.

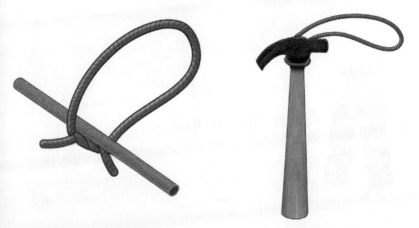

Fig. 4.7 Makeshift loop twitches.

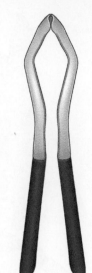

Fig. 4.8 Bulldog or pincer twitch.

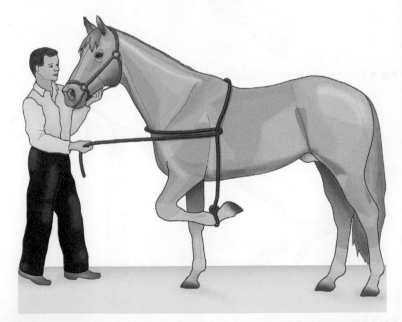

Fig. 4.9 Leg raised in roped pastern hobble.

4. Positioning
Stocks

- Gold standard for animal restraint. When available, use them.
- Site to allow easy access and pad appropriately to minimise trauma.
- Stocks limit lateral and forward–back movement but permit easy access.
- Stocks should be 'collapsible', allowing rapid release if animals go down.

Makeshift 'stocks'

- Careful positioning within the stable or yard can usefully limit animal movement against walls, corners and gates.
- Confinement in a trailer or lorry may provide the required constraint.

Rectal examination

- While use of a stable door between the man and horse is often mooted for kick protection where stocks are unavailable, the consequences are prohibitive should the animal go down.
- Ensure that the animal is appropriately restrained (bridle, twitch, raised foreleg, sedation if required) and position yourself close against the side of the animal's quarters (not directly behind) to limit the force behind any connecting kick.
- Further control over movement of the quarters may be gained by positioning the horse against the wall on the same side as the arm you will use.
- If restraint is inadequate, DON'T DO IT!

5. Restraint of Foals
Young foals

- ALWAYS restrain the dam before attempting to catch her foal.
- Quietly drift the foal towards the corner of the box (the dam's quarters can be enlisted to help confine the foal). Place one arm around the foal's chest and a second around the gaskins (Fig. 4.10).
- Small foals can be lifted clear of the ground to increase relaxation.

Older foals

- Application of a foal slip is enhanced by passing the lead rope around the gaskins.
- Slip and rope can be secured by a single handler to give control of both head and hindquarters (Fig. 4.11).

6. Chemical Restraint of Horses, Ponies and Donkeys

- Sedation/tranquillisation are important adjuncts to physical restraint for many clinical and managerial procedures, e.g. clipping and farriery.

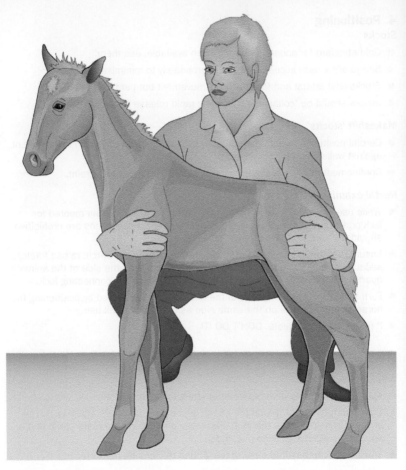

Fig. 4.10 Restraint of a young foal. (Note: raising the tail may help but can also distress the foal and cause pain.)

- Appraise each situation at outset.
- Sedatives are more effective if administered before the onset of stress or excitement and when the animal is left in peace for the full effects to develop.
- If physical restraint alone is unlikely to be sufficient, consider the suitability of sedation up front.
- Three key points to consider before sedation are:

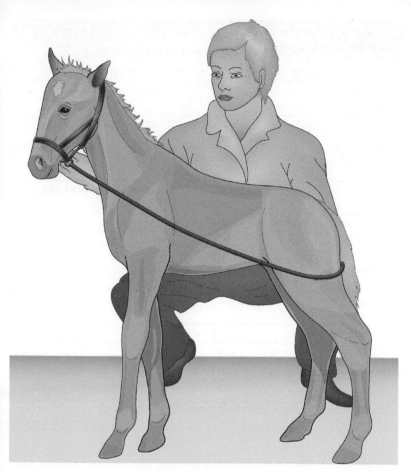

Fig. 4.11 Foal restraint with foal slip and gaskin rope.

1. *Physiological and health status* (e.g. α_2 adrenoreceptor agonists contraindicated last trimester gestation, acepromazine contraindicated in breeding animals or those with hypotensive conditions).

2. *Concurrent medication* (e.g. detomidine may cause fatal arrhythmias in conjunction with potentiated sulphonomides).

3. *Duration and depth of sedation*/tranquillisation required for the procedure.

Table 4.5 Summary of drugs and drug combinations commonly used for the restraint of horses

Drug	ACP	Xylazine	Detomidine	Romifidine
Route of administration	IV, IM, SC, PO	IV, IM	IV, IM	IV
Onset of sedation	Variable ~30 minutes	<3 minutes	<5 minutes	<5 minutes
Duration of sedation	Variable ~6–8 hours	~20 minutes	~40 minutes	~60 minutes
Dose (IV) sedative alone	10–50 μg/kg	0.5–1.1 mg/kg	10–80 μg/kg	40–120 μg/kg
With butorphanol @ 25–50 μE/kg (IV)	10–50 μg/kg	0.5 mg/kg	10 μg/kg	40 μg/kg
Sedation	Variable/unreliable	+++	++	+
Muscle relaxation	++	+++	++	+
Analgesia	–	++++	+++	+
Ataxia	Variable	+++	++	+
Common uses	Clipping	Immobility desirable, colic workup	Minor surgical procedures	Transport Farriery, pre-nerve block
Formulary page	P. 75	P. 79	P. 76	P. 78

- Large/heavy horses are relatively intolerant of α_2 adrenoreceptor agonists. Use low end of dose range.
- Oral administration of ACP (0.13–0.26 mg/kg as 25 mg tablets or paste) may aid restraint of intractable/'un-catchable' animals but the effect is slow in onset and unreliable.
- If physical restraint is insufficient for intravenous injection:

Detomidine	20 μg/kg	Composite	Leave for 30 minutes
ACP	30 μg/kg	Intramuscular	In quiet to obtain
Butorphanol	50 μg/kg	Injection	Maximum effect

7. Chemical Restraint of Foals

- Less than 4–6 weeks:

    Tranquillisation with benzodiazepines (diazepam, 0.1–0.25 mg/kg, IV only) is generally satisfactory but recumbency is inevitable.

- Healthy foals when benzodiazepines are ineffective:

    Detomidine 5–40 μg/kg, IV

    Romifidine 20–70 μg/kg, IV

    Butorphanol (50–200 μg/kg) can be added to enhance sedation/analgesia.

Section 5
Ageing

The ageing of horses from dentition alone is a very difficult (not to say hazardous) task! All *estimates* of age should be just that. Where practical and especially when documentation is required, the veterinary surgeon MUST state in writing (with a signed/dated certificate) the basis for his/her estimate. This is particularly important for examinations on behalf of a purchaser and for insurance purposes. A form for ageing is available from the Veterinary Defence Society.

It is probably wrong to decline to comment on the age of the horse when performing these examinations because the prospective owner will expect some rational advice as to the likely age of the horse. If veterinary surgeons do not do this someone else will (usually based on nothing at all by way of education and training). There are important reasons for an owner wishing to have a guide as to the age of a horse including the commercial value (older horses tend to be less valuable), the use to which it is put (very young horses may need to be worked less severely while older horses have less available performance potential in some disciplines such as racing) and its insurability (many insurance companies do not provide insurance coverage beyond a defined age). The *de facto* position at the present time is that veterinary surgeons should be able to provide an informed estimate with stated caveats. Whenever possible horses should be aged accurately at a very young age (preferably by establishing a date/year of birth before the animal is beyond the stage of accurate estimation). All such events should be accompanied by a detailed and correct, full description of the animal. When examining the age of an animal with the help of documentation the veterinary surgeon should be particularly careful to correlate the identification documents with the animal first.

There is an increasing use of passport-type identification certificates and subcutaneous microchips coupled with freeze marking/branding. These will usually provide both the year of birth and definitive identification and so it is possible to avoid any need to age such an animal. The identification needs, of course, to be verified at the time of the examination. Under no circumstances should the veterinary surgeon be drawn into making a casual estimate, especially when led to do so by an unscrupulous owner/agent.

Table 4.6 Dental eruption times

Tooth	Milk/deciduous	Permanent
Central incisor	0–1 week	2½ years
Lateral incisor	2–4 weeks	3½ years
Corner incisor	7–9 months	4½ years
Canine/tush	n/a	3–4 years[a]
Premolar 2 (cheek tooth 1)	2–8 weeks	2½ years
Premolar 3 (cheek tooth 2)	2–8 weeks	3 years
Premolar 4 (cheek tooth 3)	2–8 weeks	4 years
Molar 1 (Cheek Tooth 4)	n/a	1 year
Molar 2 (Cheek Tooth 5)	n/a	2 years
Molar 3 (Cheek Tooth 6)	n/a	3½ years

[a]*Geldings and stallions – seldom present in mares.*

- Remember that horses are aged in years from January 1st (northern hemisphere) or August 1st (southern hemisphere).
- DO NOT fall into the trap of making closer estimates than the year – even though the eruption times are reasonably accurate they can be very misleading.
- A major source of error occurs between horses aged 2 years (with a full set of in-wear incisors) and a 5–7-year-old horse with a full set of permanent incisors in wear.

WEAR PATTERN OF INCISOR TEETH

After the incisor teeth erupt, they continue to grow and lengthen until each lower-jaw incisor meets its opposite number in the upper jaw, approximately 6 months after eruption. This is known as coming into wear. The incisors, therefore, come into wear at 3, 4 and 5 years of age. The wear pattern of the incisor teeth is very unpredictable but this, together with the occlusal incisor angle, provides the best opportunity of estimation of an approximate age. Some horses have shallow infundibuli and others deep. Some have prominent pulp cavities, which appear as a linear mark at the buccal margin of the tooth at an early age, while in others it is delayed. It is wise to use every available indicator before making an *estimate* of the age (*a range should always be given*) (Fig. 4.12).

The following drawings are designed to provide a rough guide to help the clinician establish the major features. Each age shown carries a range marker that corresponds to the most likely range of age for the given parameters/appearance.

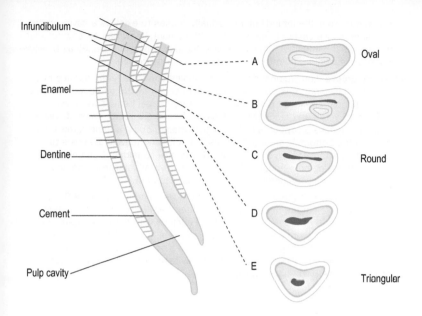

Age (years) for lower incisors

	Central	Lateral	Corner
A	5–6	6–7	7–9
B	8–9	9–10	10–12
C	11–12	12–14	13–15
D	13–15	15–18	16–20
E	> 20	> 25	> 25

Fig. 4.12 Wear pattern of incisor teeth: age (years) for lower incisors.

Remember that you should record your findings and the reasons for your estimate in a bound book as well as on the certificate.

Dental ageing forms are available from the Veterinary Defence Society. These have considerable advantages in that they provide an accurate record of the findings and an error of interpretation cannot then be viewed as any form of negligence. An example is shown in Figure 4.27.

Occlusal angle: The angle at the caudal aspect of the upper and lower central incisors. This is almost vertical (180°) when recently erupted and progressively decreases with age, approaching 90° at 20 years.

Infundibulum or 'cup': The cavity in the occlusal surface produced by the invagination of enamel. Later, as the deeper sections of the tooth are exposed to wear, the infundibulum gradually ceases to exist as a cavity and is represented by a circle of enamel filled with cement, known as an enamel *spot* or *mark*. As the infundibulum disappears, the pulp cavity is exposed as a yellow-brown transverse mark in the dentin, known as a *dental star*.

Galvayne's groove: Longitudinal depression running down the labial surface of the upper third incisors. It is often stained a dark colour by the cement it contains. It is traditionally believed to appear at 10 years of age, be half way down the tooth at 15 years and reach the occlusal surface at 20 years. From 20 years of age the groove disappears at the gingival margin and gradually 'grows' out reaching the bottom at around 30 years (i.e. it is said to take 10 years to appear fully and 10 years to grow out). This is now considered an unreliable method of ageing horses but it does add to the overall interpretation and should always be considered in the overall assessment.

Seven-year hook: When the upper and lower incisors come into wear, at 5 years, the dental tables of the upper teeth are longer than those of the lower teeth. The caudal parts of the upper teeth do not occlude with the lower teeth and, therefore, are not worn away, creating a hook. This is most obvious at 7 years and then gradually disappears. It reappears in a second cycle, when it is most obvious at about 13 years. It is now generally regarded as being an inaccurate indicator of age (Figs 4.13–4.26).

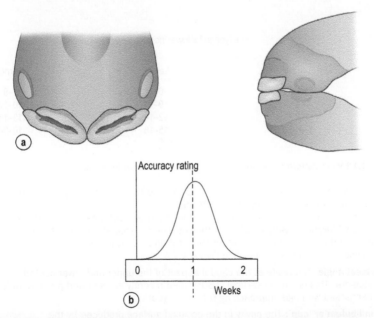

Fig. 4.13 (a) Wear pattern of incisor teeth – 1 week. (b) Accuracy rating – 1 week.

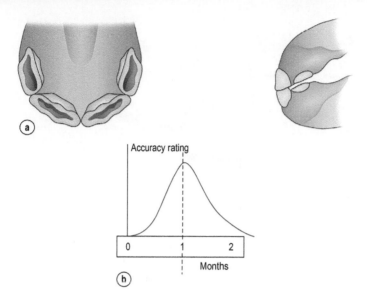

Fig. 4.14 (a) Wear pattern of incisor teeth – 1 month. (b) Accuracy rating – 1 month.

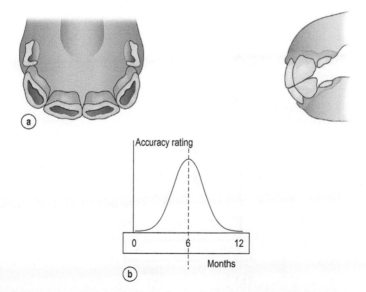

Fig. 4.15 (a) Wear pattern of incisor teeth – 1 year. (b) Accuracy rating – 1 year.

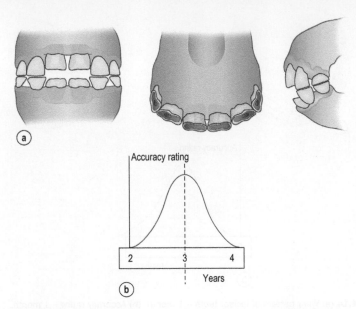

Fig. 4.16 (a) Wear pattern of incisor teeth – 3 years. (b) Accuracy rating – 3 years.

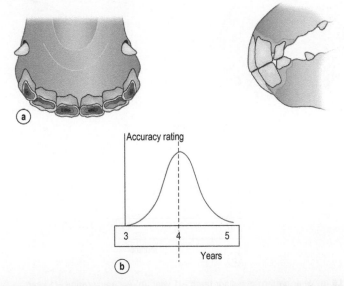

Fig. 4.17 (a) Wear pattern of incisor teeth – 4 years. (b) Accuracy rating – 4 years.

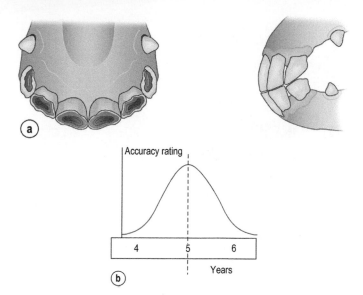

Fig. 4.18 (a) Wear pattern of incisor teeth – 5 years. (b) Accuracy rating – 5 years.

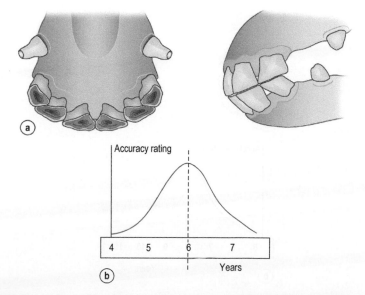

Fig. 4.19 (a) Wear pattern of incisor teeth – 6 years. (b) Accuracy rating – 6 years.

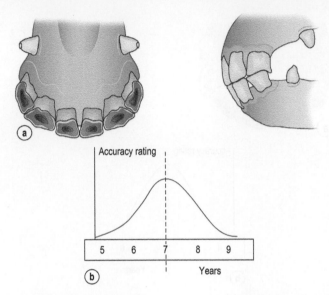

Fig. 4.20 (a) Wear pattern of incisor teeth – 7 years. (b) Accuracy rating – 7 years.

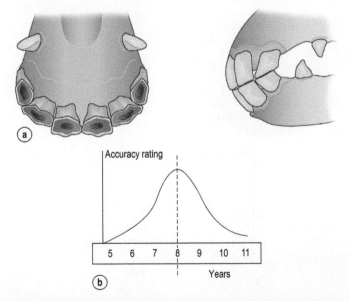

Fig. 4.21 (a) Wear pattern of incisor teeth – 8 years. (b) Accuracy rating – 8 years.

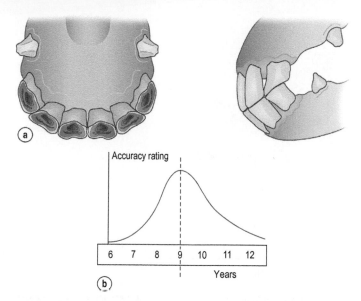

Fig. 4.22 (a) Wear pattern of incisor teeth – 9 years. (b) Accuracy rating – 9 years.

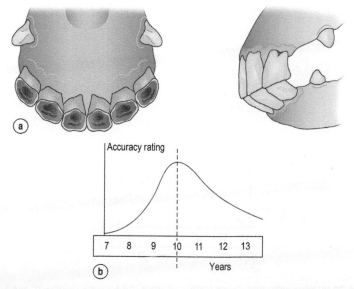

Fig. 4.23 (a) Wear pattern of incisor teeth – 10 years. (b) Accuracy – 10 years.

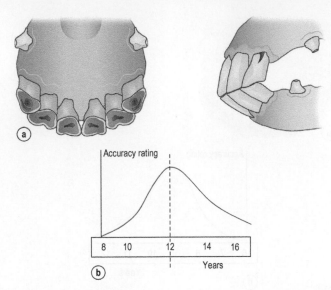

Fig. 4.24 (a) Wear pattern of incisor teeth – 12 years. (b) Accuracy rating – 12 years.

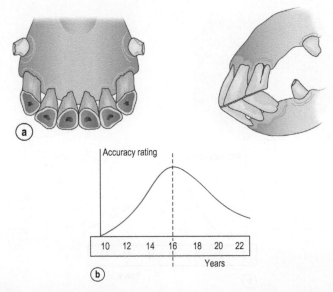

Fig. 4.25 (a) Wear pattern of incisor teeth – 16 years. (b) Accuracy rating – 16 years.

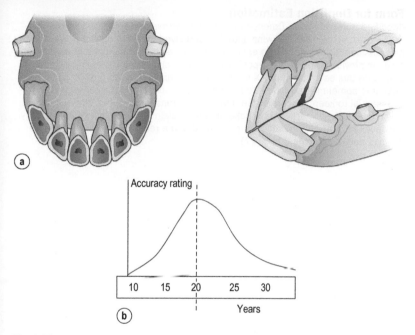

Fig. 4.26 (a) Wear pattern of incisor teeth – 20+ years. (b) Accuracy rating – 20+ years.

Form for Dentition Estimation

(Modified from Veterinary Defence Society with permission.)

The risks of litigation following actual or perceived errors in ageing of horses are considerable. Whenever an estimate is provided it is essential that a sensible range is provided. The *de facto* position is that veterinarians are the right people to provide this estimate and it is not helpful to simply refuse to provide some help. It is sometimes advisable to seek a second opinion from a colleague but it is essential to keep a record of the dental appearance upon which the estimate was made. It is not negligent to make an error – claims for negligence are virtually impossible if a true examination is performed and a record is kept of both the findings and the opinion (Fig. 4.27).

RECORD OF APPEARANCE OF TEETH

Incisors (temp/perm)	Central		Lateral		Corner	
Erupted	Y/N		Y/N		Y/N	
In wear	Y/N		Y/N		Y/N	
Infundibular cavity gone	Y/N		Y/N		Y/N	
Infundibular mark wearing out	Y/N		Y/N		Y/N	
Dental Star	Y/N		Y/N		Y/N	
Shape of incisor tables						
Hook-corner incisor	Left	Y/N		Right	Y/N	
Galvayne's groove extent	Left	....		Right	....	
Angle of occlusion	....					
Abnormal wear	....					
Tushes present			Y/N			
Wolf tooth	Left	Y/N		Right	Y/N	
Molars	....					
Vendor's stated age	....					
Documented age	....					
Approx age	....	Range	....			
Name	....					
Address	....					

Horse's name ....
Colour .... Sex ....
Certificate ref ....

Remember to emphasise that estimates of age are imprecise and unreliable.

Ages up to 6 years are reasonably definitive. For ages between 7 and 10 years an allowance of 2 years either way may be acceptable and in certain circumstances 3 years. From 10 years onwards estimates of age based on teeth are even less well correlated with true age.

Fig. 4.27 Form for dentition estimation (courtesy of the Veterinary Defence Society).

Section 6
Humane destruction

Euthanasia is possibly the most demanding of the tasks an equine veterinary surgeon is asked to perform. Reputations have been made and destroyed by how this is carried out. Remember that owners will be upset and possibly even irrational – do not 'lose your cool'! A quiet, efficient and sympathetic approach enhances your reputation.

Remember that you are the veterinary surgeon and that in the event that an animal is suffering and requires (in your opinion) to be killed immediately on humane grounds you should perform this with all due speed and efficiency. If possible you should have a competent witness to the event and you should take pains to explain what you intend to do and why. In such circumstances you have no responsibility for the financial implications of what you do – carcass disposal costs/insurance arrangements, etc., are irrelevant. It is advisable to have a police officer with you at road accidents, etc., where the owner is not known or cannot be contacted, in case of future problems.

Prerequisites
Ensure that:

(a) owner(s) is(are) aware of what you intend to do and the reasons for it – the term 'putting to sleep' can be misinterpreted with disastrous results. The term 'kill' (or destroy) is brutal but not open to misinterpretation.

(b) a signed concession form is obtained from the owner or responsible agent.

(c) all appropriate arrangements have been made beforehand (unless circumstances dictate otherwise), e.g. knacker wagon, disposal.

(d) you keep an accurate written description of the horse and details of method, place and reason for euthanasia. These should be kept in a bound notebook and should be recorded immediately. DO NOT rely on recollection at some later date.

(e) *suitable*, responsible and understanding assistance is available to restrain the horse. It is very difficult and possibly dangerous to attempt to kill a horse entirely on your own.

- Death is taken to be when all reflex activity and all spontaneous cardiac and respiratory function have ceased.
- Death may appear to have intervened but some muscular activity may still be present for up to 10–15 minutes.

DO NOT LEAVE THE HORSE WITHOUT ENSURING THAT:

1. **DEATH IS FINAL AND COMPLETE.**

(Always check the full complement of reflexes, respiration and cardiac activity with stethoscope very carefully.)

2. **APPROPRIATE ARRANGEMENTS FOR DISPOSAL HAVE BEEN MADE.**

Consent Form for Euthanasia

This consent form (Fig. 4.28) has two sides and must be completed in most circumstances and especially where there is some sense that litigation might follow.

Methods of Euthanasia Available

1. Shooting (free bullet/captive bolt) (with/without sedation).
2. Chemical destruction (with/without sedation).
3. Aortic severance and electrolyte solutions (sometimes combined with barbiturates).

1. Free Bullet Euthanasia

Notes:

- It is NOT SAFE to employ a captive bolt weapon for destruction of horses.
- Use of the captive bolt may be effective in skilled hands and pithing or rapid exsanguination is a compulsory procedure after its use. In a public place, both procedures are completely unacceptable.
- It may even be illegal to use these on horses except in slaughterhouses except in particular circumstances (e.g. in an aircraft).
- Shooting (as opposed to stunning) is also very distressing to onlookers.
- There is little excuse for the shooting of horses in modern practice given that the carcass disposal is always problematical anyway.
- It is accepted, however, that shooting is very efficient in skilled hands.

Noah's Arc Practice
Ashfield under Willow

EUTHANASIA CONSENT FORM

I ... . , being the owner/owner's
representative of the horse described overleaf, hereby give consent for the
animal to be destroyed.

I have been fully informed of the reasons for euthanasia and understand that
the horse is to be killed. The method of euthanasia and the disposal
arrangements for the body have been fully explained to me.

I agree to the proposed arrangements.

I accept that the costs of the procedure and disposal of the body are my
responsibility.

The horse is/is not insured.
 • The insurance company has/has not been informed.

A post mortem examination is/is not to be carried out.

 • **The costs and implications of this decision have been explained to me.**

Signed:	Signed:
Owner/Agent	Veterinary Surgeon
Date: Place:	Signed: Witness Name:

Fig. 4.28 Euthanasia consent form.

(Continued)

Description of horse:

Name: Age: Sex: Breed:

Colour: Freeze Mark: CHIP No:

Markings:

• <u>Head:</u>

• <u>RF:</u>

• <u>LF:</u>

• <u>LH:</u>

• <u>RH:</u>

• <u>BODY</u>:

• Acquired Markings (scars, etc.):

❖ **Reason for Euthanasia:**

❖ **Method of Euthanasia:**

❖ Body disposal arrangements:
   Burial/Knacker/cremation/cremation (ashes return)

ARRANGEMENTS MADE? Yes / No   If yes by whom:

....

Signature of Veterinary Surgeon
Name:
Address:

Practice Stamp
Da te :

Fig. 4.28, cont'd

In the UK, all persons using firearms for any purpose are required by law to hold a *valid Firearms Certificate* (Firearms Act, 1982). Veterinary surgeons are exempt from the prohibition to the owning and using of Schedule V firearms (handguns greater than 0.22 calibre). This exemption does not mean that veterinary surgeons do not need a firearms certificate! All schedule V firearms are subject to strict licensing procedures. Currently, sound-moderated (silenced) single-shot pistols are required for use on racetracks or at official events. Silenced weapons require particular licensing permissions, including a separate license for the sound moderator.

Before using any weapon, the veterinary surgeon has a responsibility to ensure that he/she is in possession of a valid firearms certificate for the weapon itself and has the necessary skill/experience to use it. Under no circumstances should a person (including veterinary surgeons) own, handle or use a Schedule V weapon for which they themselves have no certificate. Shotguns can, however, be used by a person without a certificate for the weapon with the permission of the certificate holder and in the presence of the certificate holder.

Suitable Third-Party Liability Insurance MUST be in force at the time.

- **All possible precautions MUST be taken to ensure that human lives are not risked when using firearms.** Take particular care to clear the area behind the horse. UK police guidance suggests that a clear distance of 2 km must be available in the direction of the shot. No dwellings, vehicles or other animals must be within this distance. This effectively limits shooting severely in the UK. It is hard to visualise a circumstance when these requirements could be achieved in any public place. However, a hill or a barn of straw is an effective and accepted 'backdrop'.

- **Shotguns and rifles are difficult to handle and use effectively.**

- **DO NOT attempt to shoot a horse from a distance unless you have a suitable weapon and experience.** Professional stalkers and marksmen can be used but may require guidance.

- **The minimum acceptable calibre of weapon is 0.320** using a heavy, soft-nose bullet with a strong charge rating. **DO NOT use a 0.22 calibre weapon –** very experienced people can use these effectively but there are serious risks and there will be no insurance coverage if something goes wrong!

Site for humane destruction of horses

- The **ideal site for destruction** is just above the point of intersection of lines drawn from the medial canthus of the eye to the middle of the opposite ear (see Fig. 4.29). The intersection point represents the lowest acceptable site.

- A useful quick method for locating the ideal site is to measure from the base of the forelock with: two fingers width for ponies <14 hh; three fingers width for larger ponies and small horses (14–16 hh); or four fingers width for horses >16 hh.

- The muzzle is placed just below this level in the midline.

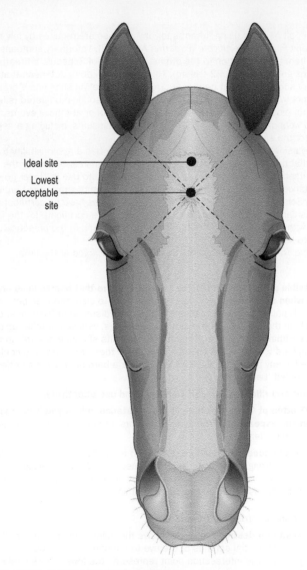

Ideal site

Lowest
acceptable
site

Fig. 4.29 Location of ideal sites for destruction.

- Aim slightly down into the brain stem and the occiput (i.e. not at right angles to frontal bone (too low)).
- **Remember that, if using a silenced weapon, you will need to reduce the fingers by one (the silencer adds about 1 finger-thickness to the barrel of the weapon).**
- **DO NOT LEAVE YOUR FINGERS THERE!!**
- Significant problems are encountered if the position selected is too low (bleeding is severe and the horse may not die!). If it is too high death may be violent. If it is off-centre the result is very unpredictable.

UNDER NO CIRCUMSTANCES SHOULD A HORSE BE SHOT FROM BEHIND THE HEAD OR IN THE EYE
The muzzle of the pistol should be held a few millimetres away from the skull. However, in the event of uncertainty, the muzzle may be rested gently on the skin but do not press firmly.

It is sometimes helpful to blindfold/sedate (or even anaesthetise) the horse.

IF YOU ARE UNCERTAIN OF THE METHOD, DO NOT SHOOT THE HORSE: USE ANOTHER METHOD!

2. Chemical Euthanasia
Method 1: High-dose pentobarbitone

- Using 1 mL/5 kg bodyweight the solution (usually 200 mg/kg) is preloaded into as many 50 mL syringes as required.
- A reliable assistant should restrain the horse with a headcollar/halter (do not wind the rope around the hand).
- A 14 gauge intravenous catheter is placed in the jugular vein (clipping and local anaesthetic may be helpful).

  If necessary, consider sedation using an α_2 agonist at full sedative dose. Subsequent collapse may be delayed by 10–15 seconds or more if premedicated with sedative.

- The full volume of barbiturate solution is injected as fast as possible.
- Collapse is expected after 35–40 seconds.
- Firm head restraint and pulling the head down and slightly forwards may help to make the horse take a step backwards.
- Death usually occurs by 1.5–2.5 minutes after collapse. Occasional gasping may be seen after collapse.

Problems/Complications

(i) Failure to inject volume fast enough:
  - Delayed, sometimes violent collapse, violent movement/panic may be encountered.

(ii) Failure to restrain adequately:
- Violent, uncontrolled collapse
- Often rearing and going over backwards.

(iii) Inadequate dose:
- Prolonged time to death, repeated gasping.

Method 2: Muscle relaxant, thiopentone (thiopental) and pentobarbitone

- Restrain with headcollar or halter.
- Pre-place 14 gauge jugular catheter.
- Sedate if required.
- Administer 10 mg/kg thiopentone (thiopental) as 10% solution as fast bolus and immediately follow it with suxamethonium (succinylcholine) at 0.1 mg/kg.
- Collapse expected in 25–40 seconds (associated with localised or extensive, fine or coarse muscular tremors and prolapse of third eyelid).
- Immediately after collapse (when safe) administer 5 mg/kg pentobarbitone (200 mg/mL strength) as fast as possible.
- Sedative premedication delays responses.
- Death usually within 3 minutes of collapse.

Problems/Complications

(i) Multiple syringes:
- Important to keep protocol in mind and label the syringes.

(ii) Muscle tremors may be distressing.

(iii) Carcass disposal is problematical.

Notes:
- It is possible to kill a horse with thiopentone (thiopental) alone. The horse should first be induced with a large overdose of thiopentone (thiopental) and, after induction, a dose of four times the calculated induction dose should be given intravenously.
- It may be necessary to repeat this dose again if by 3–4 minutes death has not intervened.

Method 3: Cinchocaine and quinalbarbitone (secobarbital)

- Restrain with headcollar/halter.
- Pre-place 14 gauge jugular catheter.
- Clip and use local anaesthetic if indicated.
- Sedate if required.

- Inject calculated volume of proprietary mixture *over 10–15 seconds* from single syringe. For horses under 145 cm (14.2 hh) use 25 mL (unless very fat/overweight or stocky). For horses over 145 cm (14.2 hh) use 50 mL (very large horses may need 75 mL).
- Collapse occurs at 35–45 seconds after the start of injection.
- Restrain by firm hold on head and pulling head downwards.
- Death usually within 2 minutes of collapse.

Notes:

- The solution is thick and slightly viscid so do not use a thin needle – the kits contain a suitable wide bore catheter. Test it during syringe loading. Use of a narrow-gauge needle will inevitably lead to a slow injection or the syringe might burst creating an embarrassing situation.
- Premedication with sedatives delays collapse by 10–20 seconds.
- **Do not use xylazine (may be violent convulsions after collapse in some cases).**
- Corneal reflex is often retained for up to 2–3 minutes after all others have ceased.
- Occasional gasping and muscle movement (particularly in the upper limb) sometimes occurs; observers should be warned of this possibility.

Problems/Complications

(i) Too slow injection:

- Normal collapse time but death delayed – possibly indefinitely.
- Possibly violent collapse and sometimes recovery to standing within a few minutes.
- The animal is effectively anaesthetised and the heart continues to beat.

(ii) Too rapid injection:

- Normal or delayed collapse followed by violent collapse/convulsions (heart stopped but inadequate barbiturate delivered to brain).
- Reflexes may be sustained until death follows from cardiac arrest alone.
- Some of these animals will recover after some hours.

3. Alternative Methods

If you find yourself in a position where a horse must be euthanised and you have nothing to do it with, do not attempt anything heroic. Take control of the situation and wait for the arrival of someone equipped to do the job! The police are very reluctant to help and in any case do not be tempted to use a police firearm – you have no certificate to handle it and so you will immediately render yourself liable to prosecution ... the police may bring the prosecution even if they have asked for your help! Attending police officers have no authority to issue 'temporary' firearms certificates.

If the owner of the horse cannot be located and the horse must be destroyed immediately on humane grounds, explain to a police officer or other responsible person why it needs to be done and then write down the circumstances and ask for the witness(es) to sign the document. Given a reasonable degree of professional competence this will always be sufficient.

Aortic severance
This method is far more difficult than it sounds and can be EXTREMELY dangerous – DO NOT ATTEMPT THIS. Severance is sometimes accompanied by violent hind leg spasms – particularly if one or more of the pelvic nerves are severed at the same time.

> **If this is the only option open then it is essential that the horse is either anaesthetised or very heavily sedated before any attempt is made.**
> **It remains a dangerous procedure whether the horse is standing or recumbent.**

Potassium chloride, magnesium sulphate and other combinations of electrolytes and anaesthetic agents
These are all more or less unreliable or sometimes can be positively dangerous/ inhumane in the conscious horse and MUST NOT BE USED. They may, however, be used on anaesthetised horses.

> **Note:**
> ● It is virtually impossible to destroy a horse solely with ether, chloroform or halothane, etc., and killing anaesthetised horses with these volatile agents is also very expensive, time-consuming and difficult. It should never be attempted no matter what the circumstances.

Part 4 CLINICAL AIDS

Section 7
Bandaging techniques

All the required dressings and equipment should be readily to hand before starting any bandaging. Allow for some dressing loss (especially if horse is resentful or in pain). One of the most effective measures for the relief of pain is a firm bandage that is logically and sympathetically applied. Even horses with fractured legs will find relief in immobilisation with a firm bandage and splint.

Tips

1. Use cotton wool rolls NOT Gamgee tissue – the latter is almost impossible to apply without kinks and folds. Recent development of a narrower thickness of Gamgee tissue is more useful in the tertiary layer and is easier to manage than cotton wool.

2. Never apply high pressure if bandage is to be left on for >2–3 hours.

3. Pressure necrosis of skin following inappropriate bandaging (or casting) is a nightmare to treat and is often more serious than the original injury – tendon involvement is particularly unpleasant.

4. Any suggestion that the bandage is not comfortable MUST be viewed with concern and appropriate measures taken to replace or reposition the bandage.

5. There is a strong tendency to use heavy dressings where these are not really required. A light dressing may be better tolerated than a heavy one that restricts movement and is hot.

BANDAGE LAYERS

(a) Primary wound dressing.

(b) Secondary wound dressing (designed to retain the primary dressing in position) (e.g. soft cotton bandage such as 'Soffban' (Smith and Nephew UK)).

(c) Tertiary dressings: Designed to cover and support the secondary dressing.

- Cotton wool layer.
- Conformable gauze bandage layer.
- Absorbable, stretchable fabric (Vetrap).
- Adhesive semi-elasticated bandage.

(d) Supportive bandage to ensure the dressings do not slip or move during natural (restricted) movement.

1. Bandaging the Foot and Fetlock

Notes:
- Bandage may 'ride up' so ensure top layer of adhesive is crossed under heels/foot.
- A single layer of elastoplast-type adhesive tape should be applied over the top of the dressing to avoid bedding, etc., falling into/under the dressing.
- Consideration must be given to the waterproofing of the dressing. Contamination with urine, faeces and soil/mud can significantly affect prognosis. Do not apply heavy-gauge polythene bags to the foot over dressings.

2. Bandaging the Carpus (Knee)

Any excessive pressure over the accessory carpal bone and the medial styloid process of the radius should be avoided because these are often the site of bandage sores that fail to heal. The use of elasticised 'zip-up' ('Pressage') bandages should be considered on cost and convenience grounds where support can be limited, e.g. skin wounds, etc. Firmly applied bandages over the knee and exercise do not mix well as the bandages tend to fall or become distorted. A single layer of adhesive bandage (elastoplast) applied to the skin at the top and bottom is sometimes helpful in keeping the bandage in position. A stable type bandage applied below the dressing may also keep it up.

3. Bandaging the Tarsus (Hock)

Any excessive pressure over the point of the hock and the common calcanean (Achilles) tendon and the medial malleolus of the tibia must be avoided. Pressure wounds are common at these sites and they are invariably problematical during healing – many take months or never heal satisfactorily. These are the sites of many disasters in bandaged horses. Elasticised 'zip-up' bandages ('Pressage' bandages) should be considered on cost and convenience grounds where only limited support is required. Horses with firmly applied bandages over the Achilles tendon in particular should not be given any significant exercise – the bandages tend to fall or become distorted. A single layer of semi-elasticated adhesive bandage applied to the skin at the top and bottom is sometimes helpful in keeping the bandage in position (Figs 4.30–4.33).

1. Left lateral view

Begin secondary
dressing below
fetlock and work
proximally

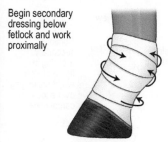

2. Left lateral view

Continue distally
and bring around
and under bulbs
of heel

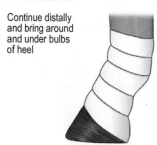

3. Dorsal view

Work proximally
to distally and
over heel bulbs

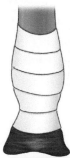

Palmar view with limb flexed

Lift foot and bring bandage
over palmar 1/3 of sole.
Wrap tertiary dressing over
bandage covering limb and
underneath foot

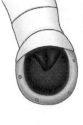

Left lateral finished appearance

4. Palmar view with limb flexed

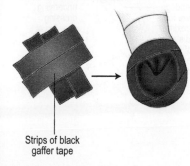

Wrap strips of waterproof
adhesive (gaffer) tape
over hoof wall, with a
cross net of tape over
the sole

Strips of black
gaffer tape

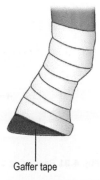

Gaffer tape

Fig. 4.30 Bandaging the foot.

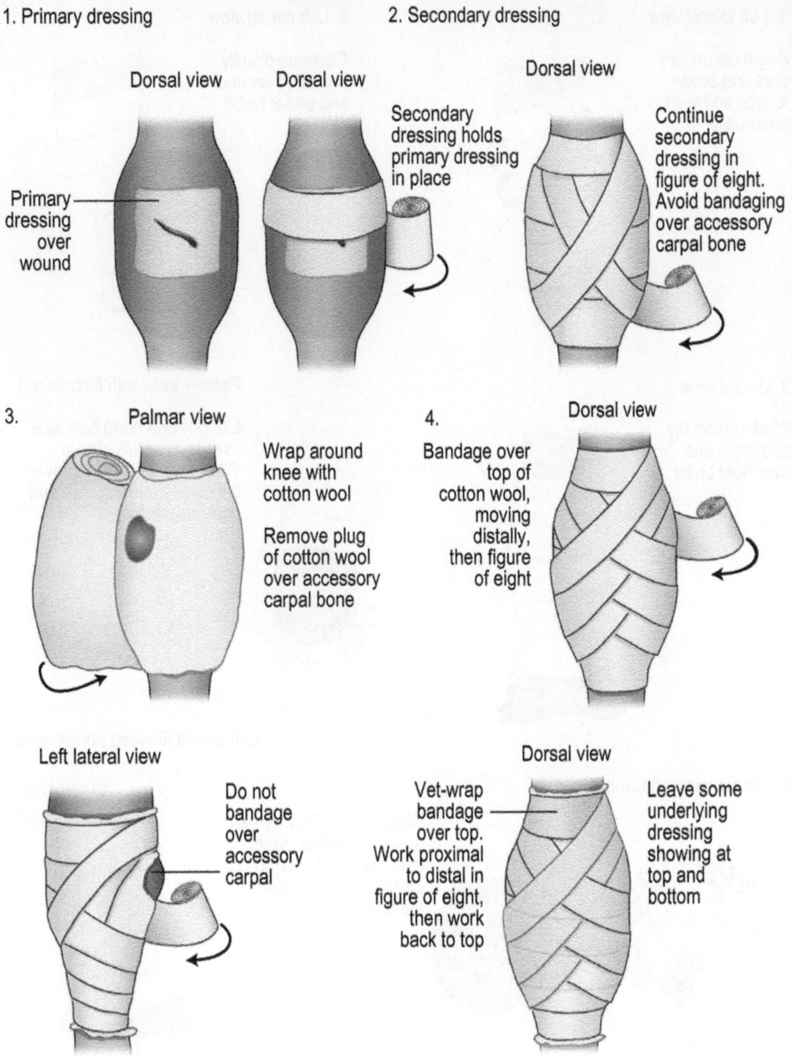

1. Primary dressing

Dorsal view   Dorsal view

Primary dressing over wound

2. Secondary dressing

Dorsal view

Secondary dressing holds primary dressing in place

Continue secondary dressing in figure of eight. Avoid bandaging over accessory carpal bone

3.   Palmar view

Wrap around knee with cotton wool

Remove plug of cotton wool over accessory carpal bone

4.   Dorsal view

Bandage over top of cotton wool, moving distally, then figure of eight

Left lateral view

Do not bandage over accessory carpal

Dorsal view

Vet-wrap bandage over top. Work proximal to distal in figure of eight, then work back to top

Leave some underlying dressing showing at top and bottom

Fig. 4.31 Bandaging the carpus (knee).

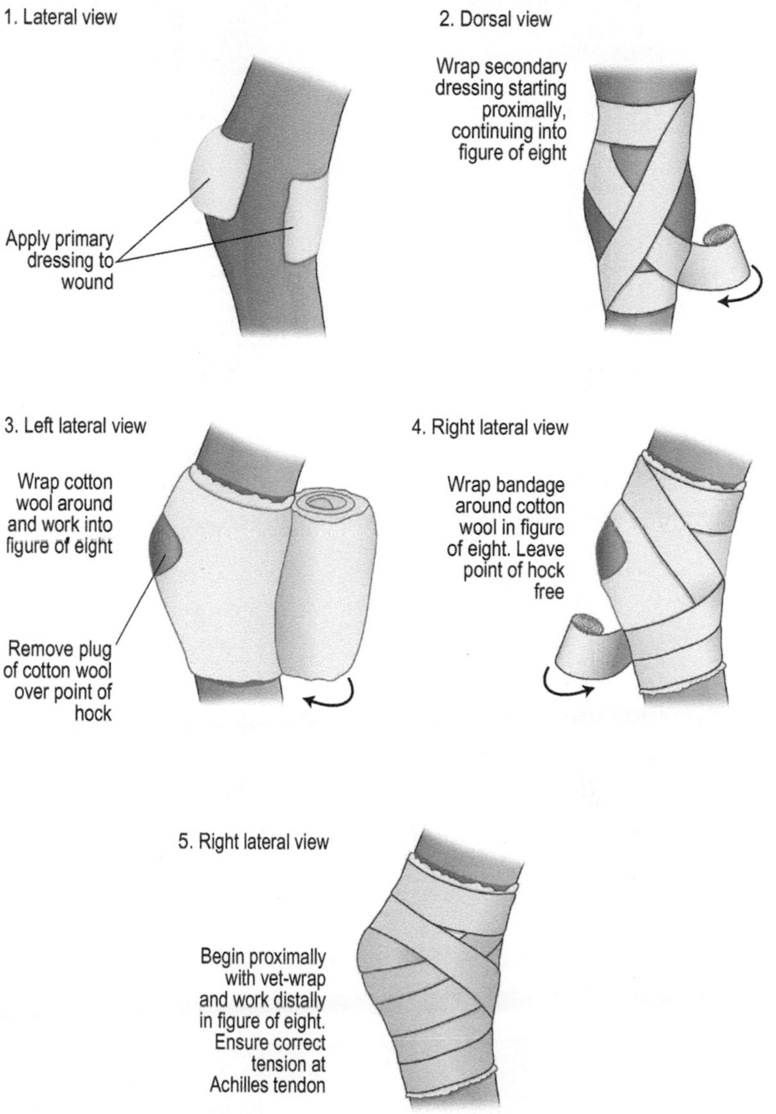

1. Lateral view

2. Dorsal view

Wrap secondary
dressing starting
proximally,
continuing into
figure of eight

Apply primary
dressing to
wound

3. Left lateral view

Wrap cotton
wool around
and work into
figure of eight

Remove plug
of cotton wool
over point of
hock

4. Right lateral view

Wrap bandage
around cotton
wool in figure
of eight. Leave
point of hock
free

5. Right lateral view

Begin proximally
with vet-wrap
and work distally
in figure of eight.
Ensure correct
tension at
Achilles tendon

Fig. 4.32 Bandaging the (tarsus) hock.

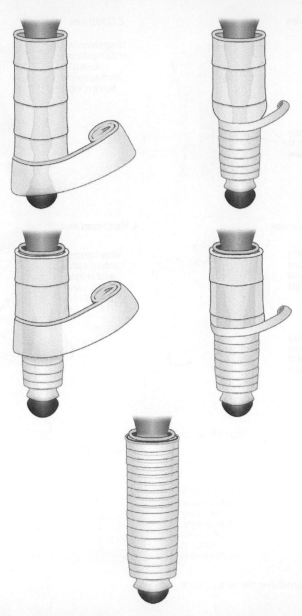

Fig. 4.33 The Robert Jones bandage.

4. The Robert Jones Bandage

This was developed to produce temporary immobilisation of human limbs and has several indications in equine practice:

- To provide first aid support for a fractured limb or disrupted suspensory apparatus giving stability and soft tissue protection.
- To provide pain relief and relieve anxiety.
- To control severe post-trauma limb oedema by application of even pressure.
- To support a limb following removal of a more rigid external or internal fixation device.
- To protect implants and soft tissues during recovery from anaesthesia.

The principle of the dressing is compression of air-filled cotton wool to increase rigidity and spread pressure evenly. To achieve this, the Robert Jones bandage has to be multi-layered and bulky. Each layer of cotton wool, approximately 2.5 cm thick, is kept firmly in place with a gauze bandage, each layer being wrapped more tightly. It is important that the layers are built up carefully so that the pressure is uniform and there is no folding and distortion of the resulting 'tubular' support. Layers are applied until a total diameter of approximately three times that of the normal leg is achieved (20–25 cm for an adult, 15–20 cm for a foal).

Method

1. Cotton wool is rolled onto the leg, first over the narrower portions, i.e. the cannon and pastern, to establish the initial base of the uniform tube that is critical to the strength of the bandage overall. The outer cotton bandage over this layer should not be pulled firmly but simply establish and stabilise the base layer.
2. Two layers of cotton wool are applied over the entire length to be incorporated with a firm cotton bandage applied over each, *avoiding pressure points*. The bandages are pulled progressively tighter with each layer. It is important to avoid the major pressure points during the early layers.
3. Further layer of cotton wool over entire length (*including pressure points*).
4. Further bandages applied over entire length.
5. Successive layers of cotton wool and bandage to provide at least 4–6 layers.
6. Top layer of elastoplast or broad nylon tape (carpet tape is effective and strong) – this must never be used on the lower layers.

The completed Robert Jones bandage should be hard and should respond like wood to a firm flick with the finger. The bandage can be reinforced with splints of wood applied on the outer layers.

5. Bandaging for Other Body Regions

Splint application

Splints are applied over the Robert Jones bandage with non-elastic adhesive tape to prevent shifting of the splint material within the bandage. Non-elastic tape does not expand and, therefore, increases the rigidity of the outer shell of the bandage. The tape should be applied as tightly as possible ensuring that the splint does not move during application.

The splinting materials that can be used include any lightweight, relatively strong, rigid material. Wood or plastics (such as guttering) are ideal although lightweight metal such as aluminium or flat steel also work well (Fig. 4.34).

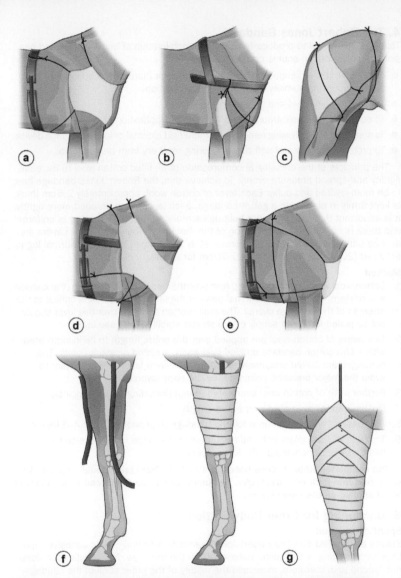

Fig. 4.34 Bandaging upper limb regions. (a) Shoulder dressing; (b) elbow dressing; (c) buttock dressing; (d) breast and shoulder dressing; (e) breast dressing; (f) upper forelimb dressing showing a retention mechanism; and (g) upper forelimb dressing retained by sutures and a support strap.

Rigid Limb Immobilisation by Means of Cast Application

This protocol relates to the use of Dynacast Pro (Smith and Nephew). The author is grateful to Dr C.M. Riggs and to Smith and Nephew Ltd. for their permission to base these notes on their pamphlet: 'rigid immobilisation of the equine limb – application of Dynacast optima' by Dr C.M. Riggs BVSc, PhD, DEO, DipECEO, MRCVS, University of Liverpool.

Cast application is difficult in the standing horse and an optimal job is impossible unless the animal is motionless and relaxed. Where possible, casts should be applied under general anaesthesia.

> **A CAST OF ANY SORT SHOULD NOT BE APPLIED UNLESS THERE IS AN IMMEDIATELY AVAILABLE METHOD FOR ITS REMOVAL.**

Indications

- Fracture fixation (sole or as support for internal fixation).
- Joint luxation/ligament damage (unstable joint/ruptured ligament).
- Support for damaged soft tissues (e.g. tendon/ligament strains).
- Severe distal limb lacerations/partial hoof avulsion.
- Correction of developmental or acquired limb deformities.

Types of cast

- Foot only.
- Half limb (cast to proximal cannon) – commonest form used (easy to manage and monitor from day to day, best tolerated of extensive casts).
- Full limb (cast to proximal radius/tibia) – very difficult to manage and poorly tolerated in most cases.
- Tube cast (foals) (proximal fetlock to proximal radius/tibia).

> **Note:**
> - There is a significant difference in the application of an *orthopaedic* (rigid limb) cast and a *bandage* cast that is commonly used to provide some degree of immobilisation for a wound site. The latter is simply a sympathetically applied casting bandage over a properly constructed wound dressing.

Equipment required

- Hoof knives, drill bit and length of wire, antibiotic aerosol spray, clippers, electric hair dryer.
- Oscillating cast saw and cast splitters (**don't forget you have to remove the cast so do not put one on unless you know how it is to be removed!**).
- Wound dressings (as required) including:
  - Allevyn® foam (Smith and Nephew) for vulnerable pressure points.
  - Stockinet of suitable diameter.

- 2–4 rolls of Soffban® (Smith and Nephew).
- Orthopaedic padding (Smith and Nephew).
- Orthopaedic felt (adhesive).
- Towel clips.
- Casting material such as Dynacast Optima (3 rolls 7.5 cm, 3 rolls 10 cm).
- Thermoplastic mesh (2 rolls) (Vetlite®).
- Synthetic resin (Technovit®).
- Gloves and protective apron.
- Suitable anaesthesia/sedation (as appropriate).

Technique of cast application

- Carefully prepare wounds, etc. (cover with suitable sterile dressings).
- Clip limb to remove coarse hair likely to cause bunching.
- Clean and prepare foot – spray sole/frog with antibiotic aerosol.
- Drill holes in distal margins of heel and pass wire through (creates a handle for easy limb extension).
- Apply Allevyn Pad® to pressure points – the accessory carpal bone, calcaneus and cranial aspect of the hock for full limb casts. Padding over the fetlock or coronary band is generally not necessary.
- Apply two rolls of Soffban®, taking care to avoid wrinkles and excessive pressure – aim to get an even, smooth bandage.
- Measure and prepare stockinet so each half of the length is rolled onto itself towards the middle. Apply two layers of stockinet over Soffban® with a twist at the toe (the two free ends should now be above the site of the top of the cast).
- Carefully measure and apply a single fitted thickness of adhesive felt around the proximal end of the cast length. Avoid any overlap and excessive tension (clip in position with towel clips).
- Establish and fix limb in required position (assistant holds limb by wire loop and supports length).
- Comfort support foam can be placed if desired – even pressure should be applied, avoiding any wrinkles. Each turn should overlap the previous one by half the width of the foam. Only one layer is needed.
- Apply casting material (read instructions carefully first to ensure ideal timing and handling). Use 7.5 cm rolls first (better conformation to limb). Apply immediately, starting at proximal end of cast, taking care to:
  - apply even pressure
  - avoid wrinkles/folds
  - overlap each layer by half the width of the tape
  - take special care over fetlock and back of cannon
  - apply subsequent rolls continuously without pauses or rests

- fold over the top half of the felt pad at the top of the cast and include it in the final layers (to produce a soft collar)
- gently and continuously massage the cast with the palm of the hand (NEVER WITH POINTED FINGERS)
- bubbling indicates curing of the resin
- always include the foot (in figure of eight pattern) and remove wire handles once cast is partially set.

- Cover open top of cast with one to two layers of Elastoplast®.
- Apply hot, malleable thermoplastic (Vetlite® (hot)) to foot (form wedge at heel to correct foot position).
- When dry, apply layer of Technovit® to toe and solar surface to provide a very hardwearing, bearing surface.

Management of horse with a cast

- Box confined with support bandaging of contralateral limb (be very careful not to over-constrict this limb).
- Keep top of cast protected from ingress of hay/shavings water, etc. – elastoplast collar.
- Twice daily checks on cast (walk a few paces, temperature (hot/cold), smell, exudate, swelling at proximal end, evidence of pain/dullness, etc.).

Removal of cast

- Sedation or general anaesthesia (as appropriate).
- Plaster saw is essential – score first and then cut to full depth in small bites.

Do not try to remove the cast until it can definitely be removed in one move (especially if the horse is conscious).

Complications

- Pressure sores.
- Cast movement.
- Cast fracture/instability.
- Vascular obstruction (gangrene).

TRANSPORTATION OF EQUINE FRACTURE PATIENTS

Emergency first aid measures of fracture patients should be directed at minimising further damage to the injured limb and maintaining it in a condition that permits repair. Protective splints should be applied immediately before further diagnostics (radiography) are carried out to lessen the risk of further damage. If possible, the joint below and above the fracture should be immobilised:

- Probably the most effective analgesic for a fractured limb is immobilisation.
- Immobilisation must take account of the biomechanics of the fracture.

Incorrectly applied 'support' can make matters worse and a treatable fracture can become untreatable during transport to the specialist hospital and so careful attention must be paid to the specific needs of the fracture – even where the exact nature of the injury may not be known.

EMERGENCY ORTHOPAEDIC FIRST AID

Introduction

Any veterinary surgeon may be faced with an acute equine trauma case, whether in equine practice or not. Knowledge of how to apply first aid care to such cases will have a profound influence on their final outcome.

Initial Evaluation

Initial assessment of the emergency needs to address:

1. Immediate risks to personnel.
2. Risks to other animals.
3. Risks of exacerbating injury to animal.
4. Life-threatening risks to injured animal(s).

Immediate action may be necessary in order to extricate all involved from imminent danger (for instance from the edge of a busy road) before the injuries to any individual case can be attended to. Some Fire and Police services are trained to help and may be willing to do so, but take precautions that they do not, themselves, get injured.

> **Conduct brief clinical examination (within possible limits) to establish presence/absence of life-threatening condition(s). Respiratory and cardiovascular function must be assessed.**

Note:
- Horses behaving in an uncontrollable manner may require sedation – this should be avoided if possible. Xylazine (0.5–1.0 mg/kg) intravenously (or intramuscularly if IV not possible) is the sedative of choice. **Acepromazine should be avoided because of its hypotensive effects.**

Once the initial situation has been brought under control, specific injuries need to be examined and managed accordingly. Certain injuries carry a hopeless prognosis and warrant immediate humane destruction of the animal. These include:

- fractures of long bones associated with severe soft-tissue injury
- contaminated open fractures
- complete fractures of the femur or tibia in adults
- complete fractures of the humerus or radius in horses over 300 kg without breeding potential
- severe cranial or spinal cord trauma.

Some apparently hopeless soft-tissue injuries (such as open luxation of the fetlock joint) carry a reasonably good prognosis, as do some fractures of more distal long bones. If you are in doubt over the chances of successful treatment and/or the welfare implications of transporting the horse to a referral hospital, do not hesitate to call the referral establishment for advice.

Some fractures can be difficult to diagnose – auscultation for bone crepitus (grating of bone fragments) with a stethoscope can be helpful.

The financial implications of any treatment need to be considered and discussed with the owner (if possible) *before* subjecting the horse to a harrowing journey.

First Aid Treatment

Acute orthopaedic injuries are broadly divided into four anatomical categories:

1. Skeletal.
2. Musculo-tendinous.
3. Synovial structures.
4. Neurological.

Note:

- Probably the greatest contribution to pain and anxiety relief is achieved by immobilisation of a fracture or injured limb. The principles behind this are fundamental to emergency management.

Fractures of Long Bones

The major limiting factor for the successful treatment of fractures is often the soft tissue damage sustained at and/or after, the initial injury. A horse with a fractured long bone may attempt to weight-bear on the affected limb, despite even gross instability. Resultant forces generated at the site of fracture will cause movement of bone fragments relative to one another and to surrounding soft tissues. Consequently, a relatively simple fracture (with a good prognosis for surgical repair) may quickly be converted to a comminuted, open fracture associated with massive damage to surrounding soft tissues (and a hopeless prognosis).

The principal objectives of first aid for a horse with a fracture are:

1. to restrict further soft tissue injury
2. to prevent penetration of the skin by a bone fragment
3. to stabilise the limb:
   - preventing further bone damage
   - relieving the anxiety that accompanies an uncontrollable limb in a horse
4. to limit the risk of contamination through existing skin damage.

These objectives are best achieved by prompt application of appropriate bandages and splints to stabilise the limb. Practical field techniques for achieving optimal stability of various fracture configurations rely on the use of readily available materials, are economical and may be applied with relative ease to the standing (sedated) horse.

Splinting the Equine Limb

When considering the most appropriate method for achieving optimum stability through the use of bandages and splints the limbs may be divided functionally into four anatomical segments (Fig. 4.35).

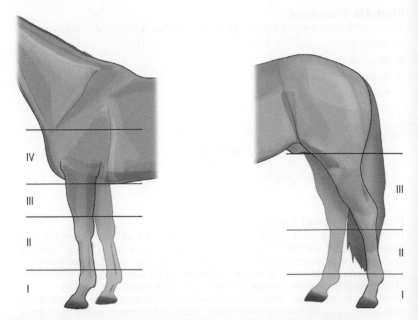

Fig. 4.35 Regions of the limb divided according to different splint requirements.

Forelimb

REGION I: DISTAL EXTREMITY TO DISTAL THIRD OF THIRD METACARPAL BONE
Includes fractures of the first and second phalanges, the proximal sesamoid bones and the distal condyles of the third metacarpal bone (common sites for fractures among racehorses).

Biomechanics

- The region is dominated, biomechanically, by the angle of the fetlock joint.
- If a fracture occurs in this region, there is a risk that the limb will bend around the fracture instead of the fetlock joint (Fig. 4.36).

Splinting

- Aims to eliminate bending forces at fetlock (and hence fracture) by straightening the limb so that the dorsal cortices of the bones are all vertical and in axial alignment (Fig. 4.37).

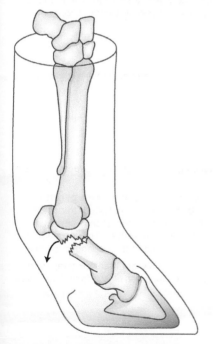

Fig. 4.36 See description in main text.

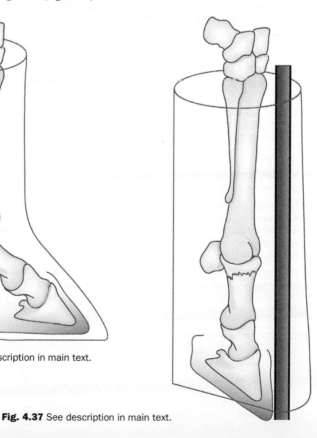

Fig. 4.37 See description in main text.

Application

- An assistant supports the leg under the distal forearm so that it hangs with the fetlock straight and the toe pointing vertically.
- Two light layers of cotton wool are bandaged to the limb, from the proximal metacarpus to the ground.
- A splint (consisting of wooden board or plastic guttering and extending from the carpus to just proximal to the tip of the toe) is then firmly taped to the dorsal aspect of limb, fixing the phalanges and metacarpus in axial alignment.
- Further support bandages or even casting tape (e.g. Dynacast Optima, Smith and Nephew) may then be applied over the splint.

> Care should be taken not to apply excess bandage between the limb and splint as this will compress and allow movement of the splint around the limb. The top of the splint must be carefully padded to prevent it from digging into the leg.

REGION II: FROM MID METACARPUS TO DISTAL RADIUS
Includes fractures of the mid-shaft and proximal metacarpus, carpus and distal radius.

Splinting

- The objective is to utilise the proximal and distal limb to attach a splint that can immobilise the fracture.

Application

- A Robert Jones bandage is applied extending from the ground surface to as far proximal as possible (the elbow).
- The Robert Jones bandage must be applied in multiple, thin layers of cotton wool, each of which is firmly compressed by an elastic bandage (if the cotton wool layers are too thick they will squash as the horse 'uses' the limb and the whole bandage will loosen and the leg will become unstable). The diameter of the final bandage should be roughly three times that of the unbandaged limb.
- Rigid splints, extending from the ground to the elbow, are then firmly taped to the *lateral* and *caudal* aspects of the bandage using *non-elastic tape* (Fig. 4.38).

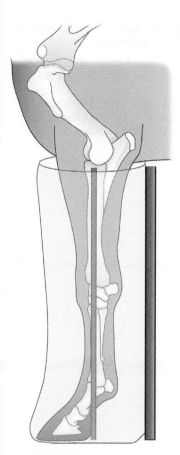

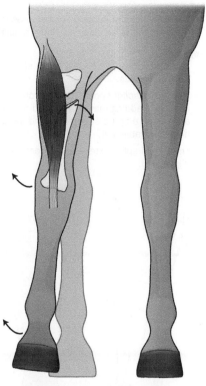

Fig. 4.39 See description in main text.

Fig. 4.38 See description in main text.

REGION III: FROM DISTAL RADIUS TO THE ELBOW JOINT
Includes fractures of the shaft and proximal aspect of the radius.

Biomechanics

- The principal musculature of the distal limb lies on the lateral aspect of the leg. When a fracture occurs in this region, the muscles no longer have an intact skeleton on which to act and they become abductors of the limb rather than effectors of extension or flexion.

- The medial side of the radius has no muscle cover and hence, when the limb is abducted, the skin is easily penetrated by the distal radial fragment as it rotates inwards (Fig. 4.39).

Splinting

● The objectives of support for fractures in this region are to prevent abduction of the limb and to achieve maximum stability at the fracture site.

Application

● A Robert Jones and caudal splint should be applied to a limb as described for Region II above.

● The *lateral splint* should extend from the ground to the level of the horse's mid-scapula. Padding may be required around the splint as it overlies the rib cage and taping a figure of eight around the body to hold the free end of the splint helps to stabilise it.

● The lateral splint extension prevents the distal limb from being abducted (Fig. 4.40).

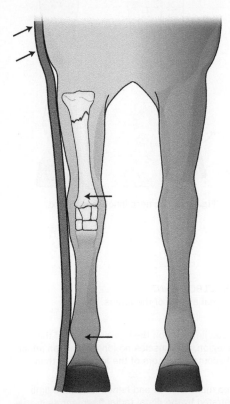

Fig. 4.40 See description in main text.

REGION IV: PROXIMAL TO ELBOW

Fractures of the humerus, ulna or neck of scapula.

Biomechanics

● Fractures of these bones are well protected by muscle cover and are closely attached to the body on their deep surface. This minimises the need to protect the actual fracture.

● However, fractures in these locations disable the triceps apparatus, making it impossible for the horse to fix the elbow for weight bearing. This results in the horse being unable to control the limb.

Splinting

● The objective is to fix the carpus in the extended position so that the horse has greater control over the limb and can use it to balance with.

Application

● A simple padded bandage and a splint placed down the caudal aspect of the leg, with the carpus taped to the splint, is sufficient to maintain the carpus in an extended and locked position for weight-bearing support.

Hindlimb

REGION I: DISTAL TO THE DISTAL THIRD OF THE THIRD METATARSAL BONE

Application

● Can be treated in the same way as the forelimb.

● The dorsal splint can be difficult to apply and the horse may require sedation to prevent it from snatching the limb up while it is being handled.

● The leg is best held under the hock in slight extension by an assistant while the dorsal splint is applied.

● Care must be taken so that the proximal limit of the splint does not dig into the hock.

REGION II: FROM DISTAL TO PROXIMAL METATARSUS

Application

● A lighter Robert Jones bandage is applied than in the forelimb (because it is more difficult to bandage the tarsus and the splints are more likely to slip).

● Splints are applied to the caudal and lateral aspect of the limb, using the *tuber calcis* as the proximal limit.

REGION III: THE TARSUS AND TIBIA

Biomechanics

● Under normal circumstances, the reciprocal apparatus causes the hock to flex and extend in unison with the stifle.

● Following fracture of the tibia or tarsus the reciprocal apparatus will act on the fracture – flexion of the stifle causes overriding at the fracture site instead of hock flexion.

- The stifle cannot be fixed but the distal limb can be stabilised to minimise trauma to the fracture site.
- As in the forelimb, the principal musculature is located on the lateral aspect of the limb and hence the distal limb tends to be abducted.

Application

- A Robert Jones bandage is applied from the ground surface as far proximal as possible.
- The most stable splinting arrangement utilises a lightweight metal bar, bent to form a loop which follows the contours of the limb on its cranio-lateral and caudo-lateral aspects, firmly fixed to the surface of the Robert Jones bandage (Fig. 4.41). A thin, concrete reinforcement rod or similar provides appropriate splinting material.
- It may not be possible to fabricate a splint as described above and a simple alternative is to position a straight splint over the lateral aspect of the limb, extending diagonally from the ground, across the hock to proximal to the stifle (Fig. 4.42).

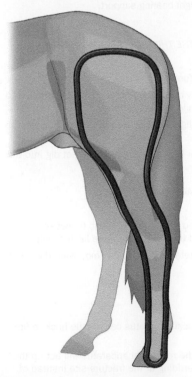
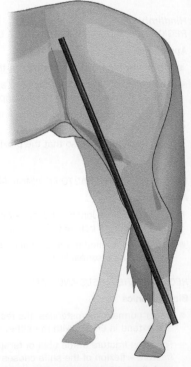

Fig. 4.41 See description in main text.   **Fig. 4.42** See description in main text.

REGION IV: FEMUR

It is not possible to immobilise fractures of the femur by external splinting. However, the vast overlying muscle mass will provide a large degree of natural stability and will allow the horse to maintain some functional control over the limb.

Other actions

- Support must be provided for the contralateral limb, which will have to bear double the load and hence will be at greater risk of injury. A firm support bandage, extending from the proximal metacarpus/metatarsus to coronary band, should be applied.

The risk of infection must be minimised by appropriate management of any open wounds and administration of systemic antibiotics.

- Open wounds should be carefully debrided of obvious contaminants and lavaged with sterile saline or Hartman solution. (A 1 L bag of fluids with a small hole cut at the nozzle provides a useful means of lavage.)

- A sterile, hydro gel (Intrasite, Smith and Nephew) or antibiotic ointment should then be lightly applied to the wound. Sterile, non-adherent dressings (Allevyn, Melonin, Smith and Nephew) should be laid over the wound.

- If penetration of the skin has occurred, broad-spectrum antibiotic coverage should be started. A combination effective against Gram +ve and Gram –ve bacteria should be used (e.g. benzyl penicillin, 15 mg/kg and gentamicin, 3 mg/kg, by intravenous injection).

- Analgesia should be provided in the form of non-steroidal anti-inflammatory drugs, alpha-2 agonists (e.g. xylazine) or opiates (e.g. butorphanol, 0.1 mg/kg, Torbugesic, Willows Francis). It is a good idea to discuss the choice of drug with the accepting referral centre as it may affect their anaesthetic protocol.

- Arrange referral to an appropriate centre.

- Make contact by telephone *before* sending case.

- Check on the requirements for transport.

- Write a brief referral note with details of all medication clearly described.

- Instruct owners to contact insurance company as soon as possible.

Transportation

- Horses will sometimes panic when first attempting to move after a large bandage and/or splints have been applied, especially to the hindlimbs. They need to be given additional support at this time and someone holding the tail, in addition to one or two assistants on the head will greatly increase its stability.

- The horse should be moved the minimum distance (i.e. the transport vehicle should be brought as close as possible to the animal). Foals should be carried wherever possible.

- Lorries tend to provide a more stable ride than trailers but usually have a higher and steeper ramp. If loading/unloading facilities are available this should not be a problem. If a trailer is used it should be of the wider variety, ideally have rear- and front-loading doors and should have long, gently sloping ramps.

- **Horses with an injury to a forelimb should be loaded facing rearwards and those with a hindlimb injury, forwards** (during transportation acceleration of the vehicle is more controllable than braking and hence the forces tend to be greatest on the forward-facing limbs).

- During transport, the horse should be strictly confined with chest and rump bars or chains and partitions to squeeze it into as limited space as possible. This will minimise the effort required by the horse to maintain its balance and may provide it with an opportunity to rest. The horse should be tied with a generous length of free lead rope to allow it to use its head and neck to maintain balance.

- Modern ambulance trailers are becoming more readily available. These have the good features described above together with a broad belly-band to provide additional support for the horse in transit.

Tendon Lacerations

- Partial or complete severance of tendons is a relatively frequent complication following lacerations to the distal limb in the horse. The tendons are relatively exposed and the surrounding soft tissues afford little protection. Such injuries most frequently occur at exercise and may be the consequence of interference between limbs or contact with a sharp object such as a flint or wooden stake, etc.

- Damage to extensor tendons carries a relatively good prognosis and usually requires standard wound management with no attempt being made to repair the severed tendon.

- Lacerations to flexor structures (superficial digital flexor tendon (SDF), deep digital flexor tendon (DDF) or suspensory apparatus) are far more serious and carry a guarded prognosis. These structures are an essential component of the load-bearing apparatus of the limb and their failure may result in its partial or complete collapse.

Signs

- Clinical signs vary depending on the structures affected.

- The size of the skin wound correlates *poorly* with prognosis: a penetrating object which creates only a stab in the skin could well result in complete severance of both superficial and deep digital flexor tendons.

- When vital flexor structures have been involved, lameness is usually severe (with the horse reluctant to bear weight on the limb).

- The stance adopted by the limb will reflect the structures involved (Fig. 4.43).

First aid

Continued attempts by the horse to bear weight on the affected limb will result in increased tension in the damaged structures leading to further injury. First aid is directed towards minimising these detrimental forces.

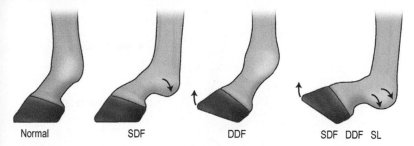

Fig. 4.43 Position adopted by digit in various traumatic injuries involving the supportive structures.

By straightening the distal limb so that the dorsal cortices of the phalanges are all vertical and in axial alignment all weight-bearing loads are removed from the flexor structures.

Application

- Open wounds should be managed as described above.
- The limb should then be bandaged and splinted as described for Region I above.
- Antibiotic and analgesic therapy should be administered as described previously.

It should be noted that attempts to reduce strains in the flexor structures by raising the heels of the foot are misdirected and contraindicated (Fig. 4.44).

Penetration of Synovial Structures

- Diarthrodial joints, tendon sheaths and bursae rely on the lubricant properties of synovial fluid to achieve their functional requirements. Consequently, they exist as separate compartments lined with a synovial membrane to produce and contain synovial fluid.
- Synovial fluid provides a medium within which many bacteria can flourish. In addition, the relative avascularity of synovial cavities renders bacterial infections within them functionally protected from normal immunological defence mechanisms.
- The inflammatory reaction that occurs within a synovial structure secondary to bacterial infection results in the production of destructive enzymes, which are extremely damaging to associated tissues (in particular articular cartilage). Unchecked, these secondary effects of infection can rapidly lead to irreversible tissue damage and permanent functional impairment of the structure involved.
- The prevention of these potentially life-threatening complications relies on *early* diagnosis and implementation of appropriate treatment (consisting of systemic

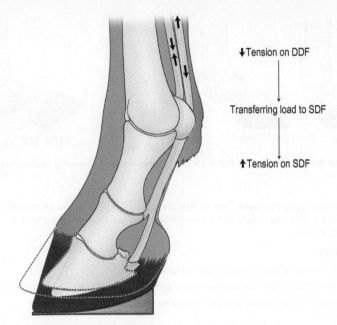

↓Tension on DDF

↓

Transferring load to SDF

↓

↑Tension on SDF

Fig. 4.44 Effect of heel elevation on the tension in the flexor tendons.

antibiotics and debridement/lavage of the structure involved). The prognosis for successful resolution decreases dramatically with increased time interval between injury and institution of appropriate treatment.

● In adult horses, the most common route of infection of synovial structures is direct contamination following trauma.

● The risk of bacterial contamination of a synovial structure (joint, tendon sheath or bursa) *must* be considered with *any* laceration or penetrating wound in its proximity.

First aid

The risk of involvement of deeper structures must be evaluated for each injury; therefore, knowledge of relevant anatomy is important.

Synovial structures more frequently affected include (Fig. 4.45):

● distal limb joints
● carpal and tarsal joints
● elbow joint
● flexor digital sheath
● flexor tarsal sheath.

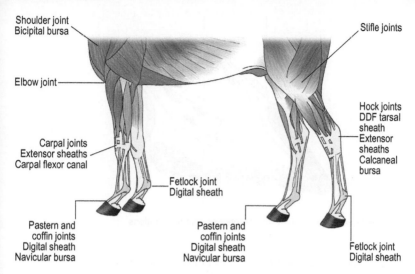

Shoulder joint
Bicipital bursa

Stifle joints

Elbow joint

Hock joints
DDF tarsal
sheath
Extensor
sheaths
Calcaneal
bursa

Carpal joints
Extensor sheaths
Carpal flexor canal

Fetlock joint
Digital sheath

Pastern and
coffin joints
Digital sheath
Navicular bursa

Pastern and
coffin joints
Digital sheath
Navicular bursa

Fetlock joint
Digital sheath

Fig. 4.45 Synovial structures most frequently involved in traumatic injuries.

Deep wounds in the proximity of these structures should be treated with suspicion. Signs suggestive of their involvement may include:

- variable lameness
- synovial fluid leaking from the wound (may be visible as a spurt when the joint is flexed)
- distension of the joint/sheath at a point remote from the initial injury
- in severe lacerations, articular cartilage or tendon within the sheath may be visible.

If there is serious concern that a synovial structure is involved, the horse *must* be admitted or referred for further investigation. Wounds should be lightly debrided, lavaged and bandaged as described previously. Antibiotic and analgesic therapy similar to that already discussed should be considered.

Puncture wounds to the sole of the foot

- Penetration of the sole of a horse's foot by a sharp object is potentially life-threatening. Contamination of the navicular bursa or distal interphalangeal joint may result in infection that is refractory to treatment and rapidly leads to irreversible damage to associated structures. Therefore, all such injuries *must* be treated seriously.
- To stage the relative risk of penetrating injury the foot can be divided anatomically into three regions (Fig. 4.46).

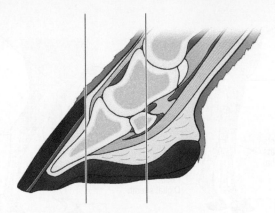

Fig. 4.46 Regions of the foot with respect to sole penetrations.

Penetrations in the *mid third* of the foot run the greatest risk of:

1. contaminating the navicular bursa
2. contaminating the distal interphalangeal joint
3. damaging the deep digital flexor tendon
4. damaging the navicular bone.

The risk of complicating injuries is determined also by depth/direction of penetration.

> **Often the owner will have removed the penetrating object (nail, etc.) before you arrive. If so, get them to keep it and to describe to you the depth and direction of penetration. If it is still in the foot, try and radiograph the digit with the object *in situ*.**

If from the site, depth and direction of penetration there is deemed to be a serious risk that a vital structure may have been affected, further investigations are indicated.

Prognosis for successful resolution of septic navicular bursitis decreases dramatically with increased interval between injury and onset of treatment. If there is serious concern that the navicular bursa or associated structures, may have been penetrated, the horse should be admitted or referred as soon as possible for further investigations.

Neurological Injury

- Traumatic injury to the central nervous system (CNS) is relatively common in the horse.
- CNS trauma can result from collisions, penetrating wounds or falls. Severe cranial trauma is more likely in falls in which the horse rears over backwards, striking its occipital or parietal bones.
- Injuries involving the brain stem may result in cardiovascular abnormalities, which can rapidly become fatal.
- Clinical signs vary widely in severity depending on the location and magnitude of the injury.
- Signs may increase or decrease in severity with time depending on subsequent pathophysiological changes within the damaged tissues. Ischaemia secondary to vascular disruption or small vessel thrombosis can lead to the release of inflammatory mediators resulting in further tissue damage, oedema and additional vascular compromise (in a vicious circle).

Evaluation

- Initial evaluation must be directed towards the most life-threatening factors: airway, breathing, cardiovascular function.
- A brief, but thorough, physical examination should be conducted for external signs of trauma.
- A neurological examination should then be performed in order to determine the location and, if possible, the extent of CNS damage.

Cranial trauma

Horses with cranial trauma should be evaluated for level of consciousness, cranial nerve deficits (especially pupil size, symmetry and response), alterations in respiratory pattern, posture and motor function:
- Coma, rigid extension of all four limbs, abnormal respiratory patterns, bilateral dilated pupils indicate a hopeless prognosis.

Spinal trauma

Following close examination of the head, horses with spinal trauma should be subjected to a systematic neurological examination including evaluation of the gait and posture, neck and forelimbs, trunk and hindlimbs and tail and anus.

- A recumbent horse should be observed for the ability to rise:
    - If only able to raise head → cranial cervical lesion
    - Head and neck but not thoracic limbs → C4–T2
    - Able to achieve dog-sitting posture → caudal to T2.
- Upper and lower motor neurone lesions should be differentiated:
    - Flaccid paralysis with hypo- or areflexia → lower motor neurone
    - Increased muscle tone, hyperactive spinal reflexes → upper motor neurone

- Spinal reflexes may be evaluated by testing the response to pinching the distal extremity and observing flexion of the joints in the forelimb and patellar and flexor reflexes in the hindlimb.
- Absence of cognitive response to pain stimulus suggests a loss of sensory pathways and is a poor prognostic indicator.

First aid

- Initial efforts should be directed to controlling life-threatening complications (although there may be little you can do).
- Sedation may be required in order to perform a clinical examination (xylazine, 0.1–0.15 mg/kg IV; 0.2–0.5 mg/kg IM).
- Convulsions may be controlled with diazepam (10–30 mg IV for foal; up to 200 mg for adult).
- Open wounds should be debrided and covered with sterile dressings.
- Broad-spectrum antimicrobial cover should be initiated as soon as possible.
- Tetanus prophylaxis must be ensured.
- Neurological case should be moved with great care – ataxia or motor dysfunction may predispose to further falls which could exacerbate the injury.
- Transport considerations are similar to those already discussed. Loading and transport of recumbent horses is really only practicable in a specialised ambulance trailer.

Part 4 CLINICAL AIDS

Section 8
Clinical techniques

ELECTROCARDIOGRAPHY

The most useful lead configuration is BASE–APEX: this arrangement is less affected by movement and respiration:

RA (right arm): Right jugular groove 1/3 up neck.

LA (left arm): Left lower thorax at apex beat (intercostal space 6).

RL (right leg): EARTH (any place remote but best to make equilateral triangle with other two, e.g. at withers).

1. Record 1 mV standard (ensure sensitivity is lowest possible at start).

2. Select speed (25 mm/second) – useful to have one section at 50 mm/second.

3. Select 'LEAD I'.

4. Select: RUN.

Table 4.7 Normal ECG duration values

		P-wave duration (ms)	P–R interval (ms)	QRS duration (ms)	Q–T interval (ms)
Horse	Mean	140	330	130	510
	range	(80–200)	(220–560)	(80–170)	(320–640)
Pony	Mean	100	217	78	462
	range	(85–106)	(209–226)	(66–86)	(420–483)

From: Hilwig RW (1987) Cardiac arrhythmias. In: NE Robinson, ed. Current Therapy in Equine Medicine, Volume 2. WB Saunders, Philadelphia.

Notes:

● Superimposed 50 mHz pattern from mains lights (fluorescent tubes, etc.) or from main supply if instrument is not effectively earthed – use 'EMG' filter and/or internal batteries.

● EARTH electrode is important. If not effective wandering of base line with/without movement and inordinate 50 Hz interference are produced.

● Ensure good gel/spirit contact at all sites (spirit contact will dry quickly).
  ● **KEEP ACCURATE RECORDS AND RELEVANT ECG TRACE.**
  ● **CLEARLY IDENTIFIED/DATED with technical data written onto trace (sensitivity/speed/power source/lead arrangement – particularly if other than normal).**

Interpretation

The following represent the parameters which are recorded at Liverpool University for routine ECG interpretation in the horse:

1. PULSE RATE = ?/min HEART RATE = ?/min
   PULSE DEFICIT: YES/NO
2. JUGULAR PULSE: YES/NO
   Description:
3. MUCOUS MEMBRANE COLOUR:
4. CRT = ?sec
5. GENERALISED SIGNS OF CHF? YES/NO List:
6. Objective questions from ECG:
   ● Is there a P for QRS?
   ● Is there a QRS for every P?
   ● Are all the complexes the same?
   ● Are F waves present?
   ● Any pauses/irregularities?
   ● Any S-T slurring/depression?
7. Comments/diagnosis:

See Figs 4.47–4.50.

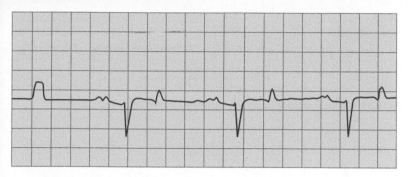

Fig. 4.47 Normal ECG trace obtained from a fit thoroughbred horse.

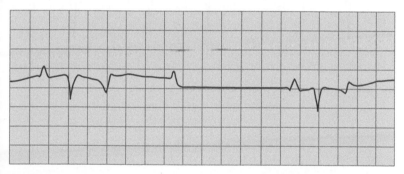

Fig. 4.48 ECG trace obtained from a fit thoroughbred horse showing common (benign) second-degree heart block.

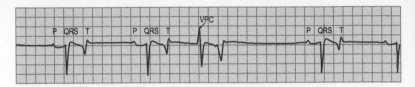

Fig. 4.49 ECG trace showing ventricular premature contractions.

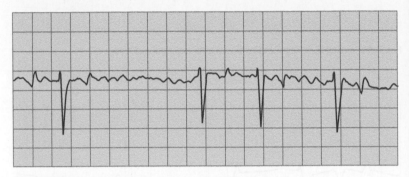

Fig. 4.50 ECG trace obtained from a case of atrial fibrillation.

Foetal Electrocardiograph

This is an effective method for determining the viability of a foal (in the later stages of pregnancy only).

It is vitally important to establish the mare's normal electrocardiographic activity before attempting this procedure. It is probably impossible to eliminate the mare's ECG from the trace and the detectable activity from the foal is usually very faint. Record this according to the method described above.

Most useful lead configuration is BASE–APEX taken across the abdomen (less affected by maternal activity):

RA (right arm): Right sublumbar fossa.

LA (left arm): Ventral midline.

RL (right leg): EARTH (any place remote but best in perineum or in left sublumbar fossa) (Fig. 4.51).

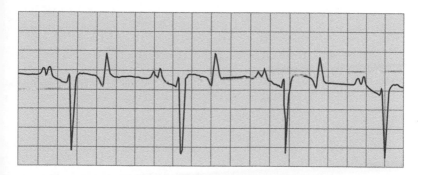

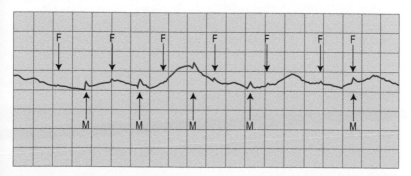

Fig. 4.51 Top: ECG trace taken from a pregnant mare in the last trimester of pregnancy. Bottom: Foetal ECG trace showing the faint recordings of the foetal activity (F) with the more obvious maternal activity (M). The foetal rate is approximately 130 bpm, while the maternal rate is approximately 40 bpm.

1. Switch on all available filters and preferably use internal battery power for procedure to avoid interference.
2. Record 1 mV standard (ensure sensitivity is highest possible at start).
3. Select speed (25 mm/second) – useful to have one section at 50 mm/second.
4. Select 'LEAD I'.
5. Select RUN.

It may be necessary to adjust the position of the electrodes as the position/location of the foal may vary – even side of pregnancy may be important.

PASSAGE OF NASOGASTRIC TUBE

There are significant risks in the process of nasogastric intubation that can be almost entirely eliminated if appropriate care and precautions are taken. The procedure can be complicated by conditions that preclude swallowing such as pharyngeal paralysis or grass sickness or when the oesophagus is obstructed or damaged.

Note:
- It is extremely difficult to pass an orogastric tube and indeed there are few circumstances when that is required.

Procedure

- The horse MUST be properly restrained (ideally in stocks). Sedation or twitching may be needed but these sometimes add to the difficulty.
- A suitable size of tube should be used for the size of the horse; also the condition may dictate the type and size of tube to be used.
- Over-small tubes may kink and may not trigger a swallow when the tube arrives in the pharynx.
- Excessively large tubes will inevitably cause nasal trauma.
- Some plastic tubes are very rigid when cold so it may be useful to warm the tube slightly. Over-softening can, however, make the procedure more difficult.
- The end of the tube must be lubricated slightly with a suitable water-soluble inert jelly.
- The tube is inserted into the ventral meatus of the nose with the curve directed in a downwards direction so that the end slides smoothly along the ventral meatus.
- Passage along the middle meatus will usually result in impact with the delicate ethmoidal region and a heavy nosebleed is the inevitable result.
- The horse's neck should be flexed as the tube reaches the pharynx and, as the horse swallows, the tube is gently but firmly advanced into the oesophagus.

  The position of the tube can be checked in the following ways:

  1. Direct observation of the left upper jugular groove – the tube can be seen readily in most normal horses as it passes down the oesophagus.
  2. If the tube is in the trachea it cannot be seen in the jugular furrow and it may rattle inside the trachea. The horse MAY also cough, although this is not a regular event.
  3. Blowing and sucking on the end of the tube is also a useful discriminator.

- The tube is correctly located in the oesophagus when the operator can blow but not suck on the tube.
- If the tube is in the trachea, the operator can blow and suck on the tube.
- If the tube is kinked, then neither blowing nor sucking is possible.

- Once satisfied that the tube is correctly located, it is advanced gently until it reaches the stomach. Gas or fluid may exit the tube – both are obviously gastric in nature.
- The tube should always be removed smoothly and slowly especially as it passes back through the pharynx.

Potential complications

1. **Resentment to passage attempts with rearing or stamping.** This should be controlled by sedation – sometimes a twitch will make matters worse in these individuals.
2. **Failure to enter the oesophagus.** This can be a part of the disease entity and is possible also if the patient is sedated. It also occurs if the tube is not handled correctly during the procedure. The neck should be flexed to ensure a suitable pharyngeal stimulus to swallowing is obtained.
3. **Nasal haemorrhage**. This occurs occasionally even with good technique but is then usually minimal. Where errors of placement result in severe ethmoid damage, haemorrhage is usually severe. Most cases will stop eventually, but it can be highly alarming and is a considerable hindrance to continued investigation. Occasionally, haemorrhage occurs when the horse moves suddenly through no fault of the operator. Haemorrhage can also occur when the tube is withdrawn too quickly.
4. **Rupture of the pharynx** is an extremely rare event and is usually associated with poor-quality tubes or with sharp, damaged tubes.
5. **Oesophageal rupture** is even more rare. Usually, if this occurs, there is existing pathology such as necrosis or severe obstruction.
6. **Pharyngeal kinking** with delivery of the tube into the oral cavity. This can result if there is an early strong stimulus to swallowing and poor timing of the tube delivery. It can also occur with use of a small-diameter tube.
7. **Gastric knotting of the tube**. This rare event can occur if an excessively long length of tube is introduced into the stomach. This is a disaster that is almost impossible to resolve. It is useful to measure the tube and to use only tubes of suitable length for the horse.

PLACEMENT OF A SUBPALPEBRAL LAVAGE SYSTEM

Placement of a subpalpebral lavage system is an extremely useful therapeutic procedure. It permits medication of a horse with a painful eye or when there is patient resistance/objection and also precludes any rough handling that might be detrimental to the health of the damaged eye. It is a simple procedure that is under-utilised in practice.

Procedure

- Sedation is essential in all cases.
- Motor nerve blockade of the upper lid via an auriculopalpebral nerve block prevents blepharospasm of the upper eyelid and allows the eye to be examined without any force being applied.

- Sensory nerve block of the upper lid is essential and can be achieved by use of a frontal nerve block.

- It is essential also to anaesthetise the conjunctiva by instilling proxymetacaine or proparacaine into the conjunctival sac some 3–5 minutes before placement of the lavage system begins.

Note:
- The procedure cannot be performed without appropriate motor and sensory blockade – if necessary, a general anaesthetic may be needed.

- Once the effect of the nerve blocks has been confirmed, a plastic disposable tongue depressor is introduced into the upper fornix of the conjunctival sac to protect the eye from damage during the procedure.

- The trochar/introducer is inserted into the conjunctival sac and the sharp point is gently run outwards to locate the rim of the orbit. It is then advanced through the conjunctiva, muscles of the eyelid and skin to emerge dorsolaterally.

- Depending on the system used, the lavage catheter is drawn behind (or through) the trochar so that the footplate is pulled into the dorsolateral fornix of the conjunctival sac.

- The tube is glued to the skin of the upper eyelid and led away between the ears and down the mane (plaiting the mane provided suitable restraint for the catheter, but it is sometimes helpful to suture the catheter in position).

- The delivery port is fastened onto the end of the tube and the lavage medication introduced at appropriate intervals.

Note:
- The subpalpebral lavage systems can be fitted from the lower lid but, while this may be more convenient in some respects, the surface distribution of medications is not ideal.

Potential Complications

1. **Infection**: This should not occur but as it is almost impossible to sterilise the conjunctival sac, it does occasionally occur. Most cases are due to poor or sloppy technique.

2. **Ulceration of the cornea**: Poor placement of the conjunctival flange with a slack tube within the conjunctival sac can result in significant iatrogenic ulceration. This is an unacceptable complication and the tube should be removed and relocated.

3. **Fracture of the tube**: This may be manageable if the conjunctival/palpebral component is intact.

PARACENTESIS ABDOMINIS

Procedure

- Clip/prepare midline, midway between umbilicus and xiphoid (most dependent part).
- Identify site of fluid pocket using linear ultrasound scanner (7.5 MHz).
- EITHER:
    (a) Use 19 g 2″ hypodermic needle thrust through linea alba. Twist and withdraw slightly and/or turn hub to encourage flow.

OR:

    (b) Use guarded No 11 scalpel blade to make stab incision through skin to depth of about 1 cm into linea alba. Carefully thrust teat cannula through linea alba.
- Collect into EDTA and plain and sterile plain tubes (twisting needle/cannula often helps).
- Assess colour, viscosity and clarity immediately.
- Submit the specimen to laboratory for cytology (white cell count/differential cytology) and protein analysis (if required, sterile sample for bacteriology should be placed in biphasic (blood) culture medium immediately).

Comments

1. Sampling from very young foals can be very difficult – the intestinal wall is often very fragile/thin and is easily damaged. In these cases, it is a wise precaution to identify a pocket of fluid by ultrasonographic examination and insert the needle directly into the pocket.
2. Fat horses may be difficult to sample – may need a long needle (e.g. 7.5 cm spinal needle), but this is also much more dangerous and less controllable.
3. Horses with severe/significant abdominal distension should not be sampled – risk of abdominal puncture and leakage. The risk of leakage in normal horses is low, but is present.

Potential complications

1. **Local infection in abdominal wall**: This is simply a matter of technique and ensuring asepsis.
2. **Perforation of intestine by needle or cannula**: This is rare, but it is a significant possibility.
3. **Inadvertent entry into the gut with ingesta delivered via the paracentesis**: If this occurs, the needle must be removed and relocated. Repeated puncture is a potentially harmful situation.
4. **Bowel rupture** caused by movement of distended gut over the sharp end of the needle. This is probably unavoidable but is more likely if there is a distended viscus.
5. **Peritonitis**: This can arise from dirty technique or from bowel leakage into the peritoneal cavity.

Note:
- Most complications can be avoided by a combination of careful case selection (there is no point in performing this if the case is definitely going to surgery anyway) and by use of ultrasonographic guidance to identify a suitable pocket of fluid in a safe location.

PARACENTESIS THORACIS

Procedure

- Prepare site on *both* sides (always tap both) at 7–9th I–C space at level of point of shoulder.
- Identify suitable pocket of fluid using ultrasound (preferably sector scanner).
- Local analgesia at site and stab incision in skin.
- Use trochar and cannula or 10 gauge IV catheter or 16 gauge needle as appropriate (all with three-way tap or one-way (Heimlich) valve). Insert off anterior edge of rib.
- Collect into plain sterile, EDTA and plain tubes.
- Assess quantity, colour, clarity and odour immediately.
- Submit to laboratory for cytology, bacteriology and protein analysis. If bacteriology required, place sample in biphasic (blood) culture bottle immediately.

Comments
1. The pleural cavities of young horses are usually separated but become contiguous with age or with any degrees of pleural cavity infection/inflammation.
2. It is entirely possible that an old horse might have separated pleural cavities – therefore, both sides should always be sampled – there may be significant differences in content, which might be very useful.

Potential complications

1. **Pneumothorax**: This can be avoided by correct technique and it is unlikely to occur except when no consideration is given to the maintenance of the pleural negative pressure. Puncture of the lung can also cause some degree of pneumothorax. Repeated punctures should be avoided. (Ultrasonography may help to identify a safe location.)
2. **Infection**: This can usually be avoided by careful asepsis throughout the procedure.
3. **Haemothorax**: This is a very unusual event. Although cardiac puncture could occur, it reflects very poor placement and poor technique.

TRANSTRACHEAL WASH/ASPIRATE

Equipment

There are commercially available tracheal aspiration kits that are designed for this purpose and which include all the instruments required. Alternatively, the following can be used:

- Suitable clipping/surgical scrub materials.
- Local anaesthetic agent (e.g. 2 mL mepivacaine solution).
- 10–12 gauge intravenous catheter or a small (sheep) trochar and cannula.
- Male dog urinary catheter (suitable to pass down the IV cannula).
- Syringes and saline solution.

Procedure

- Clip/prepare site 2/3 down the neck. The trachea is usually palpable subcutaneously in the midline.
- Local anaesthetic agent (5–10 mL 2% lidocaine (lignocaine) hydrochloride, for example) is injected in/under the skin in midline and between rings at selected site (tracheal rings easily palpable under skin).
- Pass wide gauge (≥12 gauge cannula or a fine metal trochar and cannula) between rings into trachea (downward) and remove needle (be careful not to damage far side of trachea!) – leaving cannula directed downwards.
- Pass long flexible catheter (e.g. 16/18 gauge dog urinary catheter) downwards until cough induced (end of catheter now at carina).
- Introduce 20–40 mL sterile phosphate buffered saline (PBS).
- Immediately aspirate into sterile syringe while withdrawing catheter slightly (fluid accumulations at the thoracic inlet are sampled). Repeat the aspiration several times to obtain an effective harvest of fluid.
- Collect sample in plain sterile, EDTA and plain tubes.
- Submit to lab for bacteriology and cytology. (If bacteriology is required, place appropriate sample in transport medium or use blood culture (biphasic medium).)

Comments

1. Do not use a needle as a cannula, it may cut the catheter in half and leave a piece in the trachea!

2. A fine sheep trochar and cannula can also be used and has the added advantage of being firm and it cannot, therefore, be displaced/misdirected (upwards) by coughing. A stab incision through the skin with a scalpel blade is sometimes needed though!

3. Risks of procedure are minimal – localised infection at tracheal site is rare when due care is taken to ensure sterile technique.

4. Check first with laboratory on handling requirements – transport/postage causes marked degeneration of sample – laboratory may advise you to filter the sample through a gauze swab or to make smears immediately.

Potential complications

1. **Local infection** at site of catheter placement.
2. **Leakage of air from site** into subcutaneous tissues with localised emphysema.
3. **Chondroma formation** resulting from cartilage damage from poor placement.

BRONCHO-ALVEOLAR LAVAGE (BAL)

Procedure

It is common practice to sedate the horse before performing this technique. This is less distressing for the horse and reduces the risk of coughing during the procedure.

1. **With BAL catheter (Foggarty catheter)**:
   - Standing sedation (alpha-2 agonists and butorphanol are useful).
   - Pass BAL catheter ('Foggarty BAL catheter', Bivona, USA) into trachea (via ventral nasal meatus).
   - Introduce as far as possible to wedge in airway (inflate cuff if present).
   - Introduce 100–300 mL sterile phosphate buffered saline (PBS) under gentle pressure (lower volumes are now preferred).

2. **Via endoscope**:
   - This procedure is much easier but requires a very long endoscope (2 m is the minimum effective length).
   - Standing sedation (alpha-2 agonists and butorphanol are useful).
   - Pass endoscope into the trachea via the ventral nasal meatus.
   - Select the best site/side from clinical observations.
   - Introduce as far as possible to wedge in airway.
   - Introduce 100–300 mL sterile phosphate buffered saline (PBS) under gentle pressure (low volumes are now preferred).

Withdraw fluid into sterile plain, plain and EDTA tubes (expect to harvest 50% of original volume used – sometimes less). A successful BAL is indicated by the presence of froth in the aspirate. Submit for cytology and bacteriology (transport medium or biphasic (blood) culture medium).

Comments

1. Cease if coughing is severe.
2. Some horses are dull and may cough for 1–2 days following the procedure – lower volumes safer – fewer side effects.
3. Some horses are febrile for 24–48 hours after procedure.
4. May be performed using sheathed BAL catheter using an endoscope or via endoscope introduced until wedged.
5. Sterility of all equipment is important. It is very unwise to use the same apparatus for a second horse without full sterilisation first. Infectious respiratory disease can be severe if introduced directly into the lungs.
6. Check with laboratory before sending – delays may affect results and laboratory may want you to filter or otherwise prepare the sample prior to dispatch.
7. A successful washing is indicated by the presence of a foamy aspirate (suggestive of surfactant).
8. NORMAL washing contains alveolar macrophages, few degenerate neutrophils, epithelial/alveolar cells.

Potential complications

1. **Pulmonary infection** arising from non-sterile equipment or from retrograde infection during passage of catheter or scope.

2. **Many horses develop a transient fever** 24–72 hours after the procedure.

3. **Nasal or pulmonary haemorrhage** (very rare).

COLLECTION OF CEREBROSPINAL FLUID

Cerebrospinal fluid may be collected from:

- atlanto-occipital site (fluid obtained from the cisterna magna)
- lumbosacral site (fluid obtained from the sub-arachnoid space).

Collection from either site has significant difficulties and requires special precautions. Full aseptic precautions should be used at both sites. Emergency procedures should be available to control convulsions or collapse (in standing sampling).

Procedure

1. Collection via the atlanto-occipital site:

    - General anaesthesia is obligatory. The horse is placed in lateral recumbency. The area over the occipito–atlanto–axial region is clipped and prepared for aseptic surgery.

    - The site of entry is located in the midline at the centre of a triangle formed by the cranial margins of the wings of the atlas and the caudal extent of the nuchal crest (occipital protuberance).

    - A 7.5 cm (×1.2 mm) stiletted spinal needle is introduced in the midline exactly perpendicular to the long axis of the spine and parallel to the ground. It is essential that the needle is precisely placed to remain in the midline plane.

    - The needle is advanced for some 5–6 cm until a faint 'pop' is felt and resistance to introduction is much reduced. The stilette is then removed and the hub observed for egress of clear fluid.

    - If no fluid is obtained, the position should be carefully checked and the needle can be advanced slightly and rotated through 90° until fluid is obtained.

    - If no fluid is obtained after two attempts, the stilette is replaced and the procedure repeated from the start. Usually, if fluid is not obtained, the position or depth is wrong.

    - As soon as fluid is seen at the needle hub, a three-way tap is placed on the needle and closed to prevent excessive loss of pressure and fluid. A sample can then be obtained into a sterile syringe by slow aspiration. Free flow samples are usually safe as long as the intracranial pressure is normal.

    - The needle is then withdrawn.

2. Collection via the lumbosacral site (sub-arachnoid space):

- This procedure can be performed in the standing horse. Indeed, it is probably easier to perform in the standing, firmly restrained horse (stocks are essential). Sedation may be required but excessive ataxia can make accurate placement more difficult.

- The skin over the lumbosacral space is clipped and prepared aseptically. (Note: The dorsal spines of L6 and S1 are usually not palpable – they are shorter than those on either side.)

- A small dermal and subcutaneous bleb of local anaesthetic is placed at the site and a small stab incision is made with a scalpel.

- A stiletted 15 cm spinal needle (×1.2 mm) is introduced in the midline immediately caudal to the dorsal spine of L6.

- In most horses, the ideal site is on the line joining the cranial edges of the two tuber sacral and cranial to a line joining the caudal edges of the two tuber coxae.

- The needle is advanced exactly in the midline and exactly vertically (an assistant is useful in correcting the angle).

- The needle can be advanced with little resistance up to 12–13 cm (9–10 cm for ponies). A firm resistance is felt as the needle penetrates the dorsal inter-arcuate ligament.

- Loss of resistance and often a slight jerk from the horse (or tail movement) is felt and fluid usually issues from the needle as the stilette is withdrawn.

- Flow is sometimes sluggish and a needle aspiration may be helpful.

- If bone is felt or if no fluid is obtained then the needle should be withdrawn almost completely before starting again.

- The needle is withdrawn as soon as a suitable sample is obtained.

The fluid is observed immediately for evidence of colour change or cloudiness (it should be water clear). Samples of the fluid are placed in:

1. blood-culture medium (for bacteriological examination)
2. EDTA (for cytology)
3. plain tubes (for biochemical analysis).

Potential complications

1. **Infection** (avoided largely by aseptic technique).

2. **Haemorrhage** due to vascular trauma within subdural space (potentially dangerous but also complicates analysis).

3. **Rapid drop in CSF pressure with herniation of brain** (avoided by ensuring use of fine needle with tap).

4. **Convulsions on recovery** (avoided by use of anticonvulsants for recovery period and possibly over ensuing 24 hours).

BIOPSY

Bone Marrow Biopsy Aspirate

Bone marrow aspiration is under-utilised and is a useful method of investigation of non-regenerative anaemia because juvenile red cells are confined to the marrow. Reticulocytes are not present in circulating blood.

Procedure

- Full asepsis essential.
- Best site is in the midline, in the mid sternum region where the outer cortex of the sternebra is thin.
- Alternative sites include: wing of ilium, rib (both of these are more difficult).
- Use bone marrow punch (can sometimes use 12/14 gauge needle but inclined to break off) and aspirate using 20 mL syringe.
  - (i) AVOID excessive pressure for long periods.
  - (ii) Large blood flow undesirable (marrow difficult to find!).
- Collect into EDTA (with egg albumin) and make smear immediately (fix immediately with alcohol).
- For bone marrow biopsy, use biopsy needle and place bone marrow core biopsy directly into formol saline.
- Stain Giemsa (1:100 for 24 hours OR Leishman's or Wright–Giemsa).

Interpretation

- Normal erythropoiesis is suggested by a myeloid:erythroid ratio of less than 1.5 (i.e. there are three times as many red cell series cells as white).
- A regenerative response is indicated by a ratio of less than 0.5.
- Bone marrow cytology is very difficult to interpret – do not attempt this unless you have extensive equine experience in this field.
- The megakaryocyte count in the marrow is used to indicate the platelet generation status in cases of low circulating platelet numbers.

Comments

1. Discuss with clinical pathologist before performing technique to ensure suitable handling of sample (some prefer direct smears fixed with alcohol to be sent) but sometimes difficult to extract marrow from sample so suitable carrier medium and rapid transfer are important.
2. Failure to obtain suitable depth of buffy coat means excessive haemorrhage into sample.

Potential complications

1. **Infection** (osteomyelitis).
2. **Penetration through sternebrae into chest**.
3. **Haemorrhage** (especially if clotting defect is present).

Liver Biopsy
Procedure

- Full asepsis is essential.
- RIGHT SIDE is most convenient but low down on the left is also possible where the liver is small.
- Best site = centre of quadrangle formed by:
  - Line from point of elbow to point f hip.
  - Line from point of shoulder to point of hip.
  - 14th rib.
  - 10th rib.
- **Preferably locate and confirm the presence of the liver and its location (depth and direction) by ultrasonography of region (or laparoscopy). The outline of the liver may also be percussible on the right side.**
- Local analgesia of skin and intercostal muscles and pleura.
- Perform a stab incision with No. 11 blade adjacent to cranial edge of rib (BLOOD VESSELS ALONG CAUDAL EDGE).
- Insert 'Tru-Cut' biopsy instrument horizontally and through pleural space on expiration. 'Feel' each anatomical layer as instrument is advanced. Liver capsule is firm and liver usually denser than other tissues.
- Withdraw (open) cutting sheath of instrument and then advance cutting blade firmly without moving inner part.
- Remove sample in closed instrument. Usually not necessary to suture site. Administer antibiotic/tetanus cover.

Comments
1. Latest forms of Tru-Cut type biopsy instrument (Cook UK Ltd) have a spring-loaded cutting apparatus, which makes procedure much easier but they are expensive. These instruments are recommended because of the ease of use. It is better to get a suitable biopsy first time rather than have repeated attempts.
2. Older-type biopsy needles relying on vacuum are unreliable and may damage tissue sample. They are also much wider.

The site can be identified by using a long length of string held in the middle at the point of the hip (external angle of ilium) and the two ends drawn forward to the point of the shoulder and the point of the elbow. Counting in from the 18th rib is the best method of establishing the position (Fig. 4.52).

Important
The diagram should in no way remove the necessity for positive identification of the location of the liver by percussion, ultrasound or laparoscopy.

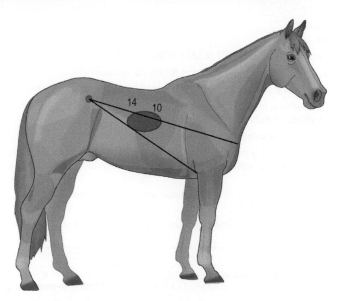

Fig. 4.52 Liver biopsy site showing major landmarks.

Notes:

- Coagulation status should be checked first.
- If chosen site is further back, then instrument needs to be angled progressively more downward and forward and length of instrument needs to be longer. Biopsy taken at the 14th intercostal space requires a much longer instrument, which should be aimed at opposite elbow.
- Ultrasound guidance should be employed if available (if not available, the case might be best referred to a specialist centre). Dubious defence if things go wrong if not used!
- Failure to obtain biopsy sample after two attempts usually means something is wrong – liver too small, instrument too short, positioning incorrect.
- Puncture of gut is a potentially serious hazard but a single clean puncture is seldom life-threatening.

Potential complications

1. **Infection** in pleural or peritoneal cavity.

2. **Abdominal haemorrhage.**

3. **Penetration of large colon** with tearing of wall or simple contamination from puncture site.

Lung Biopsy
Procedure

- Full asepsis essential. RIGHT or LEFT SIDE.
- Best site = level with shoulder joint in 8/9th rib space.
- Site can be confirmed or specifically selected with ultrasound guidance.
- Local anaesthetic in and under skin at site (anterior/cranial edge of rib – BLOOD VESSELS RUN ALONG CAUDAL EDGE).
- Stab incision with small scalpel blade.
- Insert 'Tru-Cut' biopsy instrument horizontally through intercostal muscles and parietal and visceral pleura and into lung (usually about 8 cm is enough distance).
- Withdraw and then advance cutting blade and remove sample in closed instrument.
- Place sample in formol saline (or in blood-culture medium if culture required).

> **Comment**
> Latest forms of Tru-Cut biopsy instrument have spring-loaded cutting apparatus, which makes procedure much easier but they are very expensive and are 'single use'.

Potential complications

1. **Danger of pneumothorax minimal**, but existent.
2. **Some pulmonary bleeding** is almost inevitable – transient epistaxis 1–4 hours later may be seen. Rarely significant but if severe can be life-threatening.
3. **Do not exercise horse for 48 hours (minimum).**

Skin Biopsy
Procedure

- Clip hair short but DO NOT SHAVE.
- Wash skin gently (do not scrub) and do not use alcohol-based antiseptics.
- Local analgesia (2% lidocaine (lignocaine) without adrenaline (epinephrine)) ring block (well away from selected site) or use regional anaesthesia if practicable.
- Wedge biopsy obtained using scalpel (include normal and lesion tissues). Or use punch biopsy instrument (according to requirements).
- Lesions such as skin nodules, sarcoid, granulation tissue, etc., are best biopsied in the centre.
- Shave biopsies are preferred for diagnosis of pemphigus, etc. – check with laboratory and if such samples are obtained remember to tell the lab so that appropriate sections can be cut.
- Skin scrapings and groomings (obtained by brushing with a tooth/nail brush onto a piece of cardboard or paper) are also useful for investigation of parasitic/fungal infections (place in brown paper envelope or in sterile universal bottle).
- Ensure that diagnostic tissue is obtained. Several biopsies may be required.

Comment
Some lesions are dangerous to biopsy by excision – impression smears or swab-based scrapings (squamous cell carcinoma of cornea) or fine-needle aspirates (melanoma) are better in these conditions.

Rectal Biopsy

The correlation of pathological disease of the intestine with the findings from a rectal biopsy has been questioned. Rectal biopsy is said to be helpful in the investigation of diarrhoea or weight loss syndromes or where proliferative/ infiltrative enteropathy is suspected. However, the technique is, at present, the only way a biopsy of any of the intestine can be obtained without laparotomy. The procedure is easily performed on the standing (sedated) horse.

Procedure

- Sedate and restrain appropriately. It is not necessary to use an epidural anaesthetic for the technique.
- Wash the perineum carefully with antiseptic wash and tie the tail out of the way (preferably within a tail bandage or sleeve).
- Introduce a lightly lubricated gloved hand *up to the wrist only*, into the rectum and evacuate the faeces.
- Use a sterile, endometrial, biopsy instrument (Yeoman's basket-jawed forceps or purpose-made rectal biopsy instrument) in the cupped hand within the rectum. The hand should not be inserted beyond the wrist.
- A mucosal fold of the dorsolateral rectal wall is gently grasped between thumb and forefinger and the instrument advanced to grasp the fold of mucosa just in a slightly dorsolateral position to the grasped fold.
- Taking a biopsy from the dorsolateral position avoids interference with the more prominent dorsal vasculature while maintaining the dorsal position that is an important part of the technique.
- The jaws of the instrument are closed firmly and the specimen is removed.
- Biopsy specimens required for bacteriological examination must be taken first and placed directly into Amies' charcoal medium.
- For histopathology, the specimen is placed in a container with appropriate fixative.
- Usually, formal saline is used, but Bouin's solution can be used. Advice from the pathologist should be sought if in doubt about the best fixative for the case in question.

Interpretation

- Positive changes that show definitive pathology are highly suggestive of bowel disease in the more proximal bowel but negative findings are much less helpful. A negative finding does not preclude the presence of infiltrative or infectious pathology.
- Significant findings include pathological bacteria and infiltrative inflammatory and non-inflammatory diseases.
- Many false or misleading results can be obtained, including mild eosinophilic infiltration and mild mucosal and submucosal inflammation.
- The risks from the procedure are minimal and are increased by inappropriate sedation/restraint, too deep a biopsy site and poor instrument maintenance.
- Antibiotics may be used prophylactically but they may not be strictly needed.

> **Comment**
> The instrument must be extremely sharp and well maintained.

Potential complications

1. **Rectal tears** are more liable to develop if dorsal or, more particularly, ventral biopsies are taken. A blunt instrument is more liable to cause tearing.

2. **Peritonitis** may develop if the biopsy is taken too far forward (i.e. in the peritoneal rectum).

3. **Bleeding** is a particularly unusual complication.

Ileal Biopsy

Ileal biopsy is a definitive method for diagnosis of equine dysautonomia (grass sickness) and may also be useful in other infiltrative diseases. However, biopsy requires a laparotomy (usually under general anaesthesia). There are reports of standing laparotomy biopsy but this should not be undertaken without very careful thought and surgical care.

Procedure

- The ileum is identified by tracing the ileocaecal fold from the caecum and the ileum is exteriorised.
- The proximal end of the ileum is identified as the point at which the ileocaecal fold disappears.
- An 8–10 cm length of ileum is gently clamped off with bowel clamps proximally and distally and the area packed off with saline-soaked surgipads.
- A full-thickness (transmural) biopsy of around 3–4 mm width and 2–3 cm in length is excised longitudinally midway between the anti-mesenteric border and the mesenteric border.
- The incision is closed in two layers using a Cushing's inverting suture pattern and the site irrigated copiously with warm sterile saline.
- The bowel is returned to the abdomen and after any other appropriate procedure is completed, the laparotomy is closed in the normal way.
- The biopsy is placed immediately into 10% formol saline for submission.

Interpretation

- The quality, quantity and location of the myenteric neurones are assessed.
- Interpretation requires considerable pathological skill but the results have a high specificity and sensitivity for grass sickness.

Complications

1. **Peritonitis should not occur** when this procedure is performed properly.
2. **Stricture formation may occur** if the biopsy is taken transversally (i.e. radially).

Testicular Biopsy

Testicular biopsy is indicated during investigation of reproductive failure or where obvious palpable or ultrasonographic pathology is present. Wedge biopsies can be obtained but this requires a much higher degree of invasion.

Procedure

● The procedure can be performed on the standing horse but this requires local anaesthesia and that may complicate both the biopsy and the procedure. Therefore, it is best performed under general anaesthesia using a Tru-Cut biopsy instrument.

● Full aseptic precautions are essential and simultaneous ultrasonographic guidance is helpful.

● The needle is inserted into an identified location and triggered to obtain a core biopsy.

● This is placed in Amie's charcoal medium if infection is suspected and/or into Bouin's fluid for histological examination.

Interpretation

Interpretation requires considerable pathological skill.

Complications

1. **Intratesticular haemorrhage** through inadvertent perforation of the testicular artery.
2. **Local abscessation/orchitis**.
3. **Adhesions** that prevent normal thermoregulation.

Muscle Biopsy

Muscle biopsy is indicated in some generalised conditions but also in some focal muscle disorders.

Generalised indications for muscle biopsy include:

- Polysaccharide storage myopathy (usually, semimembranous muscle is selected as a representative sample).
- Equine motor neurone disease (usually the caudalis dorsalis coccygeus muscle is chosen).
- White muscle disease.

Localised conditions for which muscle biopsy is indicated include:

- Focal muscle atrophy.

Procedure

- The skin overlying the chosen site is prepared for aseptic surgery.
- Local anaesthetic is infiltrated in such a way as to avoid direct insertion of anaesthetic agent into the chosen site (this will negate any benefit from the procedure).
- The skin is incised over the site to ensure adequate exposure of the muscle.
- Two parallel incisions are made along the length of the muscle running WITH the line of the fibres, to a depth of around 1 cm.
- The muscle is lifted from the underlying muscle belly and undermined carefully for the full length of the biopsy.
- The two ends are cut with a scalpel to release the muscle biopsy.
- The specimen is immediately placed on a cooled, saline-soaked swab for a minute or two before placing in formol saline.
- The skin incision is closed routinely in two layers.

Note:

- Biopsy instruments designed to obtain muscle biopsies via a cutaneous puncture are available but the biopsies are probably of less use.

Interpretation

Specialist muscle pathology labs must be used.

Complications

There are no significant complications.

Endometrial Biopsy

Endometrial biopsy is a routine procedure in equine stud farm medicine. It is indicated in the investigation of infertility or in the routine examination for breeding soundness. Mid-diestrus is the best stage to obtain diagnostic information.

> **BIOPSY MUST NOT BE ATTEMPTED, OF COURSE, IF THE MARE IS PREGNANT! PRIOR TO ANY INTRAUTERINE PROCEDURE, THE POSSIBILITY OF PREGNANCY MUST BE ELIMINATED!**

Procedure

- Suitable restraint is essential (stocks/chute) with or without sedation as indicated.
- The tail is wrapped and tied out of the field of view and the rectum evacuated of faeces.
- A rectal and ultrasonographic examination is performed to eliminate pregnancy as a cause of non-oestrus.
- The perineum is carefully washed. The lips of the vulva are carefully dried with a sterile paper towel.
- Using a (sterile) gloved hand introduced into the vagina the uterine biopsy instrument (Yeoman's Basket Biopsy Instrument) is introduced through the cervix into the uterus.
- The cervix may be drawn caudally with the index finger to straighten the uterine body.
- Once the instrument is located into the uterine body, the hand is withdrawn and introduced into the rectum.
- The forceps are palpated per rectum and the instrument is advanced into the previously identified location (horn, bifurcation or body) and the uterine wall is gently pressed into the open jaws of the instrument (which may be held sideways to facilitate the biopsy procedure).
- The jaws are closed firmly and the instrument is withdrawn.
- A fine bacterial swab is used to obtain a bacteriological sample from the biopsy before opening any formalin-containing receptacle in the vicinity.
- The biopsy specimen is lifted out of the basket with a fine needle (NOT forceps) and placed in Bouin's medium or formol saline.
- The specimen is submitted for routine histology.

Interpretation

- A specialist laboratory is advised.
- Interpretation can be very difficult and a full signalment and history is essential with the submission.

Complications

1. **Haemorrhage is rare**.
2. **Perforation of the uterus and/or rectum** are potential complications but are very rare if the procedure is properly performed.
3. **Intrauterine adhesions** may occur at the site.

BLOOD CULTURE

Blood culture is under-utilised in practice and is of particular value in diagnosis and management of foal (and adult horse) septicaemia, cerebrospinal fluid infections and joint infections, where conventional swabbing and culture methods are often unrewarding. The method is used to amplify the bacterial numbers in samples in which there are few organisms. Usually, a relatively large amount of blood (or synovial fluid or cerebrospinal fluid) is required to obtain a diagnostic culture and sensitivity and the blood-culture method using a biphasic culture medium offers this opportunity. As much fluid as possible should be collected. Sometimes only a few millilitres are possible.

Procedure

- The sample is obtained as aseptically as possible (to avoid contaminating bacteria). The skin should be allowed to dry thoroughly after spirit-based swabbing of the site (this will avoid false-negative cultures from the antiseptic effects of the spirit).
- The sample is transferred aseptically to the culture medium using a new sterile needle.
- The bottle is gently swirled and culture is begun in an incubator.

Interpretation

Culture results may be known by 24–36 hours but it is sometimes longer. Therefore, there is merit in instigating the process as soon as possible in the course of suspect disease.

Comment
- Blood cultures are usually negative if any antibiotic has been used prior to sampling.
- Cultures are easily contaminated unless suitable precautions are taken.

ROUTINE DIAGNOSTIC NERVE BLOCK SITES

Nerve blocking is a useful technique in diagnosing the source of pain in a lame horse and is also useful as a means of achieving analgesia. Its effective use requires knowledge of the anatomy of the limb and some basic skill and competence. Restraint of the horse during blocking is important for personal safety and use of an experienced handler and a twitch is advised. Difficult horses may require sedation with an α_2 agonist, preferably xylazine. However, sedatives can make the horse ataxic and lameness evaluation becomes more difficult; therefore, their use should be avoided where possible. All nerve blocks must be performed as aseptic procedures (Figs 4.53 and 4.54).

> **Note:**
> ● The areas of desensitisation depicted are a rough guide only and the clinician should be aware that diffusion of local anaesthetic solution might result in a greater portion of the limb being desensitised than was originally intended. The palmar digital block in particular will desensitise not only the palmar third of the foot, but also the sole and the majority of the coffin joint.

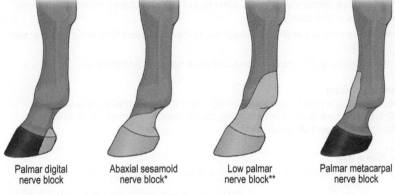

| Palmar digital nerve block | Abaxial sesamoid nerve block* | Low palmar nerve block** | Palmar metacarpal nerve block |

*   Palmar nerve block – at base of proximal sesamoid bone
** Palmar nerve block – just above fetlock

Fig. 4.53 Skin areas desensitised by diagnostic nerve blocks.

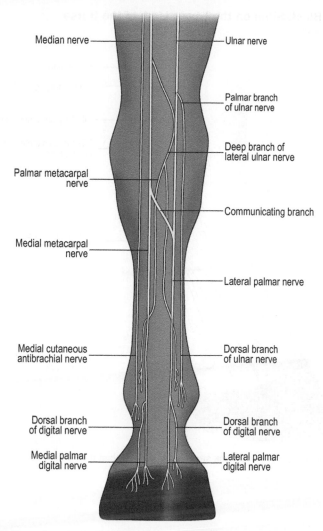

Median nerve

Ulnar nerve

Palmar branch
of ulnar nerve

Deep branch of
lateral ulnar nerve

Palmar metacarpal
nerve

Communicating branch

Medial metacarpal
nerve

Lateral palmar nerve

Medial cutaneous
antibrachial nerve

Dorsal branch
of ulnar nerve

Dorsal branch
of digital nerve

Dorsal branch
of digital nerve

Medial palmar
digital nerve

Lateral palmar
digital nerve

Fig. 4.54 Theoretical distribution of the major nerve pathways in the forelimb from the
mid-radius distally.

Nerve Block Sites on the Lower Limb of the Horse
See Fig. 4.55.

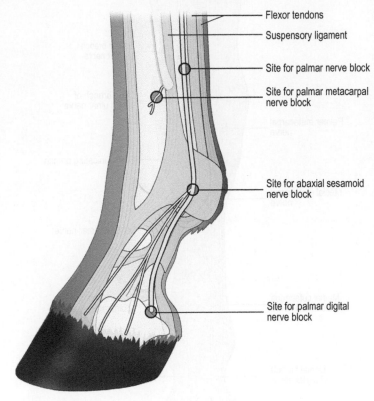

Flexor tendons

Suspensory ligament

Site for palmar nerve block

Site for palmar metacarpal nerve block

Site for abaxial sesamoid nerve block

Site for palmar digital nerve block

Fig. 4.55 Diagram of nerve block sites on the distal limb of the horse.

Palmar/Plantar Digital Nerve Block
See Fig. 4.56a–c.

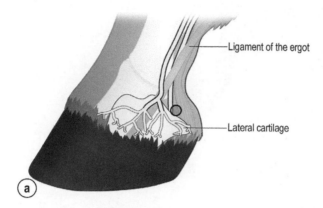

Fig. 4.56a Location of perineural (regional) analgesia of the palmar/plantar digital nerves – side view.

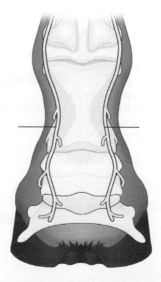

Fig. 4.56b Location of perineural (regional) analgesia of the palmar/plantar digital nerves – back view.

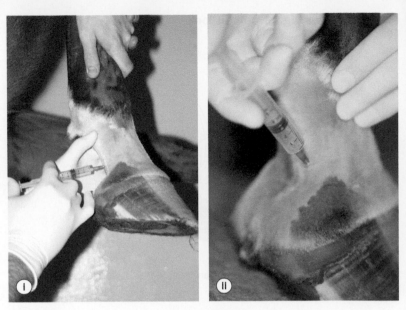

Fig. 4.56c Two views, i and ii, of a laterally performed injection on the palmar digital proximal site. Injections are also performed medially.

Aim: To block the lateral and medial palmar/plantar digital nerves at the level of the distal pastern.

The neurovascular bundle is easily palpable on the abaxial aspect of the deep digital flexor tendon (DDFT) in the pastern region of most horses. To perform a PD nerve block, a 25 gauge 16 mm needle is inserted subcutaneously over the neurovascular bundle just proximal to the collateral cartilage and 2 mL local anaesthetic is injected both medially and laterally.

Abaxial Sesamoid Block
See Fig. 4.57.

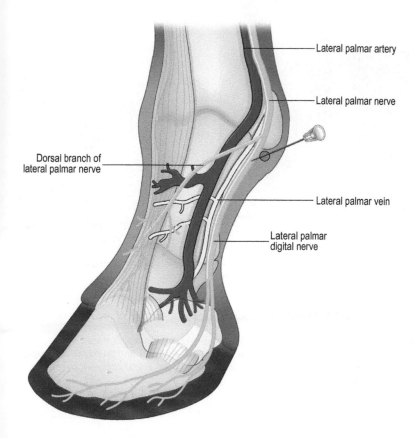

Lateral palmar artery

Lateral palmar nerve

Dorsal branch of
lateral palmar nerve

Lateral palmar vein

Lateral palmar
digital nerve

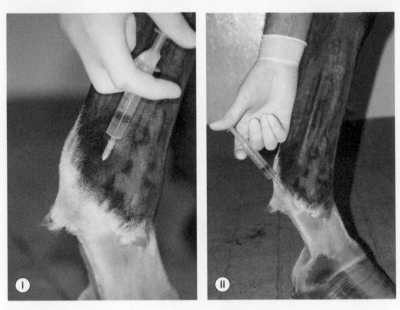

Fig. 4.57 Abaxial sesamoid block. (i) The normal abaxial site and (ii) the low abaxial site. Injections are performed both medially and laterally.

Aim: Block the lateral and medial palmar nerves at the level of the proximal sesamoid bones.

The neurovascular bundle is easily palpable on the abaxial surface of the proximal sesamoid bone and can be rolled between finger and thumb. A 25 gauge 16 mm needle is used to inject 2 mL local anaesthetic subcutaneously over each neurovascular bundle.

Low Four/Low Six Point Block
See Fig. 4.58.

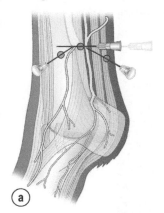

Fig. 4.58a Needles positioned for a low palmar (plantar) nerve block – lateral view.

Common and lateral digital extensor tendons

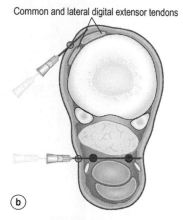

Fig. 4.58b Distal left metacarpal region demonstrating an alternative technique for low palmar (plantar) analgesia – transverse view.

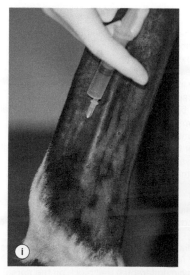

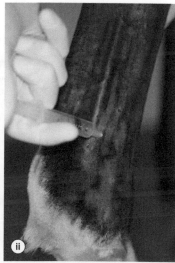

Fig. 4.58c Sites i and ii are common to front leg (low 4 point block). The hind leg analgesia receives the additional block at site iii (low 6 point block). Blocks are performed both laterally and medially.

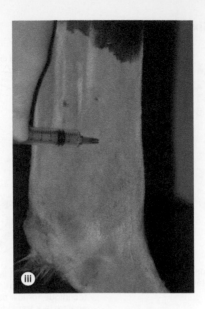

Forelimb – Low 4 point
Aim: Block the lateral and medial palmar nerves and lateral and medial palmar metacarpal nerves just proximal to the fetlock.

The palmar metacarpal nerves are blocked by injecting 2 mL local anaesthetic immediately distal to the distal button of each splint bone using a 25 gauge 16 mm needle. The palmar nerves are blocked by injection of 4–5 mL local anaesthetic subcutaneously between the DDFT and suspensory ligament using a 22 gauge 25 mm needle. The palmar nerves can be blocked either at the level of or proximal to, the level of the button of the splint. It may be advisable to block the palmar nerves at a more proximal level (e.g. mid-metatarsus region) in order to avoid inadvertent penetration of the digital flexor tendon sheath. An alternative approach to blocking the palmar nerves involves advancing a longer needle palmar to the DDFT to inject both lateral and medial palmar nerves from a lateral injection site.

Hindlimb – Low 6 point
Aim: Block the lateral and medial plantar nerves, lateral and medial plantar metatarsal nerves and medial and lateral dorsal metatarsal nerves just proximal to the fetlock.

The medial and lateral plantar and medial and lateral plantar metatarsal nerves are locked in much the same way as their forelimb counterparts. In the hindlimb, it is important to perform a subcutaneous circumferential ring block on the dorsal aspect of the metatarsus at the level of the buttons of the splint bones. This addition blocks the medial and lateral dorsal metatarsal nerves.

Subcarpal (High Palmar Nerve Block)
See Fig. 4.59.

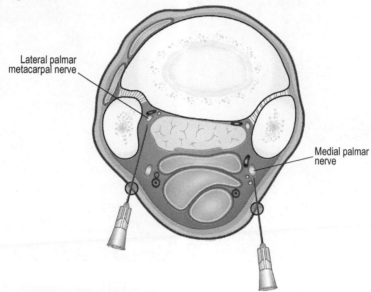

Lateral palmar
metacarpal nerve

Medial palmar
nerve

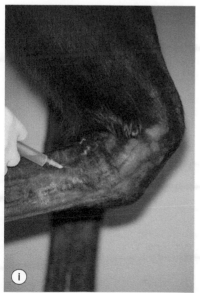

Fig. 4.59 Subcarpal (high palmar/high 4 point nerve block) – transverse view of the left metacarpal region. (i) Shows a flexed view of the high 4 point block on the right foreleg while (ii) and (iii) show the high 4 point block on the left foreleg.

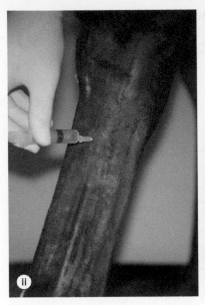

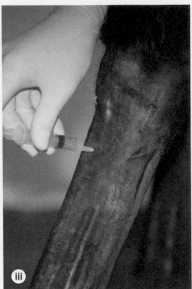

Aim: Block the lateral and medial palmar nerves and lateral and medial palmar metacarpal nerves just distal to the carpus.

The medial and lateral palmar metacarpal nerves are blocked using a 20 gauge 40 mm long needle. The needle is inserted axial to each splint bone and advanced until contact with the palmar cortex of MCIII is achieved. 5 mL local anaesthetic solution is deposited in each location.

The medial and lateral palmar nerves are blocked using a 22 gauge 25 mm needle inserted between the DDFT and suspensory ligament. 3–5 mL local anaesthetic solution is injected medially and laterally.

In some cases, it may also be indicated to inject local anaesthetic in order to locally infiltrate the origin of the suspensory ligament.

If desired, a circumferential ring block can be added to this block to abolish dorsal skin sensation (e.g. to allow suturing of wounds).

Note:
- It is important to remember that inadvertent injection of the carpometacarpal joint may also occur. Therefore, if this block is positive, the response should be compared to that after middle carpal joint analgesia.

High Plantar Nerve Block
See Fig. 4.60.

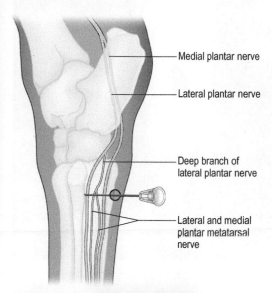

— Medial plantar nerve

— Lateral plantar nerve

— Deep branch of
lateral plantar nerve

— Lateral and medial
plantar metatarsal
nerve

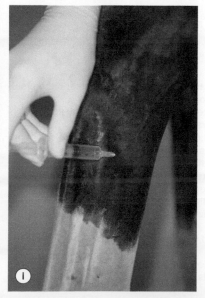

Fig. 4.60 High plantar/high 6 point
nerve block; performed both medially and
laterally. (i), (ii) and (iii) show the high 6
point nerve block technique on the right
hind leg.

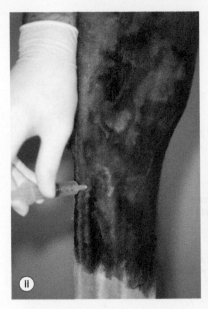

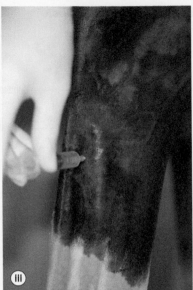

Note:
- As in the forelimb, the potential to inadvertently infiltrate synovial structures exists. Inadvertent injection of the TMT is less common than injection of the carpometacarpal joint in the forelimb, but there is a possibility of injection of the tarsal sheath. This should be considered when interpreting results.

Aim: Block the lateral and medial plantar and lateral and medial plantar metatarsal nerves just distal to the tarsometatarsal joint.

A single injection site is used on the lateral and medial aspect of the limb to block both the plantar and plantar metatarsal nerves.

A 20 gauge 40 mm needle is inserted just distal to the tarsometatarsal joint and axial to MTIV and advanced until contact is made with MTIII. 5 mL local anaesthetic is injected to block the lateral metatarsal nerve and, as the needle is withdrawn, a further 5 mL local anaesthetic is deposited in order to block the lateral plantar nerve, which lies more superficially between the DDFT and suspensory ligament. In order to block the medial plantar and medial plantar metatarsal nerves, the same procedure is repeated on the medial aspect of the limb, with the needle being inserted just axial to MTII.

In some cases, it may also be indicated to infiltrate the region of the origin of the suspensory ligament.

If desired, a circumferential ring block can be used to abolish dorsal skin sensation (e.g. to allow suturing of wounds).

Median and Ulnar Nerve Block
See Fig. 4.61.

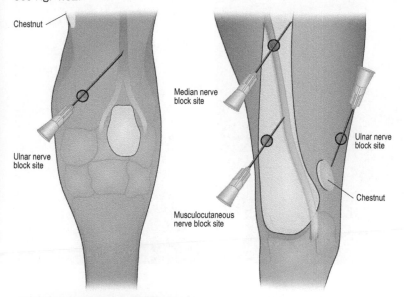

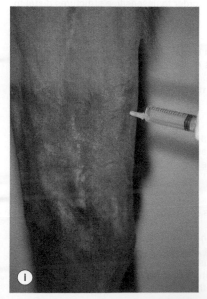

Fig. 4.61 Ulnar, median and musculocutaneous nerve block. (i) Shows the ulnar nerve block, (ii) the median nerve block and (iii) the musculocutaneous nerve block site.

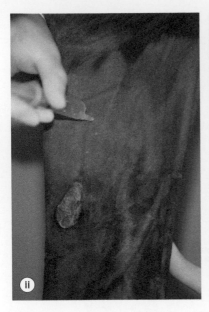 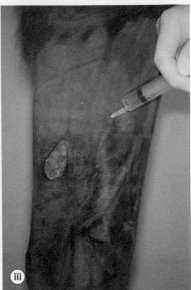

Aim: Block the median and ulnar nerves in order to desensitise structures distal to the mid-antebrachium.

Median

A 19 gauge 40 mm needle is inserted in a lateral direction 5 cm distal to the elbow joint, just below the *pectoralis superficialis m.* on the medial aspect of the limb and along the caudal aspect of the radius. 10 mL local anaesthetic is injected. The median artery and vein run caudal to the nerve and may be inadvertently punctured.

Ulnar

A 21 gauge 25 mm needle is inserted perpendicular to the skin 10 cm (one handbreadth) proximal to the accessory carpal bone in the palmar midline (in the groove between the *ulnaris lateralis* and flexor *carpi ulnaris* muscle bellies). 10 mL of 2% lidocaine (lignocaine) is used.

Musculocutaneous

Rarely and usually for therapeutic reasons, it may be indicated to block the musculocutaneous nerve.

The nerve may be blocked before it branches at a site over the *lacertus fibrosus*. The nerve is usually easily palpated and a 21 gauge 25 mm needle is used to inject 5 mL local anaesthetic subcutaneously.

Alternatively, 3 mL local anaesthetic is injected subcutaneously over the accessory cephalic and cephalic veins at the level of the mid-antebrachium.

Tibial and Fibular (Peroneal) Nerve Block
See Fig. 4.62.

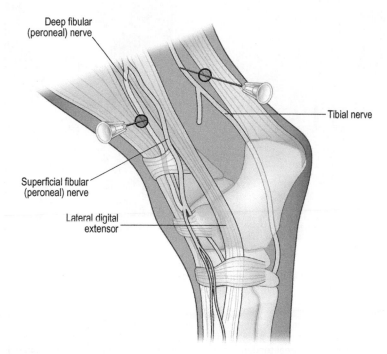

Fig. 4.62 Fibular (peroneal) and tibial nerve block – lateral view of the left crus and tarsus. (i) Shows the fibular nerve block site while (ii) shows the tibial nerve block site.

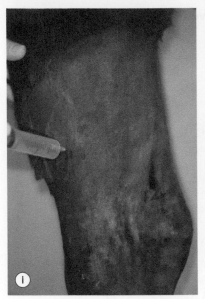
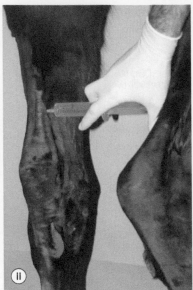

Aim: Block the tibial and fibular nerves in order to remove deep sensation from the distal hindlimb.

Tibial

A 19 gauge 25 mm needle is inserted on the medial aspect of the limb 10 cm proximal to the point of the hock, just caudal to the deep flexor tendon and cranial to the common calcaneal tendon. Approximately 20 mL of local anaesthetic should be injected at several sites in this area.

Fibular (peroneal)

A 21 gauge 50 mm needle is inserted on the lateral aspect of the limb 10 cm above the point of the hock in the groove formed by the lateral and long digital extensor muscles. The needle should be advanced until it contacts the tibia. Blood often appears at the hub and may indicate accurate needle placement. 10–15 mL local anaesthetic is injected to block the deep fibular nerve. As the needle is withdrawn, a further 5–10 mL local anaesthetic is injected more superficially to block the superficial fibular nerve.

SITES FOR SYNOVIOCENTESIS

Notes:

- Ensure all equipment is available including clipping and scrubbing – it must all be readily to hand.
- All intra-articular injection or aspiration MUST be performed with full aseptic precautions including skin preparation and surgical scrub-up with sterile gloves.
- Use only fully sterile equipment and if in doubt don't do the procedure!
- Use only preparations specifically indicated for joint injection.
- Use needle diameter/length consistent with joint (spinal needles are ideal for larger/deeper joints).
- Inject the joint with an appropriate volume of anaesthetic agent. If the horse has been sedated to allow injection, allow suitable recovery period.
- If a needle breaks off – do not panic. The risk is low if appropriate restraint is used. Locate it by ultrasound and remove it (it may need a general anaesthetic).
- Bandage the joint after the procedure (if possible) and confine the horse for a day or two.
- If a joint becomes painful, hot and swollen within 24 hours of the injection take appropriate action in case of sepsis. (Analyse synovial fluid urgently and if necessary flush joint as emergency procedure.)

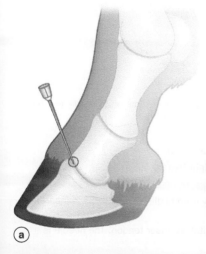

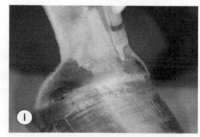

Fig. 4.63a Lateral view (see also (i)) of needle insertion in the coffin joint.

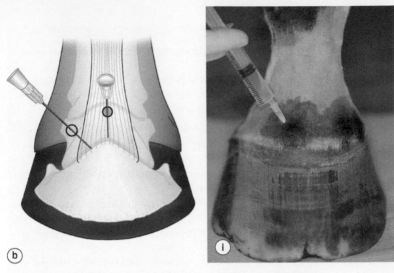

Fig. 4.63b Dorsal view (see also (i)) of needle insertion in the coffin joint.

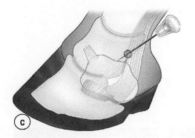

Fig. 4.63c Notch into which needle is inserted in the coffin joint.

Requirements: 20 gauge 40 mm needle (Fig. 4.63).

Difficulty: Simple – best to insert when weight bearing.

Method

1. 1–2 cm above coronary band, 2 cm away from midline. The needle is inserted distally and axially.

2. Dorsal midline through the common digital extensor tendon. The needle is angled slightly distally from horizontal.

Navicular bursa
See Fig. 4.64.

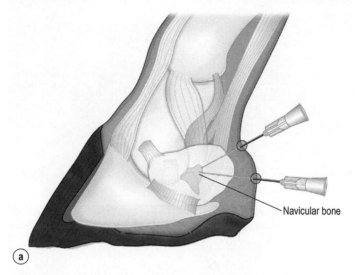

(a)

Fig. 4.64a Lateral view showing two techniques for synoviocentesis of the navicular bursa of the foot. The upper needle shows it placed in the depression between the heel bulbs and advancing the needle in a dorsodistal direction. The lower needle (and i and ii) shows the needle placed just proximal to the hairline between the bulbs of the heels using the navicular position as a guide.

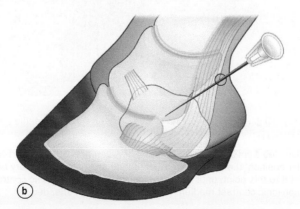

(b)

Fig. 4.64b Palmaro (plantaro) lateral view of the digit showing the approach for synoviocentesis of the navicular bursa.

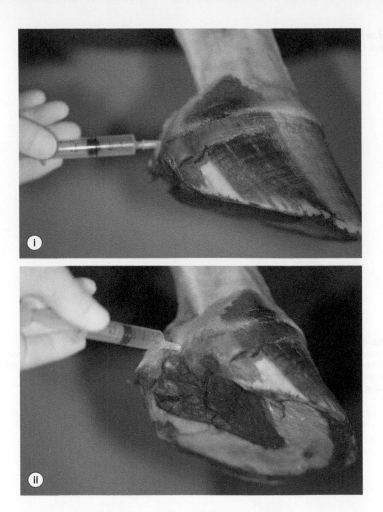

Requirements: 19 gauge 90 mm spinal needle, 25 gauge 16 mm needle (skin bleb).

Difficulty: Moderate.

Method: Skin bleb 1 cm above coronary band between heel bulbs. Insert needle to 'navicular position' (i.e. halfway between dorsal and palmar coronary band) and 1 cm distal to this point, until bone is encountered. Radiographic control and use of non-ionic contrast medium (Omnipaque) is recommended.

Pastern (Proximal Interphalangeal) Joint
See Fig. 4.65.

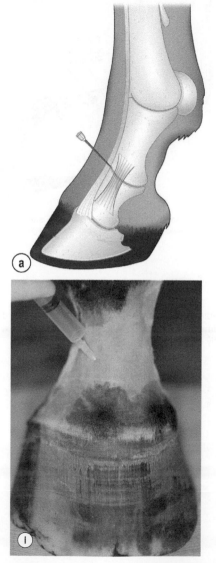

Fig. 4.65 (a) Lateral view of the nerve block site at the pastern (proximal interphalangeal) joint. (i) Shows the dorsal view at the same site.

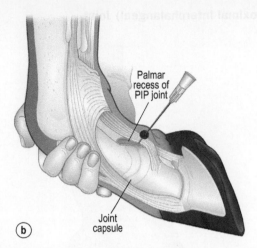

Fig. 4.65, cont'd (b) Flexed lateral view of the nerve block site at the pastern (proximal interphalangeal) joint.

Requirements: 21 gauge 50 mm needle.

Difficulty: Moderate – best to insert when weight bearing.

Method: Insert needle abaxial to the CDE tendon at a site just distal to the level of the distal palmar/plantar process of the proximal phalanx. The needle is advanced slightly distally and axially into the joint.

Note:
- Synovial fluid is only rarely retrieved.

Fetlock (Metacarpo/Metatarso-Phalangeal) Joint

See Fig. 4.66.

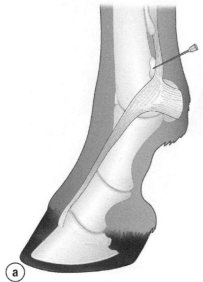

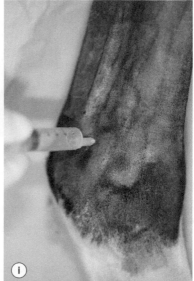

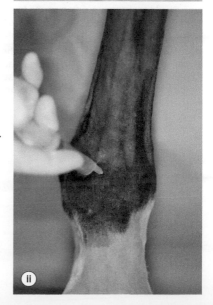

Fig. 4.66 (a) Lateral view of proximopalmar approach to the fetlock (metacarpo-phalangeal joint) (i). (ii) Shows a dorsal view of the dorsal approach to the joint. This is also performed while weight-bearing.

Requirements: 20 gauge 25 mm needle.

Difficulty: Easy (commonly injected/sampled).

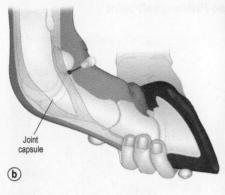

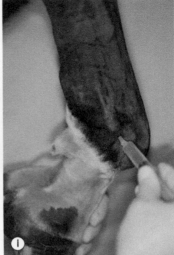

Fig. 4.66, cont'd (b) Preferred site (see also (i)) for fetlock (metacarpo/metatarsophalangeal) joint arthrocentesis in the flexed position.

Joint capsule

ⓑ

ⓘ

Method

● *Proximo-palmar approach*: Approach via lateral palmar pouch of joint capsule – located between splint button, caudal aspect of cannon and cranial to suspensory ligament. Often useful to press on medial pouch to distend lateral one. Enter slightly downwards and forwards. Injection is easy at this site, but the presence of synovial villi and haemorrhage can complicate arthrocentesis.

● *Lateral approach*: Approach between the lateral palmar/plantar surface of the cannon bone and dorsal articular surface of the lateral proximal sesamoid bone, through collateral ligament. Horse should be non-weight-bearing and the joint should be flexed. This approach results in less haemorrhage and is, therefore, ideal for arthrocentesis.

Digital Flexor Tendon Sheath
See Fig. 4.67.

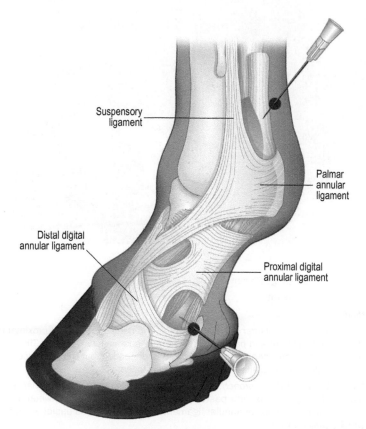

Fig. 4.67 Lateral view of the digit indicating sites for synoviocentesis of the proximal (top site) and distal (bottom site) aspects of the digital flexor tendon sheath. (i) Shows the proximal site and (ii) the distal site.

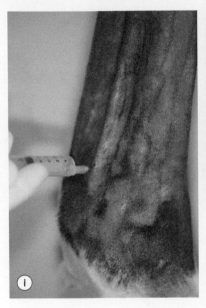

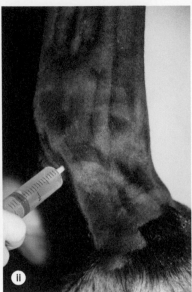

Requirements: 20 gauge 25 mm needle.

Difficulty: Easy/moderate.

Method

- *Proximal to palmar/plantar annular ligament*. The needle is inserted proximal to the annular ligament and palmar/plantar to the suspensory ligament. This is useful for injection when the proximal DFTS is distended, but the presence of synovial villi make this site unreliable for synoviocentesis.

- *Palmar/plantar distal approach*. The needle is inserted in the palmar/plantar aspect of the palmar/plantar pastern region in the outpouching between the proximal and distal digital annular ligaments. This approach is easier when a DFTS effusion exists.

- *Palmar/plantar axial sesamoidean approach*. The fetlock is held in flexion and the needle is inserted axial to the palmar/plantar border of the proximal sesamoid bone and palmar/plantar to the neurovascular bundle. Synovial fluid can usually be obtained from this site when there is no DFTS effusion.

Carpal Joints
See Fig. 4.68.

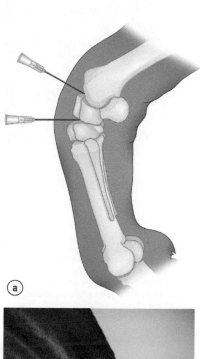

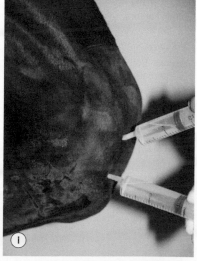

Fig. 4.68 (a) Flexed lateral view (see also (i)) indicating the nerve block sites at both carpal joints: (top) radiocarpal joint site and (bottom) intercarpal joint site.

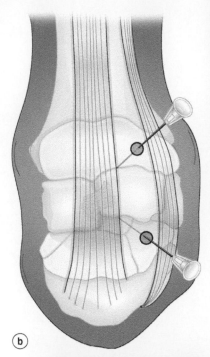

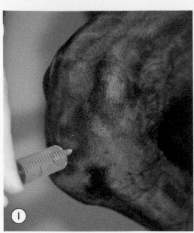

Fig. 4.68, cont'd (b) Dorsal view of the left carpus in a flexed position showing the nerve block sites of the intercarpal and radiocarpal joints. (i) Shows the site at the intercarpal joint while (ii) shows the site at the radiocarpal joint.

Requirements: 20 gauge 40 mm needle.

Difficulty: Simple.

Method: Both radiocarpal and intercarpal joints entered with knee flexed. Introduce needle midway between palpable bones between the extensor *carpi radialis* tendon (which is in midline) and common digital extensor tendon. Joint entered after 0.5–1 cm.

Note:
- Carpo-metacarpal joint communicates with intercarpal joint.

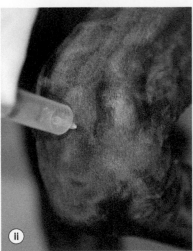

Humeroradial Joint
See Fig. 4.69.

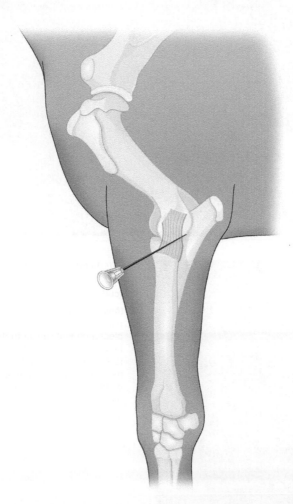

Fig. 4.69 Humeroradial joint nerve block: (i) and (ii) show the injection site at this joint.

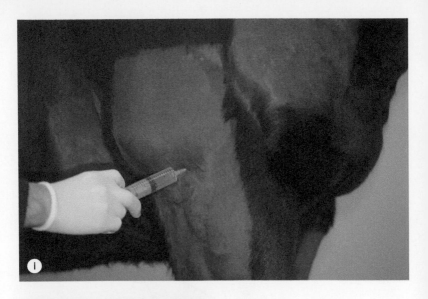

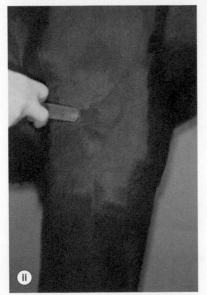

Requirements: 19 gauge 90 mm spinal needle.

Difficulty: Moderate.

Method: The needle is inserted in the palpable depression cranial to the olecranon and caudal to the lateral humeral epicondyle. The needle is advanced against the caudal margin of the collateral ligament distally, slightly cranially and medially.

Scapulohumeral Joint
See Fig. 4.70.

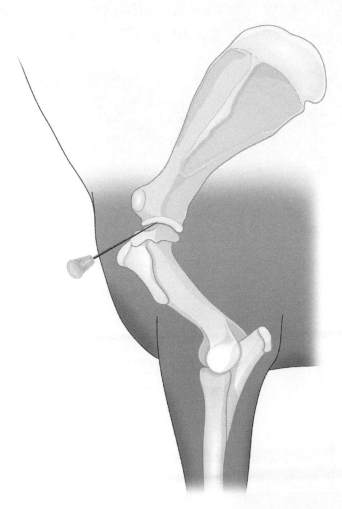

Fig. 4.70 Scapulohumeral joint nerve block: (i) and (ii) show the injection site at this joint.

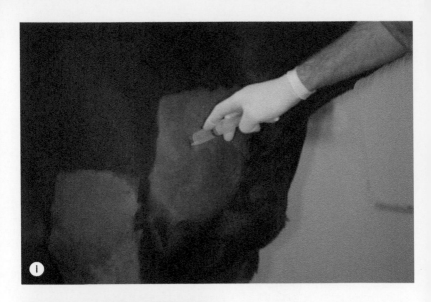

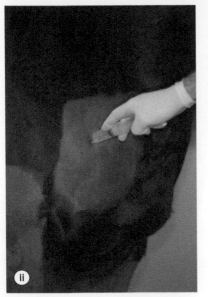

Requirements: 19 gauge 90 mm spinal needle.

Difficulty: Difficult (deep).

Method: Palpate lateral humeral tuberosity and feel the deep groove between the cranial and caudal prominences. Insert needle into this notch directed towards opposite elbow (i.e. caudomedially and distally).

Tarsometatarsal Joint
See Fig. 4.71.

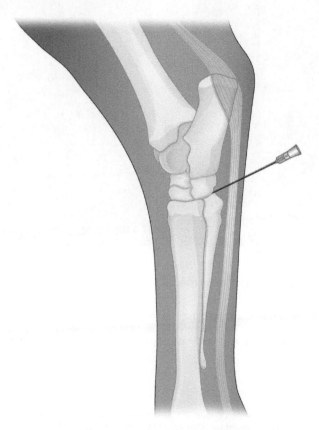

Fig. 4.71 Tarsometatarsal joint nerve block on the hind leg. See (i) which also shows the injection site and (ii) shows the same site but on the foreleg.

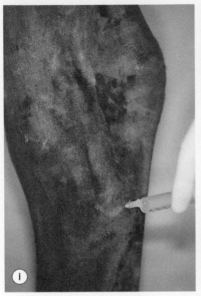
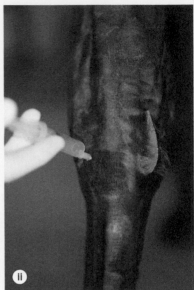

Requirements: 19 gauge 40 mm needle.

Difficulty: Moderate.

Method: The needle is inserted just proximal to the head of MTIV and in a small depression between the head of MTIV and the distal aspect of the 4th tarsal bone. The needle is angled 45° distally and 45° dorsally. First 3–4 mL enter easily.

Note:
- The TMT communicates with the distal intertarsal joint in only 8–35% of normal horses; therefore, this should be injected separately.

Distal Intertarsal (Centrodistal) Joint
See Fig. 4.72.

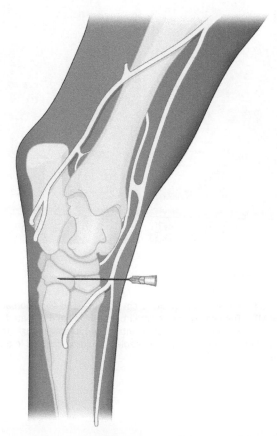

Fig. 4.72 Distal intertarsal (centrodistal) joint nerve block. (i and ii) Show two different views of the injection site at the distal intertarsal joint. The approach is made from the medial aspect.

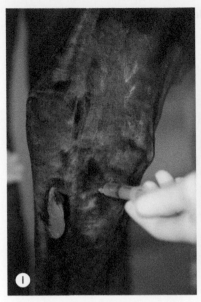 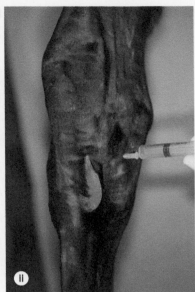

Requirements: 23 gauge 16 mm needle.

Difficulty: Moderate/difficult.

Method: The needle is inserted at a site 1 cm proximal and 1 cm dorsal to the head of MTII. The joint space is small but discernible if palpated with a fingernail in most horses. The needle is introduced at a right angle to the axis of the leg. If injection is not easy, the needle should be directed in a slightly plantar direction.

Tarsocrural (Tibiotarsal) Joint
See Fig. 4.73.

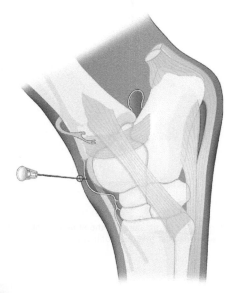

Fig. 4.73 Diagram and (i) show the tarsocrural (tibiotarsal) joint nerve block site.

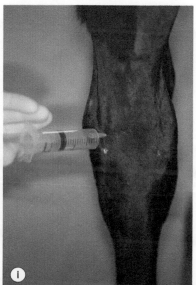

Requirements: 20 gauge 40 mm needle.

Difficulty: Simple.

Method: Enter either medial or lateral to saphenous vein 2–3 cm below medial malleolus.

Note:
● The tarsocrural joint and proximal intertarsal joints communicate in all horses.

Femoropatellar Joint
See Fig. 4.74a and b.

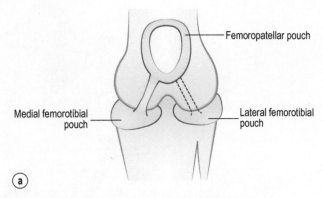

Femoropatellar pouch

Medial femorotibial
pouch

Lateral femorotibial
pouch

(a)

Fig. 4.74a Arrangement of the stifle joint showing communicating joints (femoropatellar and femorotibial).

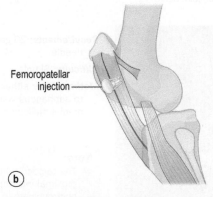

Femoropatellar
injection

(b)

Fig. 4.74b Lateral (see also (i)) femoropatellar injection site.

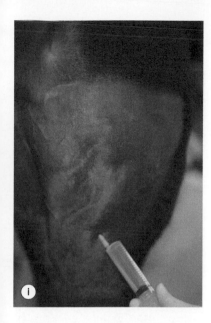

Requirements: 20 gauge 40 mm needle.

Difficulty: Moderate (resented by patient).

Method: Landmarks used are proximal end of tibial crest, medial and middle patellar ligaments and patella. Needle inserted 2.5–3.5 cm above the tibial crest, midway between the middle and medial patellar ligaments or between the middle and lateral patellar ligaments with the needle directed slightly proximally. The needle is advanced until joint fluid is obtained or articular cartilage of the distal femur is encountered.

Note:
● The three compartments of the stifle joint do not necessarily communicate and for reliable diagnostic analgesia all three compartments should be injected independently.

Medial Femorotibial Joint
See Fig. 4.74c.

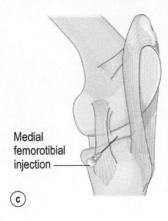

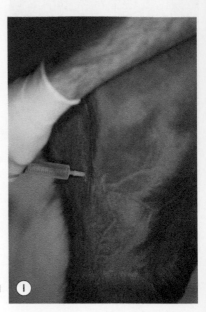

Fig. 4.74c Medial (see also (i)) femorotibial injection site.

Requirements: 20 gauge 40 mm needle.

Difficulty: Moderate (resented by patient).

Method: Landmarks used are proximal end of tibial crest, medial and middle patellar ligaments and patella. The needle is inserted perpendicular to the skin, at a site caudal to the medial patellar ligament, cranial to the medial collateral ligament and 2 cm proximal to the tibial plateau.

Lateral Femorotibial Joint

See Fig. 4.74d.

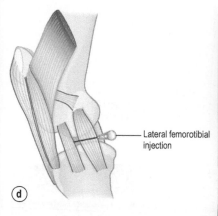

Lateral femorotibial injection

(d)

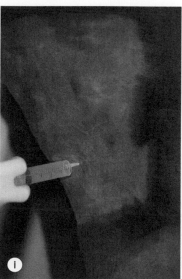

(i)

Fig. 4.74d Lateral (see also (i)) femorotibial injection site.

Requirements: 20 gauge 40 mm needle.

Difficulty: Difficult.

Method: The needle is inserted horizontally caudal to the lateral patellar ligament and cranial to the long digital extensor tendon 1–2 cm proximal to the tibial plateau. An alternative injection site is caudal to the long digital extensor tendon and cranial to the lateral collateral ligament 1–2 cm proximal to the tibial plateau.

Note:
- In contrast to the medial FT and FP joints, an effusion is rarely palpable in this joint.

See Fig. 4.74e.

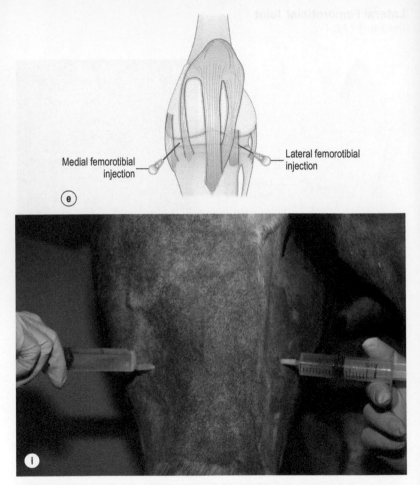

Medial femorotibial
injection

Lateral femorotibial
injection

Fig. 4.74e Dorsal view (see also (i)) of both the medial and lateral femorotibial injection sites.

Table 4.8 Local anaesthetic agents				
Agent	Onset (minutes)	Duration (hours)	Relative potency[a]	Irritancy[a]
Lidocaine (lignocaine)	5	1–2	1	
Mepivacaine	11/12	2–4	1	Less
Prilocaine	5	1–2	1	=
Bupivacaine	11/12	4–8	2–4	Less
Procaine	15	<1	0.5	=
[a]Compared with lidocaine (lignocaine) hydrochloride.				

Guide to Volumes of Lidocaine (Lignocaine) Hydrochloride (2%)/Mepivacaine Hydrochloride (2%) Used

Table 4.9 Regional nerve block	
Nerve block	mL 2% lidocaine (lignocaine)/mepivacaine
Palmar digital	2.0
Palmar	5
Palmar metacarpal	3–5
Median	10–20
Ulnar	10
Musculocutaneous	10
Superficial fibular	10–15
Deep fibular	10–15
Tibial	15–25

Table 4.10 Bursal/thecal anaesthesia

Site	mL 2% lidocaine (lignocaine)/mepivacaine
Navicular bursa	5
Digital flexor tendon sheath	10

Table 4.11 Intra-articular anaesthesia

Nerve block	mL 2% lidocaine (lignocaine)/mepivacaine
Coffin joint	5
Pastern joint	5
Fetlock joint	10
Intercarpal joint	5–10
Radiocarpal joint	5–10
Elbow joint	20
Shoulder joint	20–30
Tarsometatarsal joint	3–5
Intertarsal joint	3
Tibiotarsal joint	10–20
Femoropatellar joint	20–30
Medial femorotibial joint	20–30
Lateral femorotibial joint	20–30

Part 4 CLINICAL AIDS

Section 9
Signs of impending parturition

The majority of thoroughbred conceptions are closely monitored and the 'expected foaling date' can be readily predicted. However, 'normal' gestation lengths can vary widely (320–400 days) and some mares 'habitually' foal early or late. In paddock-bred mares, service and, therefore, foaling dates are often unknown and foaling may occur 'unexpectedly'.

Regular observation of the mare allows the owner to identify changes which indicate the proximity of foaling, enabling the attending veterinarian to be informed in reasonable time. Most foalings are normal and occur without interference but knowledge of imminent foaling allows careful observation and rapid intervention if required.

Table 4.12 Natural indicators of impending parturition

Time before birth	Signs
~3 months	**Increased abdominal size** (increasingly lateral asymmetry)
2 weeks–2 days	**Teat elongation** and mild mammary enlargement with obvious udder development usually in last 2 days
4–2 days	**Pelvic relaxation** and prominent tail base (as pelvic ligaments slacken)
2–1 day	**Teat 'waxing'** (wax candles) usually indicate imminent foaling = UNPREDICTABLE **'Milk' calcium concentrations** in excess of 10 mmol/L indicate imminent foaling (generally that night or tomorrow) = RELIABLE
Few hours	Associated with onset of **stage 1 labour: Behavioural changes** – restlessness, repeated flank watching, lying and rising, isolation, inappetence, sweating (very similar to signs of mild spasmodic colic), **colostrum leakage/ ejection**

Section 10
Neonatal assessment and scoring of foals

EVALUATION OF THE NEWBORN FOAL
Evaluation of the newborn foal is very important as it provides the first and earliest opportunity to assess its potential viability. It also allows a veterinarian to assess whether there is anything that needs to be addressed immediately (e.g. provision of oxygen, artificial (positive pressure) ventilation, blood transfusion, antibiotics, etc.)

APGAR[1] Scoring System
Foals are best scored at 1–3 minutes of age. Note, however, that foaling mares exhibit a natural period of tranquillity following the expulsion of the foal (foal usually still has hind legs in birth canal). During this stage, the foal's umbilical circulation is still very active (a pulse is still palpable in umbilical artery) and the uterus is actively contracting. This causes a progressive arterial resistance and an active return of the foal's venous blood into its systemic circulation. This is a very important stage of delivery and disturbances to assess foals at this stage may be counterproductive. Early rupture of the cord resulting from early disturbance of the mare may result in significant deprivation for the foal. Up to 1 L of circulating blood may be left in the placental circulation when rupture is rapid. Adaptation must, under these circumstances, be abrupt and this allows little scope for interference in the event of a problem.

Notes:
- Provided problems are recognised early, even some seriously depressed foals can be saved with early effective intensive care. Some conditions arise before birth so accurate history and careful clinical assessment is vital! Owners can be taught to assess the foal at birth – this does not reduce the necessity for a full examination as soon after birth as possible.

- Many high-risk foals look relatively normal at birth and up to 12–18 hours of age. Once problems develop, deterioration is usually rapid. This makes early recognition of problems an important management procedure.

- Newborn foals which are high risk or which show any evidence of respiratory or neurological (or other) compromise should be subjected to APGAR scoring system at regular intervals over the first 30 minutes. Apparently, normal foals should be scored once only and then left alone.

---

[1]Vaala WE, Sertich PL (1994) Management strategies for mares at risk for periparturient complications. *Veterinary Clinics of North America* 10:237–265.

Normal Birth Weight of Thoroughbred Foals

● 42–46 kg (primiparous mares).
● 48–52 kg (multiparous mares).

Table 4.13 Normal foal assessment at birth

Time	Temperature (°C)	Pulse (/minute)	Resp (/minute)	Notes
0–1 minute	37.0–37.5	70	70	Hypoxia/metabolic+resp acidosis
5–30 minutes	36.8–37.0	120	50	Cord rupture/shivering/righting – attempts to stand/sucking reflex
30–60 minutes	37.5–38.2	140	40	Co-ordination+ standing, maternal recognition
1–2 hours	38.0	120	35	Teat seeking, follows mare COLOSTRUM IDEAL
2–12 hours	38.0	100	35	Meconium/urine[a] passed COLOSTRUM ESSENTIAL
12–48 hours	38.0	90	30	Bonding. Closure of FO+DA NO more colostral absorption

[a]First urine usually passed by colt foals 5–10 hours; filly foals 8–12 hours.

Table 4.14 Birth (APGAR) (assessed in first 5 minutes of life)

Score/value	0	1	2
Heart rate	Undetectable	<60	>60
Respiratory rate	Undetectable	Slow/irregular	Regular >60
Muscle tone	Limp	Flexed extremities	Sternal recumbency
Nasal response	Nil	Grimace/movement	Sneeze/rejection

Interpretation
Normal foals score: 7–8
Moderate depression: 4–6
Marked depression: 1–4
Dead: 0

Methods for Measurement of IgG in Plasma of Foals Include

- Zinc sulphate turbidity test (see p. 45).
- Single radial immunodiffusion test (SRID).
- Latex agglutination test.
- Glutaraldehyde test.
- ELISA (CITE) test.
- Total protein assay electrophoresis.

REFERRAL OF FOALS TO A SPECIALIST CENTRE

Many diseases and conditions can be effectively treated on the farm but this will depend on:

- the facilities available for nursing of both mare and foal
- the number of support staff available and their ability and experience (enthusiasm is seldom in short supply – at least in the early stages of the nursing)
- the experience and facilities of the clinician
- the condition of the foal and the mare and their tolerance of transportation (e.g. some mares may not tolerate transport and so might jeopardise the foal and its handlers)
- the specific needs of the parent (e.g. splinting of a fractured leg, control of seizures, correction of hydration and electrolyte status)
- the distance to the centre and the time the journey is likely to take.

Considerations Prior to Referral of a Sick Foal to a Specialist Unit[2]

1. **An early decision** to refer is clearly better than undue delay. There is little rationale in sending a dying foal, which has little or no hope of surviving the journey, let alone the rigors of an intensive care regimen. The mare and the foal should be considered together and individually; not just the condition that is of most concern (e.g. does the foal have 'bent' legs or a septic joint, etc., which might influence the prognosis markedly).

2. **Referral should be considered seriously.** A journey may make the condition worse. It is wise to seek advice from the referral hospital early if there are doubts about the necessity to transport the foal. The referral centre will be grateful for continued contact in the early stages; they may be able to give advice and avoid transporting the foal unnecessarily. This will also give the centre useful information before the arrival of the foal.

3. **Consider whether proper care can be given on the farm.** Drugs and equipment (including laboratory support may be essential to the survival of the foal in some cases but in others minimal supportive equipment may be needed).

---

[2]Geiser DR, Henton JE (1986) Transportation of the equine neonatal patient. *Equine Practice* 8:19–24.

Table 4.15 Sepsis scoring

	Factor	4	3	2	1	0	Score
History	High-risk foaling		Yes			No	
	Pre/dys-mature (gestational days)		<300	300–310	311–330	>331	
Haematology	Neutrophils (×10⁹/L)		2.0	2.0–4.0	4.0–8.0	Normal	
	Band neutrophils (×10⁹/L)		> 0.2	0.05–0.2		<0.05	
	Toxic neutrophils (×10⁹/L)	+++	+++	++	+	0	
Biochemistry	Fibrinogen (g/L)		>6.0	4.5–6	3.0–4.5	<3.0	
	Glucose (mmol/L)		<3.0		3.0–4.5	>4.5	
	IgG (g/L)	< 2.0	2.0–4.0	4.0–6.0	6.0–8.0	>8.0	
Clinical signs	Petechiae/scleral injection[a]		+++	++	+	Nil	
	Pyrexia (°C)			>39	38–39	Normal	
	Hypotonia/coma/depression/convulsion			Marked	Mild	Nil	
	Uveitis/diarr./dyspnea/joint ill/wounds		Yes			No	
							Total score

SCORE (90% accurate): ≥11 = SEPSIS; <11 = NON-SEPSIS.
[a]*Not associated with trauma.*

The environment should be conducive to maintenance of body temperature and hygiene, for example:

- Are the correct drugs, fluids and catheters available?
- Is a suitable stomach tube or foal feeding tube available?
- Can oxygen be administered easily and safely over the full 24-hour day?
- Is a **respirator** available?
- **Assuming that all the equipment for the particular foal is present, does the clinician have experience in their use/administration?**
- Is there **suitable, experienced help** available to maintain the effort after the clinician leaves the premises?

If NO to any of these – refer immediately and expedite departure!

4. **The likely cost** of the procedure must be discussed with the owner/stud manager. Foal intensive care is a very expensive affair and the implications (win or lose) need to be considered before starting out.

5. **The nearest referral centre with known expertise and the facilities to cope should be selected**. There is no point in sending the foal to another, similarly equipped or experienced practice, just to shift responsibility for the foal to someone else.

6. **Phone and discuss** the case early (preparation is maximised and guidance can be given which might save the foal's life or may prevent an unnecessary journey).

7. **A written record of all clinical findings** and any procedures (including the timing and doses of any drugs given) should be sent with the foal. The letter should be signed by the clinician and it should include contact numbers and addresses.

8. All specimens taken (e.g. peritoneal fluid, blood or joint fluid) should be packed accordingly and sent with the foal.

9. **The placenta** should be sent if available (packed on ice in a clean, sealed, plastic bag).

10. If the mare is not accompanying the foal, **some milk/colostrum** should be obtained and sent with the foal.

11. **Interested insurance company** should be **informed**; this is often forgotten in the heat of the moment and failure to comply with policy procedures may create difficulties later on.

12. **As soon as laboratory results become available these should be sent by fax or email to the referral centre.**

TRANSPORTATION OF THE SICK OR INJURED FOAL

The most significant aspects are[2,3]:

(a) Restraint and protection from self-inflicted or other trauma:

● If the mare and foal cannot be safely transported together, consider sending the foal first and follow with the mare in another transporter.

● Physical support helps if the foal is amenable to this. Sternal recumbency is the best physiological supportive position and this should be maintained during recumbency as far as possible.

● If the foal is in pain and thrashing or convulsing, suitable medication to control pain and seizures should be given (see p. 103).

Seizure control is usually best using diazepam at 5–20 mg to effect in 5-mg increments.[4]

DO NOT USE ACEPROMAZINE or XYLAZINE.

Handlers may be instructed to administer repeat doses during travel via an intravenous catheter.

It is always wise to check the blood glucose of any convulsing neonatal foal prior to and during transportation (if possible).

(b) Prevention of hypothermia:

● Take rectal temperature before starting and take appropriate measures to restore to normal (e.g. blankets, bottles and rectal gloves filled with warm water and tied).

● Do not put the foal onto hot surfaces – application of direct heat can harm the circulation and cause skin damage/thermal necrosis.

● It is sometimes possible to have the foal in the heated cab and still within sight of the mare.

(c) Maintenance of blood glucose and prevention of nutritional depletion (energy, fluids and electrolytes are earliest and most significant requirements):

● Maintenance of normal blood glucose is particularly important for recumbent or weak foals.

● Blood glucose should be checked before departure with a dextrose stick.

● If blood glucose is less than 2.5 mmol/L and the journey is likely to be longer than 1–2 hours, it is wise to place an intravenous catheter and administer warm 5% glucose solution at 4 mL/kg bodyweight/hour. It is probably unwise to administer a large bolus of glucose intravenously at the start of the journey as this might easily induce a rebound hypoglycaemia.

[3]Cudd TA (1990) Neonatal transport. In: Equine Clinical Neonatology. AM Koterba, WH Drummond, PC Kosch, eds. Lea and Febiger, Philadelphia, pp. 763–769.
[4]Madigan JE (1997) Transport of the critically ill equine neonate. In: Manual of Equine Neonatal Medicine. Live Oak Publications, Woodland, pp. 67–69.

- Administration of 200–250 mL mare's milk or colostrum by stomach tube is helpful if the foal has not been feeding and if there is no nasogastric reflux.

(d) **A sample of the colostrum should be sent with the foal so that the specialist centre can assess its quality:**

- A sample for analysis will be especially helpful if the foal is less than 18 hours old.

(e) **If the foal has any respiratory compromise[5] it should not be left in lateral recumbency:**

- Sternal recumbency is very helpful to normal lung function.
- Oxygen should be administered if:
  - the respiratory rate is less than 30/minute or greater than 80/minute
  - mucous membranes are pale or cyanotic
  - there is any evidence of respiratory tract infection.
- A nasopharyngeal tube is easy to insert and is well-tolerated by foals. A direct oxygen line into the trachea inserted percutaneously is also available.
- Oxygen can be administered directly via a normal cylinder with a pressure-limiting valve. A demand valve can also be used.

Notes:
- A normal E size cylinder will provide a flow rate of 5 L/minute for 1 hour.
- If a facemask is used, ensure that it has a release/overflow valve or that the fit is loose enough to avoid the foal rebreathing.
- If sternal recumbency cannot be sustained, the foal should be held in sternal recumbency for at least some of the time and should be turned from side to side at 30-minute intervals.

(f) **Unless the foal is already known to be infected, it is probably wise to delay the administration of antibiotics. However, if there is any suspicion of sepsis, a suitable broad-spectrum antibiotic may be administered.**

- It may be useful to discuss the antibiotic selection with the referral centre.

(g) **The dose and time of all drugs and procedures used prior to departure and during transport should be recorded and sent with the foal!**

- It is unwise to rely on memory.

(h) **If the placenta is available, send it with the foal in a sealed, plastic bag packed surrounded with ice.**

---

[5]Kosch PC, Koterba AM (1987) Respiratory support for the newborn foal. In: *Current Therapy in Equine Medicine*. NE Robinson, ed. WB Saunders, Philadelphia, pp. 247–253.

(i) **Do not forget the needs of the mare if she is travelling with the foal or if she is to be left behind.**

Therefore:

1. Confine the foal and mare in a quiet, safe area with (preferably) no opportunity for self-inflicted trauma. Size is very important as mares may become disturbed in a close confined area and traumatise the foal. A mare that will not settle should be placed in a separate stall so that she can see and smell the foal, which should then be held all the time by an experienced handler. Sedatives can be used to calm the mare but should not be used for the foal unless there is no option. A properly fitting foal slip should be used with suitable padding if necessary.

2. Foals inclined to convulsions or uncoordinated movement need to be fully bandaged with protective padding on limbs and head to prevent injuries.

The mare should have leg bandages applied, if only to protect the foal from damaging itself and her.

Body heat should be maintained by appropriate rugging and bandaging. This is vital when ambient temperatures are below 25°C.

● 'Space blankets' are a useful emergency measure and are extremely efficient at heat retention. Sweating is very 'cooling' and, where present, an appropriate undersheet made of absorbent cotton or wool is desirable.

● Towelling the foal dry before starting the journey is useful.

● In an emergency, sleeping bags and sweaters (foals front legs through the arms and head through the neck) are good, simple measures.

● Hot water bottles and electrically heated pads can be valuable but they can cause serious skin burns especially in compromised recumbent foals.

Notes:

● THE DIRECT APPLICATION OF HEAT TO THE OUTER SURFACE CAN BE HARMFUL RATHER THAN HELPFUL.

● BEWARE OF LAYING A SICK FOAL ON AN ELECTRICALLY HEATED PAD – extensive skin necrosis can occur as the circulation is poor and compressed by the bodyweight of the foal. The skin is more liable to burn when cutaneous circulation is impaired.

● Do not transport a sick foal in an open pickup truck: heat loss and/or sunburn can be critical.

3. Prepare the box with adequate bedding over a rubber floor.

● An overlay of carpeting provides good insulation, reduces draughts and provides a clean surface.

● Shavings, sawdust or peat should not be used for young foals as they may harm the respiratory tract and the eyes in particular.

- 'Vetbed' artificial fibre blankets are excellent as they allow fluid to pass while still maintaining thermal insulation and dryness in contact with the skin.
- If the foal is standing, do not make the bed too deep (6–12 cm is enough).

4. Trailers are less desirable than boxes and estate cars.
   - Do not put a sick foal in the boot of a saloon car.
   - It is illegal, irresponsible and dangerous to travel in a trailer with the foal (use closed circuit television if necessary).
   - Equine ambulances are excellent but may not be equipped to transport a mare and foal.
   - The greater the space and the contact with handlers the better.
   - Always have at least two people with the transporter – it is unreasonable and dangerous for the driver to have to cope with every demand.

5. Avoid draughts in the transporter – but also avoid a steamy moist atmosphere by ensuring adequate ventilation throughput.

6. Stop at regular intervals unless separate staff are looking after the animals.
   - Some foals will not nurse when moving so it may be necessary to stop to allow feeding.

7. Load the foal before the mare and guide it carefully and, unless the foal can stand and coordinate normally, the mare and foal should be separated in the box.
   - It is not necessary or wise to tie the foal but a foal slip suitably padded is sometimes helpful with restraint.

8. If the foal has respiratory disease or compromised oxygen, cylinders and possibly an indwelling nasal tube with continuous oxygen should be used.
   - Fluid therapy may need to be maintained for the duration of the journey and so suitable arrangements have to be made using 'SUSI' flexible, extendible, intravenous administration set.
   - The foal should be placed in sternal recumbency but should never be forced to adopt this position (it is better to leave it comfortable than to stress it).

9. It is often helpful to make written records of any measures taken before and during transportation so that the referral centre is aware of these.
   - The vital signs, feeding regimen and frequency, rectal temperature, faecal and urinary output, details of birth and any subsequent relevant details can be supplied usefully.

Section 11
Poisons and antidotes

Poisoning is rare in horses. A diagnosis of poisoning may have considerable consequences; where this is suspected and especially where foul play or negligence is concerned, the proper recording of the events and the results of all clinical and forensic examinations must be made.

In order for a diagnosis of poisoning to be made, the following criteria must be satisfied:

- The horse must have had access to the poison.

- The horse must have ingested or otherwise contacted the poison; some poisons exert their effect by ingestion (such as lead or Ragwort), contact (such as amitraz) or inhalation (such as toxic gas, smoke).

- The poison must be found in the horse's body or the natural body fluids/ excreta.

- The clinical signs must be fully consistent with the defined effects of the poison.

- The pathological effects and morbid findings must be consistent with the known effects of the poison and the poison must be found in the appropriate distribution in clinically significant amounts within the organs of the body.

Defined acceptable (safe) or toxic concentrations of poisons are reasonably well established for most species but there is scanty information about the horse. Most legal opinion relies upon extrapolated information from other species. Drug clearance periods are not well established in horses.

If poisoning is suspected, it is highly advisable to seek support from another professional colleague and to ensure that the correct procedures are undertaken with appropriate recordings. Samples for analysis should be taken into formalin and onto ice and transferred immediately under sealed cover to the nearest forensic laboratory.

The commonest routine test for 'poisoning' in horses is the misuse of drugs to mask clinical disease during prepurchase examination or to alter performance. The Veterinary Defence Society (VDS), UK stores samples taken routinely during prepurchase examinations by their members for a defined period (usually 6 months). The Racecourse Securities Laboratory (UK) is usually empowered to analyse the samples for drug contamination on behalf of the purchaser.

Few of the genuine poisons that horses get access to have specific antidotes (see p. 254) and treatment is usually symptomatic. Treatment or antidotes usually need to be given promptly following poisoning. Ingested poisons, such as metaldehyde (slug bait) or warfarin (rat poison), may have specific antidotes that may be given when signs are detected. However, if it is known that the poison has been ingested, the Veterinary Poisons Information Service (VPIS) can be consulted. In the UK, this is a subscription organisation that is a worthwhile security investment. They provide 24-hour advice for any known poisoning. The specific name of the poison should be provided because some vary in either strength or component mixture.

General principles of treatment include:

1. **Rapid removal of the poison to prevent further contact/ingestion.**

2. **Prevention of absorption.**
   - By use of demulcents (including egg albumen) or adsorbents (such as activated charcoal at 1–3 g/kg bodyweight) if ingested.
   - By washing if skin contact involved.
   - By rapid dilution with copious water. Dilution with either acidic solutions (using cider vinegar) or alkaline solutions (using sodium bicarbonate solution) may be used to neutralise alkaline or acidic materials.
   - Emesis is not possible in horses but gastric lavage may be helpful if carried out soon enough.
   - Purgation in horses is not really effective as an emergency measure and may, in fact, sometimes create more problems than it solves. Nevertheless, there may be circumstances when a saline purge such as sodium sulphate can be helpful (e.g. as a supportive measure for the ileus that accompanies amitraz poisoning).

3. **Where specific antidotes exist, these must be given in sufficient dose by the correct route.**

4. **Symptomatic treatment may involve analgesics, sedatives, anticonvulsants and fluid therapy** (Tables 4.16 and 4.17).

Table 4.16 Known equine plant toxins in the UK

Poison	'Common' source	Clinical signs	Antidote/dose	Supportive treatment
Bracken *Pteridium aquilinum*	Pasture	Weakness/ataxia/ staggering/muscle tremors	High doses vitamin B1 (IM NOT IV!) (100 mg/day for 2 weeks+)	None needed
Ragwort *Seneccio jacobaea*	Pasture/hay/haylage	Hepatic failure	Nil	Liver support only palliative only
Yew *Taxus baccata*	Direct ingestion	Convulsions/sudden death	Nil	Nil
Mares tails *Equisetum arvense*		Weakness/ataxia/ staggering/muscle tremors	High doses vitamin B! (IM NOT IV!) (100 mg/day)	Nil
Oleander *Nerium oleander*	Plant/leaves	Sudden death	Nil	Nil
Deadly nightshade *Atropa belladonna*	Hedgerows	Ileus/mydriasis	No safe antidote Neostigmine at 0.01 mg/kg subcutaneously. Flunixin	High volume nasogastric isotonic solutions to prevent colon impaction
Foxglove *Digitalis purpurea*	Direct or contaminated hay	Bradycardia/cyanosis/ collapse	IV lidocaine 20–50 µg/min	Oral potassium chloride 25–30 g

Table 4.17 Chemical/drug poisons in the UK

Poison	'Common' source	Clinical signs	Antidote/dose	Supportive treatment
Nitrate	Pasture fertiliser	Severe depression	Intravenous methylene blue	Oxygen
Chlorate	Weed killer	Severe depression	Supportive treatment only	Fluid therapy Oxygen
Amitraz	Iatrogenic (washes)	Colic ileus	Analgesia Fluid and saline purgation Atipamezole	Remove food
Lead	Paint/batteries	Central nervous signs	Calcium edetate	Fluid therapy Sedation/anticonvulsants
Monensin	Ruminant feeds	Cardiac failure	Oral 2 g Vitamin E	REST; DO NOT USE DIGOXIN
Paraquat	Weedkiller	Progressive pulmonary oedema	Nil	Nil
Warfarin	Rodenticide iatrogenic	Bleeding	Vitamin K_1 (0.5–1.0 mg/kg IV)	Whole (fresh) blood transfusion
Heparin	Overdose	Haemorrhage	Protamine	Whole blood transfusion

Section 12
Notifiable diseases

African horse sickness (Africa, Middle East, Spain/Portugal)

Anthrax (Worldwide)

Dourine (*Trypanosoma equiperdum*) (Africa, Far East, Middle East)

Equine viral encephalomyelitis (USA/Canada/South America/Asia/Japan)

Epizootic lymphangitis (*Histoplasma farciminosum*) (Africa/Asia/Mediterranean)

Equine infectious (viral) anaemia (Europe/Africa/Asia)

Glanders/farcy (Asia/Africa)

Rabies (Worldwide)

Contagious equine metritis (Western Europe)

Equine viral arteritis (Worldwide – especially Eastern Europe)

West Nile Virus (Africa, North America, Middle East, West and Central Asia and some areas of Europe. Kunjin subtype present in Oceania.)

Note:
- In the UK, salmonellosis and Warble Fly (*Hypoderma bovis*) are reportable rather than strictly notifiable in the horse but suspect cases should be reported to Local Ministry Officials (DVO).

Section 13
Investigative methods/protocols

This section is inserted to help the new/young graduate with some of the more demanding hurdles.

REFERRAL TO A SPECIALIST/REFERRAL CENTRE

If you wish to refer a case to a colleague in a specialist or neighbouring centre you should observe all common and ethical courtesies (and you should expect them in return from the referral centre).

(a) Contact the referral centre early in the course of the disease if you think it might come to referral. They may be able to provide useful information for the further treatment/management of the case. This is particularly important for foals and other emergency referrals such as colic, painful eyes and joint infections.

(b) Consider the implications of referral – welfare, cost and likely success. Discuss with the owner early. Discuss terms of insurance policies in force.

(c) Consider reasons for referral ('passing the buck' is not a reason for referral).

(d) Consider the referral centre staff and system – record all your findings honestly and legibly (laboratory and clinical) and send with the case (fax gives some effective advance warning to the centre, etc.). Send any samples (e.g. peritoneal/joint fluids, placenta, blood samples, etc.) with the case – changes may be very significant.

(e) Ensure that suitable transport is used and that the referral centre has an estimated time of arrival. If possible, be present at loading and administer such medication and nursing care as is required (e.g. nasogastric intubation, fluids, splinting, etc.).

(f) Instruct owner/agent/driver of any emergency measures which might be needed along the way (e.g. check nasogastric tube/administer analgesics).

(g) Remind owner of the need to contact the insurance company.

CERTIFICATION

Veterinary surgeons are reminded that errors of commission and omission in certification are one of the commonest causes of litigation against members of the profession.

(a) All certificates and reports must be completed accurately and as soon as possible after the event.

(b) All certificates should include as full a description of the horse as is appropriate.

(c) All certificates must be written legibly (or preferably typed) and signed by the named veterinary surgeon on headed/official notepaper.

NEVER sign a blank certificate or page of paper – it is asking for trouble and you are likely to be disciplined in a severe fashion by both court and professional body!

The 12 Principles of Certification
(Drafted by RCVS Certification Working Party, BVA, DEFRA)
(Extracted and abbreviated from the Code of Professional Conduct, RCVS.)

1. A veterinarian should only be asked to certify those matters that are:
   - within his/her own knowledge or
   - can be ascertained by him/her personally or
   - the subject of supporting certification from another veterinarian with personal knowledge of the matters in question and is authorised to supply the supporting document(s).

Note:
- Matters not within the knowledge of a veterinarian and/or not the subject of supporting documents but known to other persons (e.g. farmer, driver and jockey) should be the subject of a declaration by those persons only. The veterinarian should be careful to avoid getting drawn into matters outside his/her knowledge/competence or which are the opinions of other people.

2. The veterinarian must not be drawn into certifying (signing) any document which he/she cannot verify him/herself. He/she should not request certifying signatures from others who have no direct knowledge or competence in the matters covered by the documents.

Note:
- The certifying veterinarian should never certify matters of hearsay or suggestion. The certificate should be a matter of verifiable fact.

3. Veterinarians should not sign a document that might raise questions of possible conflicts of interests (e.g. certificates relating to his/her own animals).

Note:
- In the event that conflicts of interest are present, an independent, second opinion/expert should be sought.

4. All certificates should be written in clear, understandable English with the minimum of technical jargon. The meaning of the certificate should be clear and unequivocal.

Note:
- Most certificates will be read by non-veterinarians at some stage and so excessive technical language should be avoided.

5. Certificates should not use words, expressions, phrases or statements that are capable of more than one meaning.

6. Certificates should be produced on a single sheet of paper wherever possible (where this is impossible, the whole document should be bound together so that it is indivisible and tamperproof). Each page should be signed. Each document should carry a unique number with copies being retained by the issuing authority/person who should be able to identify the document easily by reference to the number.

7. Certificates should be written in the first language of the veterinarian signing them. In the event of translation being required, a certified official translation should be attached.

8. All certificates should include a positive identification of each and every animal to which it refers (unless this is impractical, such as in day-old chicks). For equine certificates, this should include the normal sketch and/or narrative description. The minimum permissible identification is a full signalment and a brief written narrative description of the markings and features (see p. 442). **There are no circumstances when no descriptive identification is justified in equine certificates.**

Note:
- The basic format required is typically used on equine vaccination certificates, ID documents and passports (see p. 446).

9. Certificates should not require a veterinarian to certify that there has been compliance with the law of the European Community (or another country where appropriate) unless the specific relevant provisions of the laws involved have been provided and stated clearly and fully in the accompanying documents by the issuing authority.

Note:
- Where legal declarations are required, veterinarians should ensure that they read the accompanying documents carefully before embarking on any certification. Legal advice may be necessary or advisable.

10. Certifying veterinarians should carefully read any specific instructions required by the issuing authority before undertaking any documentation.

Note:
- This will obviate any missing matters in the certificate and eliminate any unnecessary inclusions. The document should relate to the requirements of the requesting authority and should not include matters outside this scope.

11. Certificates must always be presented in **ORIGINAL** form in a manner that is not subject to variations during copying (i.e. certificates must be completed in black, indelible ink). Photocopies and other duplicates (photographic, faxed or scanned) are not acceptable.

Note:
- However, in some circumstances, provision of an endorsed duplicate or copy may be provided. The duplicate must state categorically by endorsement that it is a duplicate/copy. In some cases, the issuing authority may not permit any form of copy.

12. The certificate should be completed on headed notepaper that provides an unambiguous identification of the place of work of the veterinarian. The signature must be accompanied by an *official (practice/authority) stamp* and *must be dated*. The signature must include the printed name and the full qualifications of the certifying veterinarian. No deletions or alterations are permitted (except where these form an integral part of the documentation). Any unavoidable alterations should be clear and unambiguous and each must be signed and dated. No portion of the certificate is left blank in such a way that it can be altered or tampered with.

   - Veterinarians providing a certificate should be satisfied that it is clear, honest and unambiguous. It should relate to matters within his/her competence and should be relevant to the matters concerned.

   - Opinions may be included provided they are clearly identified as such; indeed, many certificates include statements of opinion as to relevance or opinions relating to clinical interpretation. It is useful to include a separate paragraph/section that is headed: **OPINION**.

LITIGATION

Remember
Consult with the RCVS Code of Professional Conduct or contact the RCVS (or your governing body) as soon as you can. Early support and help has saved many careers!

You may find yourself on either side of a litigation procedure. You should conduct yourself with exemplary honesty and in a professional manner. No court will expect a witness to be perfect in every way and you may easily make mistakes and forget aspects of the matters in hand.

(a) **Expert witness**. If you are called to act as an expert witness, remember that you are not called to support or oppose either party. You are there to provide professional guidance and help for the court. Therefore, do not 'wax lyrical' when you are being questioned by 'your side' and 'clam-up' when being cross-examined. The best professional witnesses are those with whom neither side has any quarrel! That is not to say that you should not have any firm opinions – the court will decide how to interpret your statements. You are not the judge and jury!

(b) **Problems with colleagues**. Consult the RCVS Guide to Professional Conduct regularly and get to know its contents. Maintain your dignity and behave in an honest and professional manner. Consult with your governing body and, if necessary, your lawyer. Do not get involved in a 'slanging match' – leave it to the professionals. Most problems between members of the profession arise from lack of communication – so communicate and get to know your colleagues in neighbouring practices. Do not be afraid to apologise if you are wrong or have done something less than perfectly – it often cools off even the most aggressive situation.

(c) **Problem cases**. Notes must be made in a bound book at the time of identification, regarding location, reasons for procedures, examination, treatment, post-mortem examination, etc. It helps if there is a witness to the fact that contemporaneous notes are made. These should not be added to or otherwise interfered with, at any later time. Further comment can be made on additional pages after the event (e.g. laboratory results). Note should be made of the names and addresses of all witnesses and the exact circumstances of the event. The big problem is knowing which case is likely to result in legal complications. It is wise to make and keep proper records of all cases seen and procedures performed. Practice records should be kept for 5 years at least.

PURCHASE EXAMINATION

(a) ENSURE that you are being asked to carry it out for the PURCHASER.

(b) Be aware of the proposed PURPOSE/USE. Ensure your client has seen and tried the horse. Ask if there are any points which he/she has noted and wishes you to pay particular attention to (e.g. breeding potential or obvious problems such as scars, bony lumps, cough, etc.).

(c) RECORD DETAILS of the horse (age/colour/sex/height, etc.), name, address and phone number of vendor and of stable where horse is kept (if different from owner details).

(d) Check that suitable facilities and support personnel exist (darkened box/tack/suitable rider/handler/lunging facilities, exercising yard/field as appropriate). Obtain accurate travel directions.

(e) It is preferable for the prospective PURCHASER (your client or agent) TO BE PRESENT with you during the examination.

(f) Arrange APPOINTMENT WITH VENDOR (ensure horse is kept stabled overnight until you arrive – stable can be cleaned and horse fed if appropriate to time of arrival). Give specific time of arrival and arrive 10–15 minutes early!

(g) On arrival, observe yard and attitude of vendor (helpful/resentful/over-talkative, etc!). Make discrete observations into tack room/office for drug bottles/packets, needles and syringes (glance into waste bin if you get a chance!).

IN THE PRESENCE OF THIRD PARTY (if possible) ask the vendor if there is anything he/she wants to tell you. Enquire specifically about VICES, disease history (e.g. lameness, coughing, colic, etc.) and drugs either past or present. Record answers in notebook as soon as possible!

Observe horse from distance.

It is common practice (and a wise precaution) to take a blood sample from horses subjected to purchase examination (only with permission of the owner). This should include lithium heparin, fluoride oxalate and plain tubes (plasma/serum should be separated from each specimen, divided into two and stored in a freezer after being identified with owner/purchaser/name of horse and date of sampling and then sealed).

RECORD YOUR FINDINGS IN YOUR OWN NOTEBOOK as you go along.

(h) Clinical examination.

- Observe restraint/haltering and acceptance or otherwise of restraint.
- Record age, sex, type and colour.
- Full clinical examination including darkroom ophthalmoscopy and thoracic auscultation (heart and lungs including trachea). Examine arterial pulses in all available arteries and record vital signs including temperature (more to show that it can be obtained!). Examine the skin carefully.

- Carefully palpate entire body surface! Scars (e.g. Hobday, Tieback, laparotomy) and any swellings, etc., may be palpable but not visible! Record anything you find abnormal or equivocal.
- Joint and limb manipulations.
- Pick up and examine feet – test with foot tester/hammer. Feel for temperature differences between hooves. Check digital pulses (all four).
- Examine carefully for symmetry by standing the horse square and walking carefully round it observing anything unusual or non-symmetrical (left/right, front/back).
- If required, make *approximate* measurement (this is not compulsory but might be helpful to purchaser) – official height certificate can only be provided by a veterinary surgeon approved by Joint Measurement Scheme.

(i) Preliminary trot.

- In-hand walks and trot (straight line 30–40 m, circles, turns, backing).
- Sharp/tight turns left and right.
- Flexion tests (whole limb) on all four limbs.
- *Note*: Ensure handler does not affect gait or try to alter gait/behaviour, etc.

(j) Strenuous exercise.

- Tack up – observe and record type of tack used.
- Observe at all paces under saddle (ridden circle and straight line) or lunge (if appropriate).
- Listen for clarity of wind.
- *Note*: Vary exercise extent with purpose/fitness.
- Auscultate heart (record maximal rate)/lungs (including trachea and pharynx), palpate feet and legs and test symmetry of arterial pulses at end of exercise.

(k) Period *of rest* IN BOX without tack, etc.

- Observe the horse in its box (DO NOT LEAVE).
- Complete ID.
- Check cardiac rate/rhythm (take time to reach resting rate) and character of horse.
- Discuss findings (in private) with purchaser if present.

(l) Second trot and foot examination.

- Trot straight from box in straight line and test backing and turning.
- Full range of flexion tests again (full limb only).

(m) Documentation.

- Complete full VDS/RCVS approved form. DO NOT USE OTHER TYPES because they may be inadequate in some areas. The tested and legally accepted forms are the best ones to use. Ensure that you have them before you set off! (Ensure that the copy is correctly set up!) Ideally this should be typed!

- State findings on the form (e.g. 'was heard to cough once', etc.) (ALL – no matter how small/apparently irrelevant!)
- Give an honest opinion on the findings!
- Do not forget to record the results and what you have advised in your notebook at the time – even if this is done over the phone to the prospective purchaser.

It is unlikely that this examination can be completed properly in less than 1.5–2 hours unless sections of the examination are excluded (for specific reasons). If any part of the examination is not performed (for any reason) this must be stated on the form (there is usually a section for this).

Notes:
- Few horses will be perfect (if they are, it pays to be extra suspicious!).
- Remind the purchaser of the WARRANTY clause on the form regarding height, vices, ability, administration of drugs, etc. Point out what you have not done (e.g. radiographs, rectal examination, etc.) and state why.
- **DO NOT DISCUSS THE FINDINGS WITH THE VENDOR.**

If you are uncertain of the procedure for this examination, try to attend a suitable course on the matter. Purchase examination is the subject of numerous litigations against members of the profession and younger, less-experienced veterinary surgeons should be particularly careful – do not perform these unless you are certain of your ground and your ability to spot the problem horses.

IDENTIFICATION

Identification is important for the original identifier and for subsequent confirmation of identity. The method is strictly laid down by various bodies and wherever possible an approved/accepted/official prepared form of identification should be used. This is included in all purchase and insurance examination documentation and in other official identification (Equine Passports)/naming and vaccination certificates. Only a written description is usually used in letters and descriptive reports but even these have minimal requirements (age, breed, colour, sex and name). The name of the owner and the place and date of the examination should be stated in all certificates. Weatherbys, in conjunction with the RCVS and BEVA, publishes a very useful guide to the identification of horses (new edition published 2008).

Colour

Thoroughbred colours recognised by Weatherbys

Black. In a black horse, the whole coat, including legs, body, flank and head is black. Any indication of tan in coat makes the horse brown.

Brown. The mane, tail, ears and distal limbs are the same brown colour without black components.

Bay. Bay horses have black mane, tail and lower legs. If there is a difference between the black lower and dark upper limbs and body, with some tan in flanks and muzzle, the horse is bay-brown or dark bay.

Note:
- The terms light bay and dark bay should be avoided because differences often occur seasonally.

Chestnut. Variable orange to sandy colour, they can have a mane and tail which is lighter or darker than the body colour but it is not black. Lighter-coloured chestnuts may have flaxen manes and tails while darker chestnuts are called liver chestnut. Black markings such as patches can be found and should be drawn/described.

Grey. Where the coat is a varying mosaic of black and white hairs with black skin. As greys age, they tend to become lighter, approaching white in some cases. The mane may be a similar or lighter colour. Flea-bitten greys have small *groups* of chestnut hairs distributed through the coat.

Roan. Rarely encountered in thoroughbreds. The basic body colour has variable quantities of additional white hairs distributed throughout. The quantity of these hairs varies with the season. Qualification of the description 'roan' (e.g. red) is acceptable; however, these horses tend to be going grey. Some greys have chestnut hairs scattered in the coat and some bays have white hairs scattered in the coat. These are best described in the narrative.

Colours recognised by alternative authorities

Blue Roan. The body colour is black or very dark brown with a generalised scattering of white hairs, giving a blue tinge to the coat. Head and lower limbs are usually darker, while white markings can sometimes be seen on the legs.

Red Roan. The basic colour is bay or bay-brown with generalised scattering of white hairs giving a reddish tinge to the coat. White markings can occasionally be seen.

Strawberry or Chestnut Roan. Basic body colour is chestnut with a generalised scattering of white hairs. White markings can occasionally be seen.

Blue Dun. Variable stone/slate grey colour evenly distributed, with black skin, mane and tail. Occasional line (list) down the back and/or withers stripe.

Yellow Dun. Dusty yellow colour. Other features as for blue dun.

Palamino. Rich gold colour body with blonde white mane and tail.

Appaloosian. Basic coat colour usually roan with variable, generalised mosaic of spots; may be dark on light or *vice versa,* over either part or all of the body.

Piebald. Large, irregular but well-defined patches of black and white.

Skewbald. Large, irregular but well-defined patches of white and of any colour *except* black (e.g. often brown). The line of demarcation between the colours is generally well-defined.

(Odd) coloured. Large irregular patches of more than two colours, which can be less well defined than piebald and skewbald.

Cream (cremello). Cream-coloured with non-pigmented skin and pale/non-pigmented iris.

Further coat colour terminology

Ticked. Sparsely distributed white hairs throughout the coat.

Flecked. Small patches of hairs of different colour to body unevenly distributed over part of the body. The degrees of flecking may be described (e.g. 'heavily flecked', 'lightly flecked'). Colour of the flecking should be specified.

Spots. As for flecked but patches more circular.

Patch. Any large, well-defined area (not covered by previous definitions) of hairs differing from the general body colour. The colour, shape, position and extent should be drawn and described.

Zebra marks. Where there is horizontal striping, often seen on caudal aspect of limbs but also neck, withers or quarters.

Mane and tail. The presence of differently coloured hairs in mane and tail should be specified.

Ermine marks. Black spots attached to or just above the coronary band on a white limb. Often, but not always, associated with a black hoof coloration down that region of the foot.

List. A dorsal band of dark hair extending from the withers backwards along the spine.

Whorls

Whorls are formed by changes in direction of flow of the hair. Simple whorls should be referred to as 'whorl' while other types should be further defined. They should be described as accurately as possible in relation to their anatomic position and forehead whorls in relation to dorsal midline and eye level.

Simple. A single focal point from which the hairs diverge.

Tufted. A focal point into which the hairs converge from different directions and pile into a tuft.

Linear. Two sweeps of hair converging from diametrically opposite directions along a line.

Feathered. Two sweeps of hair diverge along a line at an angle to form a feathered pattern.

Crested. As for linear, but the hair from each of the two directions rises up to form a crest.

Sinuous. Crested or feathered along an irregular curving line.

The position of head whorls should be clearly described in terms of relation to midline and eye level and to white markings.

White Markings

Star. White mark on the forehead; the size, shape, position and border should be described. A few white hairs are not described as a star but should be noted.

Stripe. Dorsal white marking down the nose and not wider than the flat surface of the nasal bones. The star and stripe are often continuous and should be described as star and stripe conjoined. If there is a gap in the stripe it is described as an *interrupted stripe*. The proximal point of origin should be described as well as the termination point. Any variation in width and direction should be described (e.g. 'broad stripe', 'narrow stripe', 'inclined to left', 'terminating at upper left nostril'.

Blaze. Dorsal white marking covering almost the whole of the forehead between the eyes and extending beyond the width of the nasal bones, often to the muzzle. Any variations in direction, markings and termination points should be stated.

White face. White covering the forehead and front of the face, extending laterally towards the mouth. The extension may be asymmetric in which case that should be described.

Snip. Isolated white marking situated between or close to the nostrils. Its size, position and intensity should be specified.

Lip markings. Size, shape, etc., should be described.

White muzzle. White covering both lips and extends to the region of the nostrils.

White limbs. White markings on limbs should be accurately drawn and described (e.g. 'white to half pastern rising to fetlock on inside'). Lay terminology must be avoided (e.g. socks, stockings, etc.).

The following descriptions should be used when describing white marks without well-defined margins:

Mixed. White marking containing varying amounts of hairs of the general body colour.

Bordered. A white mark with a mixed border (e.g. 'bordered star').

Flesh marks. Patches of unpigmented skin (e.g. often on lips, should be described as 'flesh marks').

The Sketch

The sketch forms an integral part of the definitive identification of the horse and must be completed correctly with white marks in red hatching and whorls shown as a black cross – with extensions if linear or feathered, etc.

Neck whorls. Correct position of the crest whorls and neck whorls is best achieved by dividing the neck into three parts – anterior, middle and posterior.

White markings. Outlined with diagonal hatching in red. A few hairs without distinct outline are drawn as a few diagonal hatches in red.

A bordered mark. Indicated by a double ring with hatched centre space.

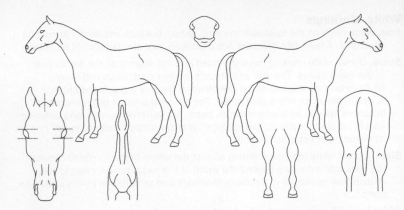

Fig. 4.75 A typical sketch outline for completion. Note that the limb descriptions must be completed from medial, lateral and posterior views. All the markings MUST be included/completed.

A mixed mark. As for white marking but stated 'mixed' in the narrative.

A spot. A white spot, if sizeable, must be outlined and hatched in red. A dark spot within a white marking (e.g. on a blaze) should be outlined and left blank.

Flesh marks. Outlined and shaded completely in red.

A bordered flesh mark. Outlined by two concentric lines and shaded completely in red.

A mottled flesh mark. Drawn as for bordered flesh mark and indicated in the narrative.

Scars. Permanent adventitious marks (i.e. not congenital marks) (e.g. marks made by tack, firing, branding and tattoo marks and surgical scars). These should be described and drawn on the sketch and indicated by an arrow.

Congenital abnormalities. Any congenital marks or other abnormalities should be clearly described in the certificate and indicated on the sketch where possible, e.g.:

- **Wall-eye.** Lack of pigmentation on iris giving a pink or silver-blue appearance to the eye.

- **Showing the white of the eye.** Where some part of the sclera shows between the eyelids.

- **The 'prophet's thumb mark.** Muscular depression seen usually in the neck, but sometimes in the shoulders or hindquarters. It should be indicated on the sketch by a triangular mark and described in the narrative (Fig. 4.75).

Limbs
Hooves. Any variation in the normal dark colour of the hooves should be noted. In the case of a grey and chestnut the colour of each hoof should be stated.

Chestnuts. The vestigial digits form the chestnuts – sometimes referred to as night eyes (USA). Chestnuts may be vestigial on or even absent from, the occasional leg. The precise shapes provide useful identification features in whole-coloured horses. They are best drawn. Common shapes include *round, oval, pear-shaped, irregular pointed* (at top, below, etc.) and *notched* (above, below, etc.).

The Description

The narrative should be typed or handwritten using block capital letters in black ink. All identification documents must be signed and stamped with an official stamp (Fig. 4.76.)

CERTIFICATE OF VETERINARY EXAMINATION
OF A HORSE ON BEHALF OF A PROSPECTIVE PURCHASER

CERTIFICATE No:
V

This is to certify that, at the request of (Name & Address) _____

I have examined the horse described below, the property of (Name & Address) _____

at (Place of Examination) _____ on (Time & Date) _____

NAME of horse (or breeding)	
RICARDO	INSTRUCTIONS 1) WRITTEN DESCRIPTION SHOULD BE TYPED OR WRITTEN IN BLOCK CAPITALS
	2) WRITTEN DESCRIPTION AND DIAGRAM SHOULD AGREE
	3) ALL WHITE MARKINGS SHOULD BE HATCHED IN RED
	4) WHORLS MUST BE SHOWN THUS "X" AND DESCRIBED IN DETAIL
BREED OR TYPE	
TB CROSS	
COLOUR	LEFT SIDE RIGHT SIDE
BAY	
SEX GELDING	
AGE by documentation	FORE REAR VIEW HIND REAR VIEW
15 yrs	
APPROX. AGE (by dentition (See Note 1 - overleaf)	
AGED	HEAD AND NECK, VENTRAL VIEW MUZZLE LEFT RIGHT LEFT RIGHT

IDENTIFICATION

Head: IRREGULAR DIAMOND-SHAPED STAR DORSAL MIDLINE, CONJOINED STRIPE TAPERING OUT MIDWAY TO MUZZLE. TRIANGULAR BORDERED FLESH MARK BETWEEN NOSTRILS, MEDIAN WHORL UPPER EYE LEVEL, WHORL LEFT OF MIDLINE AT EYE LEVEL. MIDLINE POLL WHORL ADJACENT TO MANE.

Neck: WHORL UPPER THIRD RIGHT CREST. FEATHERED WHORL MIDPOINT OF LEFT CREST. TWO THROAT WHORLS. CRESTED WHORL LOWER THIRD TRACHEA. PROPHETS THUMB MARK RIGHT JUGULAR GROOVE.

Limbs: LF WHITE TO MID-CANNON, STRIATED HOOF.
RF NO WHITE, BLACK HOOF.
LH WHITE HOOF, CRESTED WHORL PLANTAR UPPER THIRD CANNON.
RH WHITE TO PASTERN. WHITE HOOF, CRESTED WHORL PLANTAR UPPER THIRD CANNON.

Body: BILATERAL WHORLS BASE OF NECK. BILATERAL SHOULDER WHORLS WITH SINUOUS FEATHERING TO NECK. BILATERAL STIFLE FOLD WHORLS WITH FEATHERING TO WHORLS AT POINT OF PELVI.

Acquired marks/brands/microchip: CENTRAL WITHER MARKS, SCATTERED SADDLE MARKS LEFT. NO MICROCHIP.

Fig. 4.76 A typical narrative description form that is commonly included in all identification certificates such as passports, vaccination and registration documents. Note the non-technical language and clear descriptions of the markings that make the identification unique.

COLIC PROTOCOL

Do not be afraid to refer a colic horse to a specialist centre. No veterinary surgeon should feel under pressure to maintain an incorrect clinical approach and you will seldom, if ever, lose a client as a result of an early referral. The horse will be pleased with you and the owners will be satisfied that they are more likely to collect a live horse than a big bill and a dead one (Fig. 4.77)!

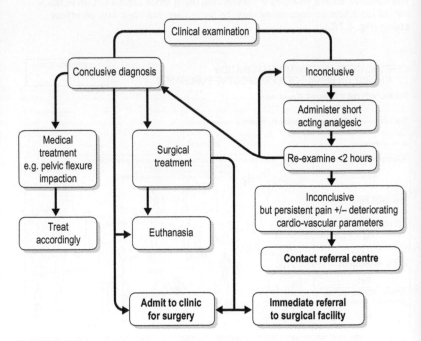

Fig. 4.77 Colic protocol.

Useful hints

- Extreme pain is usually indicative of a surgical condition (you may make an occasional mistake but it is best to err on the side of safety).
- Abdominal distension is usually surgical and an absolute emergency.
- Deteriorating C–V parameters suggest a surgical problem.
- Reluctance to move (parietal pain usually suggestive of peritonitis and possible abdominal catastrophe).
- Blood-stained peritoneal fluid suggests ischaemic/strangulating condition.

- Persistent mild pain suggests non-strangulating obstruction.
- Diarrhoea is seldom an indicator of a surgical problem unless it is complicated by secondary intestinal compromises.
- Failure to respond to analgesics suggests surgical problem.
- Extensive disruption of bedding/stable, etc., suggests prolonged/violent colic.
- Facial trauma suggests prolonged pain (may not be present at the time of examination).
- Do not subject a catastrophic case to the further stress of transport – be prepared to kill the horse immediately if this is indicated.
- NEVER ignore blood on a rectal sleeve!

  The *single most important factor that mitigates against the survival of colic horses is procrastination.*
  GB Edwards, 1987.

LAMENESS PROTOCOL

Lameness investigations should be carried out when the animal is lame, with the typical circumstances present (e.g. shod/unshod, after rest and after/during exercise). This is particularly applicable to referral cases. Referral centres do not appreciate having to try to identify lameness in animals receiving analgesics and/or when they are not actually lame. If you are in doubt about the management of a referral case, discuss it with your colleagues and with the referral centre specialist (Fig. 4.78).

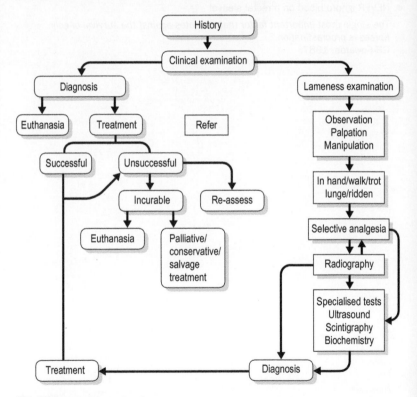

Fig. 4.78 Lameness protocol.

Section 14
Equipment for equine practice

FIRST AID KIT (FOR RACES/EVENTS, ETC.)

Always arrive promptly (events usually cannot get underway until the full complement of emergency services are present).

Remember to ensure that the organisers know you are present and where you will be found (radio may be used). Stay where you are unless the organisers are informed otherwise. DO NOT be afraid to refer cases off the course to a hospital (use ambulance if necessary).

Note:
● All items should be clearly labelled and checked regularly (at least before every event). It is best to have the items marked (*) in a small suitcase/box, which can be easily carried. It should remain with the veterinary surgeon throughout the event.

1. **EUTHANASIA GUN** (and appropriate ammunition)* (only if you are licensed and prepared to shoot horses), injectable solutions* sufficient to kill at least two horses (more if large event, far away from practice or you are the only vet) (e.g. Somulose® , Arnolds, UK (recommended), pentobarbitone (200 mg/mL)).

2. **DRESSINGS**: Melolin*, cotton bandage*, cotton wool*, Elastoplast*, Vetwrap*, Vaseline gauze, Intrasite gel.

3. **HARDWARE**: Scissors* (straight, curved), stethoscope*, SUTURE KIT* (see below), BLEEDER KIT* (clamps, tissue forceps, tourniquet/Esmarch bandage), twitch*, tracheotomy tube*, safety razors (disposable), stomach tube.

4. **SPLINTS/CASTING MATERIALS**: Wooden foot wedges and axial splints (gutter/2″×2″ wooden battens) or Equine Emergency 'Ski' Boot. At least 10 rolls of casting material (e.g. Dynacast Optima® , Smith and Nephew) with suitable orthopaedic felt.

5. **DISPOSABLES**: Syringes (60/20/10/5/2/1)*, needles, cannulae* (10–24), suture materials*, paper towel*, sterile swabs*, sterile gloves*, disposable aprons/boiler suits (in case of contagion).

6. **DRUGS**: Local anaesthetics*, butorphanol*, detomidine*, xylazine*, acepromazine*, thiopentone* (thiopental), water for injection*, tetanus antiserum, surgical scrub. Possibly antibiotics. Adrenaline (norepinephrine).

7. **STATIONERY**: Headed paper* and notebook, red/black pens*, invoicing equipment (your practice cannot afford to give the drugs, etc., away – check practice policy before event). You are there to provide FIRST AID not full investigation/treatment.

8. **CLOTHING**: Suitable protective clothing/overalls, boots.

PRACTICE 'CAR BOOT' LIST

This is not a definitive list – individuals may need/want to alter some or all of this – but it may help you over the first few days in equine practice! You might even get the nurses to ensure it is all there at the start of every week!

KEEP ALL EQUIPMENT (yourself/clothing AND YOUR CAR) CLEAN – the quality of your work is reflected in the way in which you look after all of these and they are expensive to replace – your annual salary increment may rely on it! Additionally, carefully maintained equipment functions better and is always available when you need it. If something gets broken – get it repaired as soon as possible.

Hardware

1. **Handling equipment**: Twitch, rope halter, headcollar, leading rein, Chiffney bit. Usefully kept together in a cotton bag.

2. **Farrier**: Hoof knives (steel/file/oilstone), hoof tester, hammer, buffer, nail pullers, pincers, hoof cutters, rasp, apron. Usefully kept together in a compartmentalised leather bag or tray.

3. **Clinical**: Thermometer (mercury or digital), stethoscope, plexor/pleximeter, ophthalmoscope (with spare batteries), pen torch, TORCH (rechargeable from car), stomach tubes (foal/medium/large), funnel(s), scissors (curved and straight), tooth rasps (straight/angled), Hausman's gag, stirrup pump, parturition gown, flutter valve.

4. **Other**: RUBBISH BIN and sharps container. Waterproof marker pens/pencil. Practice stamp/pad, headed paper (in closed polythene container).

   - Purchase Examination/Insurance Examination and Slaughter Certificates, RED and BLACK pens. Vaccination certificates. LVI stamp. Pads and pens are usefully kept inside the car in a polythene box.

   - **GUN (locked in case/box fixed to floor of boot or under seat) (fewer police authorities are happy with firearm use by vets and they do not condone thefts or accidents!).**

5. **Surgical**: Disposable safety razors (or rechargeable clippers with car charger).

   - SUTURE PACK (sterile) (scalpel handle, scissors, forceps (rat/plain), suture needles, two to four pairs artery forceps, needle holders, swabs, scalpel blades).

   - Sterile and non-sterile gloves.

   - Suture materials (catgut, nylon, Vicryl). Penrose drains.

   - Wolf teeth extractor (Burgess Wolf-Tooth Kit useful).

   - CASTRATION KIT (*sterile*: Serra emasculator, scalpel handle, two to six large artery forceps, blades, suture needles, suture material).

Disposables

1. Roll of paper towel, rectal gloves, sterile gloves, swabs.

2. Syringes (1/2/5/10/20/50 mL sizes STERILE), needles (disposable) (22×1″, 20×1″, 19×1.5″, 18×1.5″), IV cannulas (18/16/14/12/10), Vacutainer holders/needles (19×1.5″).

3. Blood sampling tubes (EDTA/Fl-ox/Li-hep/Plain) (preferably Vacutainers – 'mini' are excellent), microscope slides (in clean, sealed container) and slide carrier, bacterial/viral swabs (transport medium), faecal and urine pots, sterile universals/bijous. Universal bottles with 10% formol saline.

Diagnostics
Fluorescein strips, proxymetacaine (needs to be kept refrigerated!) or amethocaine (stable at room temperature), urine Dipstix.

Drugs
1. **Euthanasia solution(s)**.
2. **Anti-infective agents**: penicillin (crystalline, procaine), TMS (parenteral/oral – powder and paste), chloramphenicol eye ointment, gentamicin eye drops, povidone scrub/solution/ointment, surgical spirit.
3. **Analgesics, etc.**: butorphanol (CD), buscopan, xylazine, ketamine, atropine (eye drops).
4. **Anti-inflammatory drugs**: phenylbutazone (parenteral, oral powder/paste), flunixin (oral and parenteral).
5. **Dressings**: Elastoplast, Vetwrap, absorbent cotton, cotton bandages, melolin/allevyn, silver dressings. Poultices. *Dynacast Optima* (carry 6–10 rolls in a sealed plastic bag), orthopaedic felt.
6. **Other**: saline (1×5 L+4–5×1 L), Hartman solution (5×5 L minimum – more may be required according to the type/grade of the event and the local climate), liquid paraffin (5 L minimum), Duphalyte (×2), WATER FOR INJECTION. Saline (4×250 mL and 500 mL sterile pack).

CLIENT FIRST AID KIT CONTENTS

A minimal client first aid kit should contain:

1. *Hardware*:
   - Scissors (straight and curved)
   - Thermometer
   - Mills wound irrigator
   - Plastic bowl
   - Disposable gloves
   - Paper towel
   - Razor blade (disposable)
   - Teaspoon
   - Nose twitch
   - Penknife
   - Pen torch

2. *Wound management materials*:
   - Cotton wool (1/2×500 g rolls)
   - Sterile gauze swabs (3 packs of 10)
   - Sterile saline in bag (2×500 mL, 1×250 mL)
   - Hydrogel (e.g. Intrasite Gel, Smith and Nephew, UK)
   - Wound antiseptic (e.g. Chlorhexidine scrub, Hibiscrub)
   - Salt (100 g in sealed container)

Note:
- An approximately physiological saline can be made from 1 flat teaspoonful of salt in a pint of lukewarm, previously boiled water.

3. Dressings
   - Absorbent dressings (e.g. Allevyn, Smith and Nephew, UK) (adhesive and non-adhesive in various sizes)
   - Plastic film dressing (e.g. Melolin, Smith and Nephew Ltd, UK)
   - Soft cotton roll (6–8 rolls) (Soffban, Smith and Nephew Ltd, UK)
   - Non-elastic conforming bandages (12×10–12 cm size)
   - Semi-adhesive bandage 4–5 rolls (Co-Plus Smith and Nephew Ltd, UK)
   - Adhesive bandage (Elastoplast, Smith and Nephew Ltd, UK)

4. *Instruction booklet with personal details and emergency information* including next of kin and doctor's name, address and telephone number (in the event of an accident) *and details of veterinary practice* (name, address, telephone numbers).

CLIENT FIRST AID KIT CONTENTS

A typical client first aid kit should contain:

1. Instruments
   - Scissors (straight and curved)
   - Thermometer
   - Mills wound irrigator
   - Plastic bowl
   - Disposable gloves
   - Paper towel
   - Razor blade (disposable)
   - Tourniquet
   - Nose twitch
   - Penknife
   - Pen torch

2. Wound management materials
   - Cotton wool (1/2 × 500 g rolls)
   - Sterile gauze swabs (3 packs of 10)
   - Sterile saline in bag (2 × 500 ml, 1 × 50 ml)
   - Hydrogel (e.g. Intrasite Gel, Smith and Nephew, UK)
   - Wound antiseptic (e.g. Chlorhexidine scrub, Hibiscrub)
   - Salt (100 g in sealed container)

   Notes
   An alternative to the Intrasite Gel saline can be made either by boiling tap water or a salt in 2 l (1 pint) flask of previously boiled water.

3. Dressings
   - Absorbent dressings e.g. Allevyn, Smith and Nephew, UK, adhesive and non-adhesive in small sizes
   - Plastic film dressings e.g. Melolin, Smith and Nephew Ltd, UK
   - Soft cotton roll (e.g. Soffban, Smith and Nephew Ltd, UK)
   - Non-elastic conforming bandages (2.5, 10, 15 cm size)
   - Semi-adhesive bandage (e.g. Orabind (Orabine, Smith and Nephew Ltd, UK)
   - Adhesive bandage (Elastoplast, small and medium, 10 cm)
   - Permanent marker with practical notes and emergency coordinator supply name of vet and doctor's name, number and telephone number in the event of an accident and details of vet's, doctor (name, address, telephone number).

Part 4 CLINICAL AIDS

Section 15
Anaesthesia

FIELD ANAESTHESIA

Before embarking on any anaesthesia the attending veterinary surgeon MUST be satisfied that the proposed method is both safe and effective. The duration and depth required will depend on the procedure being performed.

Sedation of Unhandlable Horse in a Field

If possible, withhold water for 2 days – then add 3–6 g/45 kg of chloral hydrate (30–60 g total for the average-sized horse) to a gallon of water in a bucket.

The mixture tastes very bitter and it is unlikely even a thirsty animal will drink it all, but hopefully it will drink enough to sedate the horse.

Chloral hydrate is a 'pro-drug' and has to be metabolised to its active form in the liver. Therefore, be patient and allow up to 30 minutes before disturbing the horse. If you have estimated the weight wrongly and have overdosed the horse it may become recumbent.

Depending on the level of sedation from the chloral hydrate you may want to 'top-up' the degree of sedation with a more familiar drug.

> **Note:**
> ● Chloral hydrate does not provide any analgesia – so remember to give an analgesic if you are going to do anything that will cause pain.

SEDATION OF PREGNANT MARES

Late term pregnant mares in particular can be a challenge to sedate or anaesthetise.

Many physiological parameters in the mare change with pregnancy, others (e.g. ventilation and circulation) are affected by the massive bulk of the uterus. Metabolic and hormonal changes also occur.

Most of the drugs we normally use will pass the placenta and will be found in the foetus as well. This is mainly a concern in late pregnancy or Caesarean section.

The aims during sedation or anaesthesia in non-obstetric surgery are to:

1. maintain foetal oxygenation
2. maintain uterine blood flow
3. prevent premature foetal delivery

4. maintain maternal homoeostasis

5. ensure rapid recovery.

If it is absolutely necessary to sedate the mare, it helps to stick to a plan in order to keep time of sedation/anaesthesia as short as possible and least stressful for you:

1. Prepare all the requirements you need for the procedure beforehand.

2. Try to keep the mare quiet and pre-oxygenate if possible by mask or nasopharyngeal tube.

3. If the mare is hypovolemic (sweating, not drinking over some period, etc.) place a catheter to administer fluid electrolytes (2–10 mL/kg/h).

4. Sedate with *romifidine 20–80 μg/kg* (because it causes the least and the shortest intrauterine pressure increase and because there is no evidence that its use is linked with abortion). This can be combined with *butorphanol 0.02–0.1 mg/kg*. This provides sedation and analgesia but at high doses some ataxia may develop.

5. Provide O_2 as long as possible and let the mare recover in a quiet environment with close observation during the next few days.

For any procedure requiring general anaesthesia, the mare should probably be referred to a hospital that can provide full intensive care support and controlled anaesthesia with positive pressure facility.

FOAL SEDATION

Factors to Consider

- Foals are small and have a high surface area to body weight ratio so ensure they are kept warm and dry to avoid hypothermia.
- They have a reduced ability to metabolise most drugs so take care with dosing, especially if repeated doses are necessary.
- Cardiac output is dependent on the heart rate as the myocardium is less compliant and they are less able to increase stroke volume.
- Foals often have a patent or partially patent ductus arteriosus in the first 24–48 hours and may have physiological murmurs over the heart base for the first 3 months.
- Murmurs can also occur due to fever, anaemia or high cardiac output.
- PCV is higher in foals (43%) and will fall to normal over the first few weeks of life.
- Oxygen consumption is higher in the first few weeks of life so foals are more susceptible to hypoxaemia; if possible maintain in sternal to optimise the PaO_2.
- Fluid requirements are greater and they have a greater total body water (mainly in greater ECF volume). Ideally, foals should drink 25% of their body weight daily.
- Monitor the blood glucose levels as they are prone to hypoglycaemia (too much glucose can cause rebound hypoglycaemia when the glucose-containing fluids are withdrawn).

- May need to check IgG levels. May need to give colostrums or plasma preoperative/pre-sedation.
- Sedate the mare, especially if the foal is to undergo GA and keep her sedated until the foal recovers.

Sedation

1. **Useful to aid restraint** for procedure such as bandaging and catheter placement and to reduce stress.
2. **Diazepam:**
   - 0.1–0.2 mg/kg IV
   - Mild sedation.
   - Especially useful in younger foals and sick foals
   - Minimal cardiorespiratory depression
   - Will cause recumbency
   - No analgesia.
3. **Xylazine:**
   - 0.3–0.5 mg/kg IV
   - Sedation may last for up to 90 minutes in foals
   - Can **combine with butorphanol** 0.02 mg/kg to enhance sedation and analgesia
   - Foals will tend to become recumbent
   - Heart rate will drop and so can compromise cardiac output (the second-degree AV block seen in adults with this drug is rare in foals)
   - May cause some degree of respiratory noise due to muscle relaxation around the larynx and airway collapse.
4. **Other alpha-2 agonists:**
   - Have too long a duration of action and, therefore, side effects
   - Detomidine may prove more reliable than xylazine when given intramuscularly.
5. **ACP:**
   - Long duration
   - May enhance hypothermia due to the vasodilation caused
   - Will not provide adequate sedation for most procedures.

DETOMIDINE DRIP SEDATION

1. **Potential uses:**
   - Prolonged standing procedures such as frontal sinus trephine, thoracoscopy and ovariectomy.

2. **Advantages**:
   - No need for repeated top ups.
   - Aims to maintain an even plane of sedation.
   - Can anticipate changes in level of sedation.

3. **Disadvantages**:
   - Time taken to set up.
   - Cost.
   - Possibility of profound sedation if not observant.

4. **Procedure**:
   - Place IV catheter.
   - Sedate horse with 6 µg/kg detomidine.
   - *Note*: May take 5 minutes to achieve full effects.
   - Give an analgesic dose of butorphanol (0.05–0.1 mg/kg).
   - Add 12 mg of detomidine to 500 mL of saline.
   - For a 500 kg horse start drip rate at 4 drops per second (~0.1 µg/kg/min) – dose is adjusted for other bodyweights.
   - Aim to 'predict' requirements for deeper sedation and increase drip rate pre-emptively as there is an ~1–2 minutes lag in increasing drip rate before full effect is seen.
   - When adequate sedation is achieved, reduce to 1–2 drops per second.
   - Horse should be able to leave stocks 10–15 minutes after stopping drip.

PROCEDURES FOR EQUINE FIELD ANAESTHESIA

Pre-anaesthetic Assessment

History

In all cases, a history should be obtained. Important aspects of the history include the following:

- Has the horse been anaesthetised/sedated before? Were there any adverse reactions?
- The vaccination status. All horses undergoing surgery should be up to date with their tetanus and if not it is recommended to give tetanus antitoxin.
- Any known problems in the past (e.g. penicillin reactions, adverse reactions to sedation, etc.).
- Insurance details; this is important as most companies will need to be informed before elective procedures are carried out if the insurance is to be valid.
- Ensure you get informed consent before every anaesthetic.

Clinical examination

- This is essential in all cases. However, occasionally it may have to be restricted and a fractious animal may require sedation first to allow examination.

- The most important body systems with respect to anaesthesia are the cardiovascular and respiratory systems.
- Place a catheter before anaesthesia.

Weight
Accurately measuring or estimating the weight is very important to avoid both under- and overdosing of the anaesthetic agents.

In the field, it is often impossible to accurately weigh the horse and, therefore, girth tapes and calculated weights are very useful (especially for thoroughbred-type horses). Some weigh tapes are specially designed for larger or smaller horses and are correspondingly more accurate.

Pre-Anaesthetic Sedation
The sedation protocol will depend on several factors including:

1. the temperament and breed
2. significant findings in the pre-anaesthetic exam
3. available helpers
4. environment
5. personal familiarity with the drugs available.

Route of administration is important and will vary according to the horse's temperament, the drug involved and the ease of administration.

If ketamine is to be used as the induction agent, then the horses must be well sedated to avoid the excitement that ketamine alone causes.

Acepromazine (ACP)
- 10 mg/mL (Large Animal Solution).
- Dose:

0.1–0.25 mg/kg per os (in UK only the paste form is licensed, the tablets are not licensed for horses).

0.03–0.1 mg/kg IM.

0.01–0.05 mg/kg IV.

- Onset 30–40 minutes irrespective of the route of administration, so adequate time should be allowed before induction.
- Only about 70% of animals respond and further top ups can prolong the duration of the side effects or lead to excitement and increased locomotor activity.
- Generally, will not cause adequate sedation if ketamine is to be used.
- Mental calming effect can be improved by the addition of opioids.
- Hypotension by vasodilation, especially a problem in hypovolaemic animals.
- May cause profound hypotension and even collapse in very excited animals (treat with phenylephrine, not adrenaline (epinephrine)).
- Minimal effects on respiration.

- Spasmolytic, anti-arrhythmic.
- Muscle relaxation. Including the retractor penis muscle so the penis protrudes.
- *Care in stallions* as prolonged penile protrusion can lead to severe problems that may necessitate penile amputation!
- Inclusion in the pre-anaesthetic protocol reduces the risk of perioperative morbidity/mortality and may improve the quality of recovery by providing mild sedation in the recovery period.

Alpha-2 adrenoreceptor agonists

- These will normally provide reliable sedation for most horses:
  - Xylazine 0.3–1.1 mg/kg
  - Detomidine 5–20 µg/kg
  - Romifidine 40–100 µg/kg.
- Use the lower end of the dose range for the large horses and the higher end for the smaller horses.
- All will provide analgesia to varying extent; the duration of analgesia is approximately 1/3 to 1/2 the duration of sedation and, therefore, must not be relied upon as the sole analgesic agent.
- All alpha-2 agonists will cause bradycardia (can be 50% of the original heart rate) and are dose-dependent with higher doses producing more profound bradycardia.
- The blood pressure will initially rise and then fall to resting levels or just below and the duration of this depression is longer than the duration of the sedation.
- The cardiac output will be reduced due to this bradycardia and the fall in blood pressure.
- If blood samples are taken after alpha-2s, glucose levels may be high due to effects of the drug.
- They will increase the intrauterine pressure in both pregnant and non-pregnant animals and these may compromise the uterine blood flow and, therefore, possibly compromise the placental blood flow (see p. 457 for the sedation of pregnant mares).
- Alpha-2s can also cause sweating, shaking and panting.
- The effects can be reversed with atipamezole (antisedan) 25–50 µg/kg. **This product is not licensed for use in horses.**

Analgesia

> **Notes:**
> - All horses undergoing anaesthesia/a surgical procedure should receive appropriate analgesia.

- The use of butorphanol with the premedication and the alpha-2 agonists used will not provide adequate analgesia.
- The addition of a non-steroidal anti-inflammatory drug will provide longer lasting and more effective analgesia.

Butorphanol

- Provides better analgesia for visceral pain than somatic pain.
- For **analgesia, butorphanol doses are 0.01–0.1 mg/kg IV** (much higher than those used for sedation and it has a short duration of action).

Pethidine

- It must be given intramuscularly as it causes histamine release when administered IV; this will cause hypotension, excitement and convulsions.
- The dose is 3.5–10 mg/kg. Because it is a 50 mg/mL solution, large volumes need to be given and it stings in injection and has a short duration of action (30 minutes to 1 hour), but is a good spasmolytic.

Morphine

- Not licensed in horses.
- Dose 0.1–0.2 mg/kg (0.12 mg/kg is usually about right).
- Provides 4 hours of analgesia.
- May cause ileus in recovery that may cause colic.

Carprofen

- NSAID.
- Doses 0.7 mg/kg IV q 24 hours for 3–5 days.
- Useful for foal analgesia as potentially has less harmful side effects (e.g. gastric ulceration) but it is wise to always provide a gastroprotectant.

Other NSAIDs

- **Phenylbutazone** (4.4 mg/kg) for orthopaedic pain.
- **Flunixin** (1.1 mg/kg) for soft tissue pain.
- Always remember that buscopan contains the NSAID drug dipyrone and should not be given with other NSAIDs.
- Other NSAIDs – check data sheet of licensed products.

Local Anaesthesia

- This is a useful adjunct to anaesthesia and can improve the quality of anaesthesia.
- Most techniques are safe to perform and can be done easily in the field.

Induction and Maintenance of Anaesthesia

Adequate restraint must be ensured before induction of anaesthesia. There are several drugs available for induction of anaesthesia and the drugs chosen will depend upon personal preference, the maintenance regime to be used and the horse.

Thiopentone (thiopental) (see pp. 468–469 for doses)

- Given as a bolus injection following premedication with ACP, an alpha-2 or no premedication.
- Will produce cardiovascular depression and transient apnoea.
- Often used with GGE for induction of anaesthesia.
- Top-up doses cannot be used for the maintenance of anaesthesia due to thiopentone's cumulative effects, producing a hangover effect and prolonged recovery from anaesthesia.

GGE (see p. 469 for doses)

- A centrally acting muscle relaxant with no analgesic or anaesthetic properties.
- See Part 3 Section 1, p. 89 on GGE for more information.

Ketamine (see pp. 468–469 for doses)

- Dissociative anaesthetic agent.
- Direct myocardial depressant; however, this is counteracted by an increase in sympathetic tone leaving an overall neutral effect on the cardiovascular system in healthy animals.
- Must be given following sedation to prevent excitement.
- Muscle hypertonus can occur following ketamine and the addition of a benzodiazepine or other muscle relaxant (α_2) will help counteract this.
- Can be used for the maintenance of anaesthesia but beware prolonged administration as an active metabolite (norketamine) has 1/4 of the potency of the parent compound and can prolong the recovery from anaesthesia.
- Will provide excellent analgesia.

Benzodiazepines

- Will provide sedation only in foals under 4 weeks of age.
- They are used as adjuncts to ketamine anaesthesia to provide muscle relaxation to aid induction and intubation with minimal cardiovascular side effects.

TOTAL INTRAVENOUS ANAESTHESIA (TIVA)

TIVA is the induction and maintenance of anaesthesia using only intravenous methods. It is based on the combination of two or three different types of drug, usually a muscle relaxant, a dissociative and a sedative.

The ideal combination of drugs would have identical half-lives, short elimination and no active metabolites. Xylazine and ketamine have similar durations of action and, therefore, work well together; the other alpha-2s have longer durations of action and can, therefore, become cumulative if used in top-ups or triple drip with ketamine. This can prolong the horse's recovery and this means an increase in your time.

The extra expense of xylazine compared to the other alpha-2s may be offset by this increase in recovery time.

Advantages

- TIVA is easy to do in the field and there is less need for complex equipment than with inhalation anaesthesia.

- The cardiovascular depression caused by these combinations is usually less than that caused by the inhalational methods and arterial blood pressure may be better maintained.

- There is less stimulation of the stress response to anaesthesia with TIVA; therefore, it is regarded as a physiologically better method of anaesthesia than inhalation anaesthesia.

- Allows combination of several drugs to reduce the side effects of each individual drug.

Disadvantages

- Ideally, oxygen supplementation should still be provided but this involves insurance implications for transporting O_2 cylinders in cars if horses are not to be anaesthetised on practice premises.

- Over-dosage can lead to respiratory arrest and often there is less equipment available for the supplementation of oxygen and IPPV.

- Extended procedures will have prolonged recoveries and excitement due to the accumulation of active metabolites over time, especially if the procedure takes longer than anticipated.

- Once administered, the agents cannot be taken back, whereas inhalation agents can be rapidly removed using IPPV in 100% O_2.

- Anaesthetic depth may be harder to monitor.

- Not ideal for surgery of the eye or upper airway due to maintenance of the cranial nerve reflexes.

Top-Up TIVA

- This is the maintenance of anaesthesia with bolus doses of anaesthetic agent. The use of top-ups is easy to perform in the field but will produce an undulating plane of anaesthesia in the horse.

- Top-ups of ketamine are usually used, as thiopentone (thiopental) is unsuitable for repeat administration if using a total dose of less than 10–15 mg/kg thiopentone (thiopental) (i.e. 5.0–7.5 g total dose in a 500 kg horse).

- The top-up doses must be timed on the clock when using ketamine as it takes 1–3 minutes to start working following intravenous injection and if the top-up doses are administered when signs of lightening anaesthesia start, then this is too late and the horse will become too light.

- It is advisable to have top-up doses prepared before anaesthesia and also to have a dose of thiopentone (thiopental) available for the horse that becomes light quickly or starts moving, so that the plane of anaesthesia can be swiftly deepened with minimal risk to personnel.

- This method should not be continued for more than 90 minutes due to the accumulation of norketamine and prolonged recovery times. (See pp. 468–469 for doses and regimes.)

Triple Drip

- This is continuous infusion, total intravenous anaesthesia. The triple drip can be used for induction of anaesthesia or another method of induction can be performed. If the surgery is expected to last for more than 1 hour, it is advisable to have an alternative method of induction so the maximum dose of GGE is not reached too early.

- There is a limited amount of time available when using the triple drip method, so the cases on which this is used should be carefully selected and an alternative method of maintenance of anaesthesia should be available.

- Infusion rates may be lowered if the visual and auditory stimuli are reduced (e.g. stuff the ears with cotton wool and cover the eyes).

- Monitoring horses on triple drip is different from those maintained with inhalation methods. The horses maintained with triple drip are receiving large amounts of ketamine. These horses may appear to be light (e.g. nystagmus, movement, changes in respiratory pattern) when they are actually too deep. If the drip rate is increased to attempt to deepen the anaesthesia, the horse may appear even lighter due to increased amounts of ketamine.

- GGE is also cumulative. Too much central muscle relaxation can make the horse weak in recovery and prolong recovery or reduce the quality. Catechol is a metabolite of GGE and when it builds up it causes excitement and can lead to the horse looking too light when in fact it is too deep.

- Triple drip must be used immediately after it is made up. Any remaining solution must be thrown away and not used the next day; hence, it can be wasteful and expensive for very short procedures.

Monitoring Under TIVA Anaesthesia

- Monitoring should be as any anaesthetic with a pulse rate and respiratory rate.
- As horses have a large cardiac reserve they do not need to increase heart rate to increase cardiac output (they just increase the stroke volume and, therefore, blood pressure), so heart rate is not a good indicator of a lightening plane of anaesthesia in horses.
- Horses also have a large respiratory reserve (unless they have respiratory disease); therefore, they will not increase their respiratory rate with a lightening plane of anaesthesia. However, they will often change their respiratory pattern; this is often a sudden deeper breath. Equine respiratory patterns may change when they are too deep (e.g. ketamine can cause periodic breathing – which is several small breaths followed by a long pause).
- Remember that the use of ketamine will not abolish the cranial nerve reflexes; they should have palpebral and gag reflexes and may twitch, so monitoring their depth can be difficult.
- The depth of anaesthesia will undulate and top-ups should be given by the clock, even without the signs of a lightening plane of anaesthesia.
- Eye position is an unreliable indicator of the plane of anaesthesia in horses; the sign of a lightening plane of anaesthesia is nystagmus.

EQUINE FIELD ANAESTHESIA RECIPE BOOK

Ingredients

- Appropriate location (no water, flat surface, non-slippery).
- Padded headcollar and rope.
- IV catheter (preplaced).
- Ideally, source of oxygen (e.g. demand valve and endotracheal tube).
- Drugs for induction.
- Drugs for maintenance.
- Heparin-saline flush.
- Top-up drugs if patient moves during procedure: have 1 g thiopentone (thiopental), 500 mg ketamine and heparin saline ready to use in preloaded syringes.
- All other perioperative medication (e.g. analgesics, antibiotics, tetanus antitoxin).
- Sedatives for recovery.

Premedication

Table 4.18 Drugs for premedication		Dose (/kg)	Route	Notes
ACP (acepromazine)		0.03 mg	IV/IM	Takes 30–40 minutes to work, 'protective' during anaesthesia. DO NOT USE IN STALLIONS.
Alpha-2 Agonists	Xylazine	1.1 mg	IV	10–20 minutes sedation
	Detomidine	5–20 µg	IV	Up to 80 minutes sedation
	Romifidine	40–100 µg	IV	Minimum 80 minutes sedation
'Magic' mix	Detomidine	0.02 mg	IM	IM sedation for the ill-tempered horse
	ACP	0.03 mg		Leave unstimulated for 30–40 minutes (1 mL of mixture for 100 kg of horse)
	Butorphanol	0.05 mg		

Induction

● Choose location carefully, plenty of room, flat, clear of debris, no bystanders, no water or roads.

● Pad headcollar with foam or jumper.

● Once induced, position patient with dependent front leg pulled forward and, if possible, legs parallel with ground (especially if a longer procedure is anticipated).

● Remove headcollar after induction to prevent pressure on the facial nerve.

● Covering the eye can reduce stimulus while the animal is under anaesthesia as well as cotton wool in their ears, but remember to take it out!

Table 4.19 Drugs for induction	
Ketamine	2.2 mg/kg after an alpha-2 agonist is given IV
Ketamine + benzodiazepine	2.2 mg/kg + 0.05 mg/kg diazepam/midazolam after alpha-2 premedication
Thiopentone (thiopental)	5–8 mg/kg after alpha-2 premed. 10–15 mg/kg after ACP premedication
Thiopentone (thiopental) + benzodiazepine	5–8 mg/kg thiopentone (thiopental) + 0.05 mg/kg benzodiazepine post-alpha-2 premedication 10–15 mg/kg thiopentone (thiopental) + 0.05 mg/kg benzodiazepine post-ACP premedication

Maintenance

Table 4.20 Top-up anaesthesia	
Ketamine + Alpha-2 agonist	Top up every 10–15 minutes (on the clock). Give ⅓–½ the induction dose of ketamine and alpha-2 agonist If using *xylazine* top up every 10–15 minutes with ketamine and xylazine If using *detomidine* premed, give ½ initial dose at 30 minutes (i.e. with 3rd top-up of ketamine) If using *romifidine* premed, give ⅓–½ initial doses at 1 hour or one-sixth dose every top-up or ½ dose for recovery. Ketamine is slightly cumulative, therefore, increase your intervals after 3rd top-up Can add benzodiazepine at 0.025 mg/kg every 20–30 minutes (after 3 doses extend duration to 1 hour)
Thiopentone (thiopental)	0.5–2.5 mg/kg top ups as required Be careful total dose does not exceed 10–15 mg/kg Works quickly; therefore, excellent for movement Can add benzodiazepine at 0.025 mg/kg every 20–30 minutes (after 3 doses extend duration to 1 hour)

Note: Thiopentone (thiopental) can be used after a ketamine induction and ketamine after a thiopentone (thiopental) induction.

Intravenous Infusions

- Induction as previously described.
- Make sure catheter is secure in vein after induction (and preferably placed down the vein).

Note:
- GGE is extremely irritating if injected extravascularly.

- All infusions are given 'to effect', on average 1 mL/kg/h or roughly 3 drops per second for a 500 kg horse, from a 20 drops/mL giving set.
- Horses should seem to be in a 'light' plane of anaesthesia with spontaneous blink and swallow responses.
- The plane of anaesthesia (and the infusion rate) should be a reduced dose over time and should not exceed a total anaesthesia time of 2 hours.
- Always keep a top-up dose of either ketamine or thiopentone (thiopental) for movement.
- Don't forget about patient positioning with field anaesthesia!

Drugs and doses

- GGE 15% (150 mg/mL)+xylazine (1.5 mg/mL)+ketamine (3 mg/mL) (i.e. 500 mL bottle of 15% GGE); add 750 mg xylazine+1500 mg ketamine (£52.06 cost price mix).

- GGE 15% (150 mg/mL)+romifidine (0.06–0.075 mg/mL)+ketamine (3 mg/mL) (i.e. 500 mL bottle of 15% GGE); add 30–37.5 mg romifidine+1500 mg ketamine (£30.70 cost price per mix).

- GGE 10% (100 mg/mL)+xylazine (1 mg/mL)+ketamine (2 mg/mL) (i.e. 500 mL bottle 10% GGE); add 500 mg xylazine+1000 mg ketamine.

- GGE 10% (100 mg/mL)+detomidine (0.02 mg/mL)+ketamine (2 mg/mL) (i.e. 500 mL bottle of 10% GGE); add 10 mg detomidine+1000 mg ketamine.

- GGE 10% (100 mg/mL)+romifidine (0.05 mg/mL)+ketamine (2 mg/mL) (i.e. 500 mL bottle of 10% GGE); add 1000 g ketamine).

- GGE 5% (50 mg/mL)+xylazine (0.5 mg/mL)+ketamine (1 mg/mL) (i.e. 500 mL bottle of 5% GGE); add 250 mg xylazine+500 mg ketamine.

Recovery

- Recoveries after total intravenous anaesthesia in horses are generally a lot more controlled, taking fewer attempts to stand and once standing a lot less ataxic.

- Generally, if left to their own devices, they will stand beautifully without assistance.

- To assist in recovery a lunge line can be attached to the headcollar allowing control of the direction of the head, while also allowing to move well clear of the animal (they can, however, cause a problem if let go and the line gets caught around the legs).

- Downward pressure on the tail as the animal attempts to rise can also aid in steadying the patient.

Part 4 CLINICAL AIDS

Section 16
Current requirements concerning drug usage and passport regulations in the UK

(As of September 2011: Modified from DEFRA Web site.)

Horses and other equidae are considered to be food-producing species in the European Union (EU). Veterinary medicines used to treat animals, including horses, fall within the scope of Directive 2001/82, as amended and the national legislation that transposes the EU legislation into national law. The VMR transpose Directive 2001/82/EC into UK law. In accordance with Commission Regulation 504/2008, horses can be declared as either intended for human consumption (food-producing horse) or not intended for human consumption (non-food-producing horse) in the horse passport. This declaration determines what products can be administered to the animal and, therefore, consideration of what medicines may be used must be taken. Horse passports: All horses and ponies are required to have a passport identifying the animal. All horses born after July 2009 must be microchipped. Horse passports contain information relating to: horse's appearance, which is illustrated in diagram called a 'silhouette', micro-chip details, age, breed/type, all the medications administered (if the animal has been declared 'intended for human consumption').

Medicines for horses

All horses should be treated with veterinary medicinal products (VMPs) which have a UK marketing authorisation (MA) for use in horses as the first choice. However, if there is no suitable authorised product available, the veterinary surgeons may prescribe a medicine under the cascade for use in the animals under his care.

Under the cascade, a horse that is signed off from the food chain can be treated with any veterinary medicine authorised in the UK to treat another animal species or another condition in the horse. If there is no suitable veterinary medicine authorised in the UK, a UK-authorised human medicine or veterinary medicine authorised in another Member State (MS) may be imported for use with permission from the Veterinary Medicines Directorate (VMD). The last option is to prescribe a medicine specially prepared for that animal by a veterinarian, a pharmacist or a person holding a manufacturing authorisation or a medicine imported from a Third Country.

The prescribing cascade, explained above, also applies to food-producing horses. However, a food-producing horse can only be treated with a veterinary medicine that contains pharmacologically active substance(s) listed in Table 1 of Regulation EU 37/2010 for use in a food-producing species and a suitable withdrawal period should be set by the responsible veterinary surgeons.

Commission Regulation 1950/2006 established, in accordance with Directive 2001/82, a list of substances essential for the treatment of equidae: this is

European legislation that allows the use of certain substances in horses (declared as food- or non-food-producing in the passport) under the use of the cascade and with a statutory withdrawal period of 6 months.

If any substance which is not contained within Table 1 (the Allowed List) of Regulation EU 37/2010 or on the list of Essential Substances, such as phenylbutazone, is administered to an animal, that animal must be permanently excluded from the food chain and the passport declaration should be completed at Part II of Section IX by the owner or horse keeper or by the veterinary surgeon who administers the product. If the owner/keeper does not sign Part II of Section IX, the veterinary surgeon must do so.

Record keeping requirements

According to Commission Regulation No 504/2008, all vaccines administered by a veterinary surgeon must be recorded in the Horse Passport regardless of whether or not the horse is intended for human consumption.

There is no statutory requirement to record any other medicines in the non-food horse's passport; however, veterinary surgeons have recordkeeping obligations for all prescription medicines under the VMR.

Any substance on the essential substances list administered to a food-producing horse must be recorded in the passport. Recording medicines administered under the cascade in the passport is optional.

In addition to the Horse Passport Regulations, there are other recordkeeping obligations within the VMR that apply to keepers of horses intended for human consumption and to veterinary surgeons, pharmacists and Suitably Qualified Persons (SQPs) supplying medicines for horses. These are set out within the body of the guidance document, but in summary, records of use for medicines of all distribution categories must be kept for all horses that have been declared as 'intended for slaughter for human consumption' in the Horse Passport or have Part II of Section IX unsigned. It is not a legal requirement for the record to be kept in the medicines pages of the horse passport but it is acceptable for this to be done if preferred by the owner or keeper. Alternatively, a separate written record must be kept.

CHECKING THE PASSPORT

If you intend to administer, prescribe or dispense any medicinal substance for use in a horse, the following procedure should be followed:

Ask to be shown the passport for the horse if you do not have prior knowledge of its status (if you have previously seen the passport and are aware of the horse's current status, it is not necessary to see the passport before every treatment with a medicine);

Satisfy yourself that the passport supplied relates to the horse in question;

Note whether the horse is declared as INTENDED for human consumption (Section B of the old Passport/Part III of Section IX) or there is no declaration or the horse is declared as NOT INTENDED for human consumption (Section A of the old Passport/Part II of Section IX). The default position is that if Section IX contains no signature, the horse is INTENDED for human consumption;

If the document does not contain Section IX, it is not a valid horse passport.

If you do not have prior knowledge of the horse's status and a passport is not available or if you are not satisfied that the passport relates to the horse in question, follow the procedure at the section: 'If the horse is presented WITHOUT a passport'.

If the horse is declared 'not intended for human consumption'.

In this case, the horse should be treated with VMPs which have a UK MA for use in horses as the first choice. The VMD publishes a Product Information Database on its Web site, which holds information on every veterinary medicinal product authorised for use in the UK: http://www.vmd.defra.gov.uk/ProductInformationDatabase.

If there is no suitable authorised product available, the cascade may be used to prescribe an alternative medicinal product. The cascade must be used for clinical reasons.

Under the cascade, the non-food horse can be treated with any veterinary medicine authorised in the UK to treat another animal species or another condition in the horse. If this option is not available to that particular animal, then a UK-authorised human medicine or a veterinary medicine authorised in another Member State (MS) may be imported for use with permission from the VMD. Permission is granted via the issue of an Import Certificate which, in most cases, can be applied for online at www.vmd.defra.gov.uk/sis/default.aspx at no cost (a fee applies to postal applications). Products containing substances in the list of essential substances can also be used, as well as extemporaneous preparations. In exceptional circumstances, medicines may be imported from Third countries.

For further information please refer to VMGN 13 Guidance on the Use of the Cascade, which is published on the VMD's Web site.

http://www.vmd.defra.gov.uk/public/vmr_vmgn.aspx.

According to Commission Regulation No 504/2008 all vaccines administered by a veterinary surgeon must be recorded in the Horse Passport regardless of whether or not the horse is intended for human consumption.

There is no statutory requirement to record any other medicines in the non-food horse's passport; however, you should note that veterinary surgeons have recordkeeping obligations for all prescription medicines under the VMR. Further Guidance on record keeping is available in Part 2 of this VMGN and in VMGN 14 Record Keeping Requirements for Veterinary Medicinal Products, which is published on the VMD's Web site.

http://www.vmd.defra.gov.uk/public/vmr_vmgn.aspx.

If the horse is declared 'intended for human consumption' or no declaration was made.

(a) Use of VMPs in Table 1 of 'Allowed Substances' for food-producing animals

A food-producing horse should be treated with a veterinary medicine authorised in the UK for use in food-producing horses which will have a specific withdrawal period defined in the product literature and SPC.

If there is no suitable authorised product available, the cascade may be used to prescribe an alternative medicinal product. Only medicines which contain substances listed in Table 1 (Allowed Substances) of European Council Regulation 37/2010 can be used in a food-producing horse.

Another provision of the cascade is that, if there is no suitable veterinary medicine authorised in the UK, a UK-authorised human medicine or a veterinary medicine authorised for use in food-producing animals in another Member State (MS) may be imported for use with permission from the VMD. Permission is granted via the issue of an Import Certificate, which can be applied for online at www.vmd.defra.gov.uk at no cost (a fee applies to postal applications). Only a veterinary surgeon may apply for an import certificate. A wholesale dealer may also import products authorised in other MS by means of a Wholesale Dealers Import Certificate (WDIC) and retail it to a veterinary surgeon against an import certificate.

Extemporaneous preparations, that is, medicines tailor-made for a particular animal by a veterinary surgeon, a pharmacist or a person who holds an appropriate manufacturing authorisation, may be used under the cascade. In exceptional circumstances, a product may be imported from a Third Country with a VMD Import Certificate, providing that a withdrawal period can be set. These are the last options in the prescribing cascade.

Where medicines are being used under the cascade, a withdrawal period must be set by the veterinary surgeon. The minimum withdrawal period will be the statutory cascade withdrawal period (28 days for meat, 7 days for milk) or that defined in the SPC for the authorised medicine in question, whichever is longer. If a VMP has been imported from another MS and has a withdrawal period specified for horses in the SPC, then this should be observed.

Some veterinary medicines have been authorised in the UK that contain active substances in the Allowed Substances list, but are indicated for use in non-food horses only on the label. This is because the manufacturers did not intend to market these products for food-producing horses and, therefore, did not undertake the tests that would be required to provide residue depletion data. To allow label harmonisation with such products authorised in several MS, some products may state on the label:

'Treated horses may never be slaughtered for human consumption'.

This statement does not apply if the product contains a substance in Table 1 and has been prescribed by a veterinary surgeon in accordance with the cascade provisions, as explained above. In this case, a suitable withdrawal period needs to be observed, that is, at least the minimum statutory cascade withdrawal period or the withdrawal period indicated on the product's SPC for another food-producing species, whichever is longer.

(b) Use of veterinary medicinal products NOT in TABLE 1 ALLOWED substances (Regulation 37/2010)

It is recognised that the range of VMPs for horses destined for human consumption could be improved. As explained above, medicines for food-producing animals normally require an MRL for the active ingredient. However, because of the relatively small market for horse medicines, there have been some conditions for which there are no authorised medicines.

To help address this, the European Commission (EC) introduced Council Regulation 1950/2006. This established a list of medicines that were considered essential for horses and for which there is no authorised alternative. This list does not include phenylbutazone.

All substances on this list can be used in horses intended for human consumption and have a set minimum 6-month withdrawal period before horses can enter the food chain. Some substances are contained in VMPs authorised in the UK for use in other species and some may only be available as human medicines. Others may only be available if produced extemporaneously by a veterinary surgeon, pharmacist or a suitably authorised manufacturing site.

When a product containing a substance on this list is administered to a food-producing horse, the medicines record in Part IIIB of Section IX of the Horse Passport must be completed with details of the product(s) administered, including the date of the last treatment as prescribed, as this will, in effect, declare the horse as temporarily not for human consumption until the 6-month withdrawal period is completed.

The list of Essential Substances may change.

(c) Prohibited substances for food-producing animals

Products containing substances in Table 2 (Prohibited Substances) of European Council Regulation 37/2010 must not be administered to a food-producing animal. If any of these substances are administered, the horse can NEVER be slaughtered for human consumption and the declaration in the horse's passport at Part II of Section IX must be signed by the owner or veterinary surgeon as 'not intended for human consumption'. This declaration is irreversible.

The prohibited substances (as of 2011) are:

Aristolochia spp (and preparations thereof)

Chloramphenicol

Chloroform

Chlorpromazine

Colchicine

Dapsone

Dimetridazole

Metronidazole

Nitrofurans (including Furazolidone)

Ronidazole

If the horse is presented WITHOUT a passport.

If the owner or keeper of a horse does not have the passport for the horse to hand at the time of treatment and the veterinary surgeon has not previously seen it, the veterinary surgeon should presume that the horse is intended for human consumption – the veterinary surgeon is not able to ascertain that the horse is signed out of the food chain if a passport has never been presented.

In this situation, the veterinary surgeon must only prescribe/dispense/ administer medicines that are authorised for use in food-producing horses or those that are not authorised for use in horses but contain substances in Table 1 of Commission Regulation 37/2010 for use in other food-producing animals.

In Emergency Situations

In an emergency, where the health or welfare of a horse/foal is at risk and treatment with a substance that is not allowed for a food-producing animal is required (e.g. Etorphine), in order to proceed with treatment, the veterinarian surgeons must issue a document which details the medicines given and an instruction to the owner or keeper to exclude the animal from the food chain if necessary. An example of this document can be obtained from British Equine Veterinary Association (BEVA) – www.beva.org.uk. The veterinarian should retain a copy of this document.

Some scenarios are described below:

(a) *No passport has ever been issued for the animal*

The veterinary surgeon should inform the owner or keeper that a passport will need to be acquired for the animal from the relevant Passport Issuing Organisation and that the horse, if above 1 year of age, will be declared as not intended for human consumption, which will be irreversible for the remainder of its life.

(b) *Passport lost for a horse*

The horse owner or keeper should apply to the Passport Issuing Organisation for a replacement or duplicate passport which will be over stamped 'Not intended for human consumption'.

(c) *Passport exists but is not available*

As explained above, the veterinarian must issue a document which details the medicines given to the horse and instructs the owner or keeper to exclude the animal from the food chain if necessary, depending on the substances given to the horse.

Information on Phenylbutazone

The Directive 2001/82 as amended states that only products containing pharmacologically active substances listed in Table 1 of Regulation 37/2010 may be administered to food-producing animals. Medicines containing active substances included in Table 2 of Regulation 37/2010 – Prohibited Substances – are banned from use in food-producing animals.

Phenylbutazone is in an anomalous situation because neither has it been listed in Table 1 nor has it been included in the list of prohibited substances. This means that, while not a banned active ingredient, it cannot be used in a food-producing animal.

This situation occurs because data on phenylbutazone were submitted to the Committee for Veterinary Medicinal Products (CVMP) for consideration in the 1990s but they were not sufficient to establish an MRL. The applicant was given the opportunity to respond to the questions raised by the CVMP but no additional data were provided. Consequently, the CVMP did not recommend the establishment of an MRL for phenylbutazone.

The main concerns raised by the CVMP related to the possible myelotoxic effects of phenylbutazone in humans; carcinogenic, nephrotoxic and hepatoxic effects in laboratory animals; and evidence of mutagenic activity in lymphocytes in human lymphocytes (*in vitro*). No adequate data on reproductive toxicity were made available to the CVMP. This information is in the public domain (Vet Rec 23 April 2005, p. 554, letter from the EMEA – Phenylbutazone and equine research).

Phenylbutazone is a useful non-steroid anti-inflammatory drug (NSAID) for the management of orthopaedic conditions. Conscious of the needs of the veterinary profession and the equine industry, the VMD has authorised products containing this active ingredient; but, mindful of food safety issues and the obligations imposed by the legislation, we have restricted the use of these products to non-food horses only. Horses which have been treated with phenylbutazone must not enter the food chain and their passports must be signed at part II of Section IX to indicate that the animal is not intended for human consumption. This is an irreversible decision.

Recordkeeping Obligations for Veterinary Surgeons, Pharmacists and SQPs

Administration by a veterinary surgeon

If the product is administered by a veterinary surgeon, he or she must either enter into the owners or keepers records or give written notice to the owner or keeper, of the:

name of the veterinary surgeon;

name of the product; and the batch number;

date of administration;

amount administered;

identification of the animals treated;

the withdrawal period.

Supply of prescription medicines (POM-V and POM-VPS)

It is the responsibility of the veterinary surgeon, pharmacist or SQP who supplies POM-V (Prescription Only Medicine – Veterinarian) and POM-VPS (Prescription Only Medicines – Veterinarian, Pharmacist, Suitably Qualified Person) medicines on a retail basis, for both food-producing and non-food-producing horses, to keep records for at least 5 years for each incoming or outgoing transaction. The information required is as follows:

date and nature of transaction;

name of the VMP;

the batch number (except that, in the case of a product for a non-food-producing animal, this need only be recorded either on the date he receives the batch or the date he starts to use it);

quantity received or supplied;

name and address of the supplier or recipient;

and if there is a written prescription, the name and address of the person who wrote the prescription and a copy of the prescription.

Supply of medicines under the cascade

A veterinary surgeon who administers or prescribes a medicinal product for a horse under the cascade must keep a record, for at least 5 years, of the:

date of examination of the animal(s);

name and address of the owner;

identification and number of animals treated;

the result of the veterinary surgeon's clinical assessment;

trade name of the product if there is one;

manufacturer's batch number shown on the product if there is one;

name and quantity of the active substance;

doses administered or supplied;

duration of treatment;

withdrawal period.

Who can I contact about queries?

DEFRA helpline number for passports is 08459 335577 (from outside UK +44 20 7238 6951).

VMD can be contacted on 01932 336911.

British Equine Veterinary Association:

Mulberry House
31 Market Street
Fordham, Ely
Cambridgeshire
CB7 5LQ
Tel: +44 (0)1638 723 555
Fax: + 44(0)1638 724 043

INDEX

Note: Page numbers followed by f indicate figures, b indicate boxes and t indicate tables.

Printed and bound by CPI Group (UK) Ltd, Croydon, CR0 4YY

03/10/2024

01040847-0001